Operating Room Leadership and Management

Edited by

Alan D. Kaye, MD, PhD
Professor and Chair
Department of Anesthesia
Louisiana State University
New Orleans, LA, USA

Charles J. Fox III, MD
Associate Professor of Anesthesiology
Vice Chair for Academics
Director, Perioperative Management Fellowship
Department of Anesthesiology
Tulane Hospital and Clinic
New Orleans, LA, USA

Richard D. Urman, MD, MBA
Assistant Professor of Anesthesia
Harvard Medical School
Director, Procedural Sedation Management and Safety
Co-Director, Center for Perioperative Management and Medical Informatics
Brigham and Women's Hospital
Boston, MA, USA

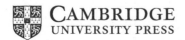
CAMBRIDGE
UNIVERSITY PRESS

CAMBRIDGE UNIVERSITY PRESS
Cambridge, New York, Melbourne, Madrid, Cape Town,
Singapore, São Paulo, Delhi, Mexico City

Cambridge University Press
The Edinburgh Building, Cambridge CB2 8RU, UK

Published in the United States of America by Cambridge University Press, New York

www.cambridge.org
Information on this title: www.cambridge.org/9781107017535

First published 2012

Printed and bound in the United Kingdom by the MPG Books Group

A catalogue record for this publication is available from the British Library

Library of Congress Cataloguing in Publication data
Operating room leadership and management / edited by Alan D. Kaye, Charles J. Fox III, Richard D. Urman.
    p. ; cm.
Includes bibliographical references and index.
ISBN 978-1-107-01753-5 (hardback)
I. Kaye, Alan D. II. Fox, Charles J. (Charles James), 1961– III. Urman, Richard D.
[DNLM: 1. Operating Rooms–organization & administration. 2. Leadership. 3. Practice Management. WX 200]
617.9′17–dc23
2012016083

ISBN 978-1-107-01753-5 Hardback

Royal Liverpool University Hospital – Staff Library

Please return or renew, on or before the last date below. Items may be renewed **twice**, if not reserved for another user. Renewals may be made in person, by telephone: 0151 706 2248 or email: library.service@rlbuht.nhs.uk. There is a charge of 10p per day for late items.

Operating Room Leadership and Management

I dedicate this book to my wife, Dr. Kim Kaye, my son, Aaron Joshua Kaye, my daughter, Rachel Jane Kaye, and my many colleagues at LSU School of Medicine and Tulane School of Medicine in New Orleans. I am honored to be a part of your lives.

ADK

I dedicate this book to my wife, Mary Beth, for her selfless devotion to our family and to our kids, Chris, Mary Elise, Patrick, Julia, Claire and Margaret who enrich our lives more than we ever imagined.

CJF

I dedicate this book to my wife, Dr. Zina Matlyuk-Urman, and our daughter, Abigail Rose; to my colleagues among physicians, nurses, and administrators at Harvard who supported my efforts in writing this book; and to all my mentors and trainees.

RDU

Contents

List of contributors   *page* ix
Foreword   xii
Larry H. Hollier

Preface   xiii
Alan D. Kaye, Charles J. Fox III, and Richard D. Urman

Section 1   Leadership and strategy   1

1   **Leadership principles**   1
Christoph Egger and Alex Macario

2   **The path to a successful operating room environment**   15
Ross Musumeci, Alan D. Kaye, Charles J. Fox, and Richard D. Urman

3   **Strategic planning**   25
Michael R. Williams

4   **Decision making: The art and the science**   32
Michael R. Williams

Section 2   Economic considerations, efficiency, and design   39

5   **Health care and economic realities**   39
Robert Lynch

6   **Influence of staffing and scheduling on operating room productivity**   46
Franklin Dexter and Richard H. Epstein

7   **Operations management and financial performance**   67
Jeffery Anderson, Seth Christian, and Richard D. Urman

8   **Reenginering operating room function**   77
Nigel N. Robertson

9   **Operating room design and construction: Technical considerations**   95
Judy Dahle and Pat Patterson

10 **Operating an ambulatory surgery center as a successful business**   108
John J. Wellik

Section 3   Surgical and anesthesia practice management   121

11 **Preoperative evaluation and management**   121
Alicia G. Kalamas

12 **A surgeon's perspective: Perioperative standards, quality, and consents**   132
Frank G. Opelka

13 **Anesthesia practice management: Core principles**   139
Sonya Pease and Barbara Harris

14 **Anesthesia staffing models, productivity measurement, and incentive plans**   151
Ashish Dabas, Dipty Mangla, Asa C. Lockhart, and George Mychaskiw II

15 **Compensation for anesthesia services**   160
Asa C. Lockhart

16 **Basics of billing, coding, and compliance**   168
Deborah Farmer and Devona Slater

17 **Surgical coding**   183
Bernadine Smith

18 **Postanesthesia care unit management**   186
Michael J. Yarborough, Henry Liu, and Sabrina Bent

19 **Pain practice management**   194
Steven D. Waldman

20 **Office-based surgery practice** 201
Seth Christian and Charles J. Fox

21 **The future of perioperative medicine** 216
Michael R. Hicks and Laurie Saletnik

Section 4 Safety, standards, and information technology 222

22 **Nursing: Organizational structure, staffing, resource management, metrics, and infection control** 222
Melissa Guidry and Lesley Bourlet

23 **The Joint Commission, CMS, and other standards** 235
Shermeen B. Vakharia and Zeev Kain

24 **Safety, quality, and pay-for-performance** 244
Richard P. Dutton and Frank Rosinia

25 **Sedation: Clinical and safety considerations** 253
Ann Bui and Richard D. Urman

26 **Medical informatics in the perioperative period** 267
Keith J. Ruskin

27 **Simulation training to improve patient safety** 274
Valeriy Kozmenko, Judy G. Johnson, Melvin Wyche, and Alan D. Kaye

Index 279

Contributors

Jeffrey Anderson, MD
Anesthesiology Resident, Department of Anesthesiology, Tulane University School of Medicine, New Orleans, LA, USA

Sabrina Bent, MD, MS
Director of Pediatric Anesthesiology, Department of Anesthesiology, Tulane University School of Medicine, New Orleans, LA, USA

Lesley Bourlet, RN, MSN, CNOR
Director Perioperative Services, Tulane-Lakeside Hospital, Metairie, LA, USA

Ann Bui, MD
Resident in Anesthesiology, Brigham and Women's Hospital, Boston, MA, USA

Seth Christian, MD
Perioperative Management Fellow, Department of Anesthesiology, Tulane University School of Medicine, New Orleans, LA, USA

Ashish Dabas, MD
Resident in Anesthesiology, Drexel University School of Medicine, Philadelphia, PA, USA

Judy Dahle, MS, MSG, RN
Education Coordinator, OR Manager, Rockville, MD, USA

Franklin Dexter, MD, PhD
Department of Anesthesia, Carver College of Medicine, University of Iowa, Iowa City, IA, USA

Richard P. Dutton, MD, MBA
Executive Director, Anesthesia Quality Institute and Clinical Associate, University of Chicago, Department of Anesthesiology and Critical Care

Christoph Egger, MD, MBA
Hospital Chief Executive Officer, Klinik Beau-Site, Hirslanden Hospitals Bern, Bern, Switzerland;

Consulting Assistant Professor, Stanford University School of Medicine, Stanford, CA, USA

Richard H. Epstein, MD, CPHIMS
Department of Anesthesiology, Jefferson Medical College, Thomas Jefferson University, Philadelphia, PA, USA

Deborah Farmer, CPC, ACS-AN
Senior Compliance Auditor, Auditing for Compliance and Education (ACE), Inc., Overland Park, KS, USA

Charles J. Fox III, MD
Vice-Chairman and Clinical Associate Professor, Tulane Medical Center, Director, Perioperative Management Fellowship, Department of Anesthesiology, New Orleans, LA, USA

Melissa Guidry, RN, MPH, CNOR
Director Perioperative Services, Tulane Medical Center, New Orleans, LA, USA

Barbara Harris, RN, MHA
Vice President of Operational Excellence, TeamHealth Anesthesia, Knoxville, TN, USA

Michael R. Hicks, MD, MBA, MS, FACHE
President and Chairman, Pinnacle Anesthesia Consultants, PA; Chief Executive Officer, AnesthesiaCare, an EmCare Affiliate, Dallas, TX, USA

Judy G. Johnson, MD
Assistant Professor, Residency Program Director, Department of Anesthesiology, Louisiana State University Health Sciences Center, New Orleans, LA, USA

Zeev Kain, MD, MBA, MA (Hon)
Professor, Anesthesiology & Pediatrics & Psychiatry, Chair, Department of Anesthesiology & Perioperative Care, and Associate Dean of Clinical Operations, School of Medicine, University of California, Irvine, CA, USA

Alicia G. Kalamas, MD
Medical Director, Preoperative Clinic and Associate Clinical Professor, Department of Anesthesia and Perioperative Care, University of California, San Francisco, CA, USA

Alan D. Kaye, MD, PhD
Professor and Chairman, Department of Anesthesiology and Professor, Department of Pharmacology, LSU School of Medicine, New Orleans, LA, USA

Valeriy Kozmenko, MD
Department of Anesthesiology, LSU School of Medicine, New Orleans, LA, USA

Henry Liu, MD
Director of Cardiac Anesthesia, Department of Anesthesiology, Tulane University School of Medicine, New Orleans, LA, USA

Asa C. Lockhart, MD, MBA
Principal, Golden Caduceus Consultants; Course Director, Certificate in Business Administration for the American Society of Anesthesiologists; East Texas Medical Center, Texas Spine and Joint Hospital, Tyler, TX, USA

Robert Lynch, MD
Chief Executive Officer, Tulane Medical Center, New Orleans, LA, USA

Alex Macario, MD, MBA
Professor of Anesthesia and of Health Research & Policy and Program Director, Anesthesia Residency, Department of Anesthesia, Stanford University School of Medicine, Stanford, CA, USA

Dipty Mangla, MD
Resident in Anesthesiology, Drexel University School of Medicine, Philadelphia, PA, USA

Ross Musumeci, MD, MBA
Anaesthesia Associates of MA, Assistant Professor of Anesthesia, Boston University School of Medicine, Boston, MA, USA

George Mychaskiw II, DO, FAAP, FACOP
Professor and Chair, Department of Anesthesiology, University of Central Florida College of Medicine/Florida State University College of Medicine, Nemours Children's Hospital, FL, USA

Frank G. Opelka, MD, FACS
LSU School of Medicine, New Orleans, LA, USA

Pat Patterson
Editor, OR Manager Newsletter, Rockville, MD, USA

Sonya Pease, MD
Chief Medical Officer, TeamHealth Anesthesia, Knoxville, TN, USA

Nigel N. Robertson, MB, ChB, FANZCA
Staff Specialist Anesthesiologist, Auckland City Hospital, Auckland, New Zealand

Frank Rosinia, MD
Chairman, Department of Anesthesiology, Tulane University School of Medicine, New Orleans, LA, USA

Keith J. Ruskin, MD
Professor of Anesthesiology and Neurosurgery, Yale University School of Medicine, New Haven, CT, USA

Laurie Saletnik, RN, DNP
Director of Nursing for Perioperative Services, Johns Hopkins Hospital, Baltimore, MD, USA

Devona Slater, CHC, CMCP
President and Senior Compliance Auditor, Auditing for Compliance and Education (ACE), Inc., Overland Park, KS, USA

Bernadine Smith, CPC, RCC, PCS
Director of Coding and Regulatory Issues, Auditing and Consulting, ACS Physician Practice Management Company, Metairie, LA, USA

Richard D. Urman, MD, MBA
Assistant Professor of Anesthesia, Harvard Medical School and Director, Procedural Sedation Management and Safety, Co-Director, Center for Perioperative Management and Medical Informatics, Brigham and Women's Hospital, Boston, MA, USA

Shermeen B. Vakharia, MD
Clinical Professor, Department of Anesthesiology and Perioperative Care, Vice Chair for Quality and Patient Safety, School of Medicine, University of California, Irvine, CA, USA

Steven D. Waldman, MD, JD
Clinical Professor Of Anesthesiology, University of Missouri At Kansas City School of Medicine, Leawood, KS, USA

John J. Wellik, CPA, MBA
Senior Vice President, Chief Administrative Officer,
United Surgical Partners International, Inc., Addison,
TX, USA

Michael R. Williams, DO, MD, MBA
Chief Executive Officer, Hill Country Memorial,
Fredericksburg, TX, USA; Executive Vice President,
AnesthesiaCare, an EmCare Affiliate, Dallas, TX, USA

Melville Wyche III, MD
Director of Simulation and Assistant Professor,
Department of Anesthesia, LSU School of Medicine,
New Orleans, LA, USA

Michael J. Yarborough, MD
Director PostAnesthesia Care Unit, Department
of Anesthesiology, Tulane University School of
Medicine, New Orleans, LA, USA

Foreword

Gone are the days when operating rooms (ORs) were dominated by bombastic surgeons or a tyrannical OR Nurse Supervisor. Personalities and prejudices are just not tolerable in a time when productivity and revenues are so important to the viability of the hospital. As the overall hospital revenue is so highly dependent on the share derived from perioperative services, a collaborative work ethic and efficiency of the unit become paramount.

High-performing teams set the standards for productivity and value in the perioperative setting. The opportunities to be derived from collaboration cannot be overemphasized. Savings in supply chain management provide the low-hanging fruit and are dependent upon the engagement of the physician staff in the minimization of variety of surgical supplies. Achieving this, however, requires leadership that is able to be inclusive of all participants in the environment of the operative theater. Throughput of cases is facilitated by a broadly understood mandate that the preoperative data be ready in advance and available to the necessary participants, from the preoperative evaluation, the financial clearance, the consents, and the anesthesia and nurse evaluations in the OR.

This book brings into perspective the need and the opportunities to bring proper and efficient management to the perioperative environment. Leadership is critical in this arena, where anxieties can run high and leadership is the calming force that directs the harmony that leads to patient safety and financial success.

Larry H. Hollier, Jr., MD, FACS
Chancellor, LSU Health Sciences Center
New Orleans, LA, USA

Preface

Currently, there is no up-to-date, evidence-based text that encompasses the "A to Z" of operating room (OR) management: metrics, scheduling, human resource management, leadership principles, economics, quality assurance, recovery, ambulatory practice, and topics specific to surgeons, anesthesiologists, and pain service providers.

Years ago, the OR stood alone, and very little attention was given to the perioperative period. This is because until the 1980s the OR generated large profits despite its inefficiency. Thus, hospital administrators allowed it a great deal of autonomy. However, today's hospital administrators realize that, although it is typically one of the biggest sources of revenue for a hospital, the OR is also one of the largest areas of expense. This, coupled with increasing requirements for cost containment in health care and a demand for accountability to the federal and state government, insurance companies, hospital administrators, surgeons, and patients, has magnified the need for an effective and efficient perioperative process. Whereas there was little centralized leadership in the perioperative period of the past, perioperative management is now a critical feature of successful hospitals.

As mentioned above, today's perioperative practice of medicine has evolved significantly and is now influenced by a vast array of factors, both medical and administrative. Because of this, knowledge of hospital economics and administration, OR mechanics and metrics, human resources, financial planning, governmental policy and procedure, and clinical perioperative management is necessary for success. A good management team must bring together these diverse components to maximize productivity.

Today there are more regulations, quality measures, and outcome expectations, which push innovation and provide additional burdens and challenges for hospitals. The need for this expensive technology, to compete with other hospitals, forces reform and new thoughts for traditional ways of the past. Staffing ratios, preoperative visits, and postoperative care will be highly scrutinized financially, while clinical and administrative "multi-tasking" is now expected. Areas such as quality data definition and collection, leadership style, simulation, and OR design will evolve quickly to create a more productive and efficient perioperative process.

We should not lose sight of the fact that the OR is where miracles happen every single day through teamwork, natural talent, hard work, and empathy. From all of this, we create game-changing and life-altering experiences for our patients. Without effective and efficient leadership from all areas – nursing, administration, surgery, and anesthesia services – we are doomed to failure. Let us also remember that we and our families one day will be patients, making a first-rate OR in the best interests of everyone.

As we have observed from all of our real-life experiences collectively accumulated over the past three decades, the science of perioperative patient care is constantly evolving. This speaks to the enormous complexities in all aspects of management and development of a winning OR. We applaud the authors for their hard work and dedication. Their chapters give straightforward information and insight into creating a successful perioperative program.

We all have challenges to make success in the OR environment. We hope any stakeholder in administration, surgery, anesthesia, or nursing services will find tools, ideas, and practical solutions in this book as we all do our best to move forward to the future.

Alan D. Kaye, MD, PhD
Louisiana State University
Charles J. Fox III, MD
Tulane University
Richard D. Urman, MD, MBA
Harvard University

Chapter

Leadership principles

Christoph Egger MD, MBA
Alex Macario MD, MBA

Evolution of leadership   1
Game theory in the OR context   6
Challenges of OR leadership   8

Summary   12
Appendix A. Characteristics of
leadership   12

Evolution of leadership

What is leadership?

As individuals move up within an organization and accept more responsibility, their interest in leadership rises as they have more people reporting to them. Leadership is about leading people, or the *capacity to lead*; specifically the behavior of an individual when directing the activities of a group toward a shared goal [1]. Akin to a conductor of an orchestra, a leader has a capacity to direct and motivate multiple professionals to perform to their peak ability while minimizing uncoordinated advances.

In our own experience, leadership is about making sure everyone feels a sense of purpose and is engaged in the future outcome of the organization. Among many other things, leaders: are role models for the values of the organization; set the optimal course; and establish priorities. Making people connect and collaborate as well as finding the appropriate style and amount of communication are formidable, but central, tasks for health-care leaders. Yet, just because a person is in a leadership position, this does not make him or her a leader [2].

The goals of this chapter are to review what is known from the published literature about leadership in general and in the context of health-care organizations, to illustrate the operating room (OR) suite as a challenging work place where different parties must cooperate or thwart each other to achieve success, and lastly, to

identify the challenges inherent to an OR leadership position.

Leadership styles

Multiple differing leadership styles have been described. Some aspects of each leadership style overlap with one another [3–6] (Table 1.1).

The mix of the health-care workforce and the complexity of the medical workplace demand a team approach to problem solving. This requires a leader who is comfortable "sharing power" by empowering people and can make decisions with a balance of idealism and pragmatism – a leadership style described as "leading from behind" [7]. This type of leader understands how to create an environment or culture in which other people are willing and able to lead. For example, the image of the shepherd behind his herd is based on Nelson Mandela's autobiography *Long Walk to Freedom* and acknowledgment that leadership is a collective activity in which different people act at a different time.

This image of leadership is backed by the idea of "Theory Y people," as described in McGregor's *The Human Side of Enterprise* [8,9]. According to McGregor, people can be divided into the two groups, Theory X and Theory Y. Theory X assumptions are:

- people are inherently lazy and will avoid work if they can;
- most people have little desire for responsibility and prefer to be directed;

Operating Room Leadership and Management, ed. Kaye A.D., Fox C.J. and Urman R.D. Published by Cambridge University Press. © Cambridge University Press 2012.

Table 1.1 Leadership styles

Authoritarian (coercive, commanding) leaders employ coercive tactics to enforce rules and to manipulate people and decision making
- Derived from the Prussian military, the command and control model is the primary management strategy.
- Believe in a top-down, line-and-staff organizational chart with clear levels of authority and reporting processes.
- Demand immediate compliance to orders and accomplish tasks by bullying and sometimes even demeaning the followers.
- Used in situations where the company or group requires a complete turnaround.
- May be effective during catastrophes or dealing with under-performing employees, as a last resort.

Pacesetting leaders set high performance standards for themselves and their followers and exemplify the behaviors they are seeking from other group members.
- Give little or no feedback on how the followers are doing except to jump in to take over when the followers lag.
- Work best when followers are self-motivated and highly skilled.
- May be effective to get quick results from a highly motivated and competent team.

Transactional leaders balance and integrate the organizational goals and expectations with the needs of the people doing the work.
- Work through creating well-defined structures, clear goals and distinct rewards for following orders.
- Motivate workers by offering rewards for what the leaders need to be done.
- Offer the appeal of employment and security in return for collaboration and assistance.

Authoritative (visionary) leaders mobilize people toward a compelling vision.
- Most effective when a new vision is needed, or when the path to that vision is not always clear.
- Although the leader is considered an authority, this type of leader allows their followers to figure out the best way to accomplish their goals.
- May be effective when changes require a new vision, or when a clear direction is needed.

Coaching leaders are genuinely interested in helping others succeed, and hence develop people for the future.
- Help employees identify both their strengths and weaknesses, provide feedback to their subordinates on their performance.
- By delegating tasks they give employees challenging assignments.
- May be effective to help employees improve their performance or develop long-term strengths.

Democratic (participative) leaders build consensus through participation.
- Give members of the work group a vote, or a say, in nearly every decision the team makes.
- A collaborative process brings a family atmosphere to the workplace and creates respect for the contributions by each member.
- When used effectively, the democratic leader builds flexibility and responsibility. This helps identify new ways to do things with fresh ideas.
- The level of involvement required by this approach (e.g., decision making), can be time-consuming.
- Appropriate for building buy-in or consensus, or for receiving input from valuable employees.

Affiliative leaders often are more sensitive to the value of people than reaching goals.
- Pride themselves on their ability to keep employees happy, and create a harmonious work environment.
- Attempt to build strong emotional bonds with those being led, with the hope that these relationships will bring about a strong sense of loyalty in their followers.
- May be appropriate to resolve tensions in a team or to motivate people in difficult situations.

Authentic leaders use a deep self-awareness to engage followers, to shape organizational environments, and eventually allow the organization to achieve persistently high performance.
- Authenticity involves both owning one's personal experiences (values, preferences, thoughts, emotions, and beliefs) and acting in accordance with one's true self.
- The ability of a leader to behave authentically as a person (authenticity of the person) positively affects his/her leadership efficacy (leadership multiplier).

Table 1.1 (*cont.*)

Transformational leaders care about human understanding – they transform and motivate followers through their idealized influence (or *charisma*) and role model, intellectual stimulation, and individual consideration.
- Aim at creating an environment where every person is empowered and motivated to fulfill his or her highest needs.
- Each member becomes a part of a collective identity and productive learning community of the organization.
- See themselves as servants to others and guide them in creating and embracing a vision for the organization. This inspires and brings forth top performance and creates a belief system of integrity. Servant leadership demands that a leader places company goals and values first, the management team and employees second, and the leader's own welfare third. In this paradigm, leaders exist to permit production and to obliterate obstacles, not acquire power, glory, wealth, or fame.

Table 1.2 Five main components of emotional intelligence

Self-awareness	Understand one's own emotions, strengths, weaknesses, needs, drives, and their effect on others
Self-regulation	The ability to control and manage feelings and moods so they are appropriate
Motivation	A passion to work for reasons that go beyond money and status
Empathy	The ability to understand the emotional makeup of other people
Social skill	A proficiency in managing relationship, building networks, and working with others

- people must be coerced, controlled, or threatened with punishment to get them to perform.

On the other hand, Theory Y postulates:
- work is as natural as play and rest;
- people are ambitious, self-motivated, and will readily accept greater responsibility;
- people will use their creativity, ingenuity, and imagination to solve problems.

In reality, a person's beliefs will fall somewhere between Theory X and Theory Y. Whereas Theory X leaders enforce the rules of behavior and punish those who violate the standards, Theory Y leaders function as a "coach" encouraging their team. They focus on developing and facilitating the team through nurturing, encouragement, support, and positive reinforcement.

Situational leadership

Goleman suggests that successful leaders employ multiple leadership styles and should be able to move between leadership styles according to a specific situation (situational leadership) [4]. Leadership in the OR requires this adaptive style because of the personalities encountered in a highly trained and demanding workplace. For example, during a cardiac resuscitation an authoritarian or coercive leadership style may be appropriate to making sure all code team members receive clear instructions. In contrast, an affiliate style

may be appropriate to resolve a conflict between two surgeons disputing over a certain OR time slot.

Goleman's situational leadership model suggests that although leaders may have a preferred style, they must identify and select the appropriate mix of various leadership behaviors in a given situation.

"Emotional intelligence" may be a better predictor of leadership effectiveness than intellectual intelligence (IQ) or technical skills [10]. Emotional intelligence is a person's ability to be aware of, manage, and use emotions appropriately in dealing with people in various situations (Table 1.2). Emotionally intelligent, person-oriented leaders may have more satisfied and committed staff members, who better attend to patient-care needs. These concepts are discussed further in Chapter 2.

Difference between management and leadership

A notion often heard is that managers are people busy with operational tasks (command and control) whereas leaders engage in strategic endeavors (vision and mission, change management). To quote Naylor, most persons have worked "with leaders who were not particularly skilled at management, but who had an ability to win loyalty and carry others with them through their clarity of vision, generosity of spirit, and 'people skills.' Ironically, then, leadership may be most obviously exerted when others follow a person who has no direct authority over them, and may be less important in strictly hierarchical organizations where managerial discipline prevails" [11].

The differences between managers and leaders then may simply be attributed to different leadership styles (e.g., transactional and transformational leadership style), or different leader positions (top executive versus middle-management position).

Significance of leadership for health-care organizations

Governments around the globe are increasingly searching for cost-containment practices to counteract mounting health-care expenditures. This has led to shrinking fees for physician and hospital services, the replacement of fee-for-service payments with prospective payment systems using case-based lump sums based on diagnosis-related groups (DRGs), and capitation and other compensation systems that shift financial risk from the payer to the service providers.

Such rapid reimbursement and technological, policy, and procedural changes intensify the challenges of health-care leadership [12].

There are unique leadership challenges inherent to health care [13]:

- health-care leaders face inconsistent, conflicting, and dynamic external (i.e., regulatory and other) demands;
- as a "human" service rendered directly by providers, health care is prone to natural variability;
- health care is a technology-intensive sector with a high frequency of innovation – such advances exacerbate tensions in balancing cost, quality, and access to health-care services;
- health-care leaders must interact with powerful and dominating professionals (e.g., physicians) who may not be employees of the organization.

The following factors contributed to the growing need for a dedicated professional as a perioperative leader:

- growing surgical caseload, exceeding regular workday shift hours;
- medical consumables included in case-based lump sum payment, which cannot be charged separately to the payer;
- multiple lines of authority causing a lack of continuity and a lack of ownership for decisions;
- increasing variety of professionals working in the OR suite;

- difficulties in recruiting health-care professionals;
- increasing number of ORs and creation of different OR suites within the same facility;
- increasing number of nonsurgical interventions outside the surgical suite with growing need for hospital-wide provider scheduling;
- lack of physician involvement in OR leadership.

Leadership in the health-care literature

In 2002, an extensive review of 6628 articles revealed that most of the health-care and business literature on leadership consisted of anecdotal or theoretical discussion [14]. Only a few articles include correlations of qualities or styles of leadership with measurable outcomes on the recipients of services or positive changes in organizations. It is still unclear which leadership attributes are important in improving either patient-care outcomes or team and organizational outcomes.

There are, however, some specific studies of leadership in health care that are noteworthy [13]. Transformational leadership style is more likely to be used by leaders in not-for-profit organizations than by leaders in for-profit organizations. In the hospital setting, transformational leadership style has been shown to be positively and significantly associated with staff satisfaction, extra effort from staff, perceived unit performance, and staff retention. Some weak evidence indicates that leadership matters more for nonprofessionals (e.g., nursing assistants, clerks, secretaries) than for professionals.

Managers with higher ranks demonstrate more transformational behavior than those lower in the hierarchy. Of note, health-care leaders may perceive the use of rewards as transformational leadership behavior, whereas in surveys among nonhealth-care leaders the use of such systems is linked to a transactional leadership style. Physician executives with management degrees are more likely to provide transformational leadership than those without training [15]. Despite evidence that supports transformational leadership theory for the health-care setting, leadership style is but one important factor in successful organizational change. Organizational structure and culture matter just as much. Participative and person-focused leadership styles are positively associated with nursing staff job satisfaction, retention, and organizational commitment.

In the health-care and hospital setting, leaders must take into account their followers' expectations

Table 1.3 Differences between clinicians and the manager/
leader

Clinicians	Manager/leader
Clinical competence	Interpersonal competence
1:1 interaction	1:N interaction
Doers	Planners
Value autonomy	Value collaboration
Reactive	Proactive
Identification with profession	Identification with company
Patient advocate	Organization advocate
Lay IT/information skills	IT/information skills power user
Informal communication	Formal communication
Leadership skills optional	Leadership skills essential
Member of a "brother-/sisterhood"	Member of the "dark side"
Micromanaging a must	Overmanaging a sure way to fail
Independent	Adaptation to a boss
Pursuit of self-interest	Trustworthiness

and understand how and why professionals respond (or not) to different leadership styles.

There exist seven recognized competency areas for effective leadership in health-service management:

- interpersonal relationship;
- communication;
- finance and business acumen;
- clinical knowledge;
- collaboration and team building;
- change management;
- quality improvement.

Managers with advanced education may be more effective in leadership roles. Junior nurse managers value clinical and communications skills more than senior managers, who value more negotiation skills and business knowledge [13]. There is, however, little evidence that more educational preparation leads to improved physician leaders' effectiveness, in particular when the authority and power from their clinical roles is factored in. Various barriers exist for physicians to take leadership roles [16]:

- identity issues – leadership roles may threaten the physicians' view of themselves as clinical professionals;
- deep-rooted skepticism about the value of spending time on leadership;
- lack of career development or financial incentives;
- lack of leadership and management training;
- risk of losing credibility with clinical colleagues and others;
- greater risk of unemployment as a leader/manager than as a clinician;
- loss of popularity as a result of tough decisions;
- the need to learn to being accountable to their organization rather than their colleagues;
- the need to overcome an "us-versus-them" mentality in physicians and health administrators.

A common myth is that a physician successful in clinical practice can easily transfer to leading an organization [17]. Physicians in the midst of the transition between clinical and managerial/leadership positions start to realize the substantial differences between clinical and managerial/leadership positions (Table 1.3).

Health care in general has been slow to adopt systematic organizationally based leadership development programs. Instead, responsibility for leadership development has been left to individuals and the profession.

Leadership is crucial in the management of perioperative services

The OR suite is a complex working environment, with different groups of individuals involved in a coordinated effort to perform highly skilled interventions. This is analogous to high-reliability organizations such as aviation, the military, and nuclear industries, in which the importance of a wide variety of factors in the development of a favorable outcome has been long stressed [18]. These include ergonomic factors, such as the quality of interface design, team coordination and leadership, organizational culture, and quality of decision making.

The role of a leader and manager is central for forming high-performance inter-professional teams. Underlying key principles for successful team building are a shared vision and mission. To align the goals of employees and physicians, the leader must convey the vision and strategies [19].

Predispositions for leaders

Trait theory, which suggests that leadership abilities depend on the personal qualities of the leader, is controversial. On the one hand, some traits are related to leadership emergence and effectiveness. Leadership emergence refers to whether and to what degree an individual is viewed as a leader by others within a work group. On the other hand, leadership effectiveness is a between-group phenomenon, and refers to a leader's performance in influencing and guiding the activities of his or her unit toward the achievement of its goals.

Five dimensions can be used to describe the most prominent aspects of personality: neuroticism, extraversion, openness to experience, agreeableness, and conscientiousness. This five-factor model of personality was also shown to be a reasonable basis for examining dispositional predictors of leadership [20]. Extraversion and conscientiousness are the most important traits of leaders, and these dimensions are more strongly related to leadership emergence than to leadership effectiveness.

The following traits are associated with successful leaders [21]: humility, courage, integrity, vigilance and passion, inspiration, sense of duty and dedication, compassion, discipline, generosity, dedication to continuous learning, a collaborative approach, and competitiveness. Personality traits of OR directors/leaders are also described in Chapter 2.

Appendix A, on page 12, has a checklist that may be a way for leaders to self-assess some of their own strengths and weaknesses as a leader. In addition, it could be used by people working in a surgical suite to evaluate the OR director.

Game theory in the OR context

The OR suite's stakeholders

A stakeholder is any group or individual who can affect or is affected by the achievement of an organization's purpose [22]. For the perioperative leader, it is important to identify the relevant stakeholders and their specific needs, expectations, and preferences. This will allow the leader to engage the various parties for common goals and to give priority to competing stakeholder interests and claims (stakeholder salience). Various individuals or groups have a specific interest in the OR suite and can affect (or can be affected by) their actions:

- patients – suffer from sickness or injury and expect high-quality medical services at no additional risk (patient safety);
- surgeons – expect maximum convenience and service, easy and fast access to OR time (especially for add-on and emergency cases), and state-of-the-art equipment – the surgeons are powerful stakeholders, as they assign the medical priority, which determines the urgency of a case;
- anesthesiologists – the OR provides a place to practice – they prefer predictable working hours;
- nurses – expect predictable working hours and an enjoyable workplace without disruptive behavior or harassment;
- suppliers – surgical support services and housekeeping – the OR must consider the concerns of its suppliers;
- executives, administrators – want efficient use of OR time, high utilization, and low staffing cost and little capital expenditure in equipment;
- owners – want to maximize the quality and reputation of their health-care organization and their return on investment as applicable.

Knowing the stakeholder's needs and expectations allows a leader to manage them better. The tools required to manage stakeholder expectations include good communication, active listening, building trust, negotiating skills, addressing concerns, and quickly resolving issues. They will, as the common refrain goes, not be able to make everybody happy. An OR leader will have to make some decisions that will make one or more parties satisfied and others less so. Depending on the combination of power, legitimacy, and urgency, the OR leader will assign priority to a specific stakeholder (stakeholder salience) [23] (in this context, power has been defined as the ability of those who possess power to bring about the outcomes they desire, legitimacy as a generalized perception that the actions of someone are desirable, proper, or appropriate within some socially constructed system of values and beliefs, and urgency as the degree to which stakeholder claims call for immediate attention, respectively). Urgency is directly related to the medical priority of a case, which is usually determined by the surgeon. Regardless of whether the information about urgency is reliable or not, high urgency of a case combined with the surgeon's power will benefit the surgeon with any decision making. Each stakeholder may attempt to manipulate the priorities of the manager, who must persistently stand by their established principles to maintain order and fairness.

Game theory concepts

Leaders in the perioperative setting should understand essential game theory concepts in order to understand and influence the interactions between individuals and groups to achieve a cohesive team with mutual goal-oriented benefits.

In game theory, players can be team players (same goals) or opponents (different or opposing goals) [24]. Players in a game can choose either to cooperate or to fail ("defect"), but none of the players is aware of the other's choice. If every player chooses to cooperate, all gain. However, if one chooses to defect, that person's individual gains are usually much bigger. If all defect, everybody loses or gains very little.

There are several dilemmas hindering participants from cooperating.

- Prisoner's dilemma: a situation in which two parties would each gain more by cooperating with each other. Instead, they each act independently, and "defect," betraying the other party. This ultimately results in a lesser gain for each of them. It also undermines any momentum toward an alliance.
- Tragedy of the commons: a situation similar to the prisoner's dilemma except that it involves more than two parties.
- Free rider: a situation that can lead to the loss of shared resources. Individuals may be able to enjoy a community resource without paying for it, but if no one voluntarily pays and everyone chooses instead to be a free rider, they all exhaust the resource.
- Stag hunt: in this situation, a group can win a massive reward if all the members cooperate with each other. However, members may elect to defect for chasing smaller but surer individual rewards.

Several outcomes of games can be observed: the zero-sum game, also known as the win–lose game, reflects a situation in which a fixed pie must be divided among participants. In this situation, the "payoff," or reward, to one player is charged to his or her opponent; thus the sum of the reward and loss is zero. In other words, if one of the participants gets more of the pie, the other loses by an according amount. In nonzero–sum games, cooperative behavior leads to a net increase in the value of the system.

Rewards and punishments depend on whether both cooperate, both choose to betray, or one player

cooperates and the other betrays. The greatest reward is given to a player who betrays his or her opponent when the opponent chooses cooperation. If both players cooperate, the individual rewards are lessened. Reward diminishes further if both players defect and is least for the player who cooperates when his or her opponent defects. If one player cooperates and one defects, the combined reward for both players is less than if they had both cooperated. No player can reliably predict what his or her opponent will do, and both will have to play the game again.

In various sciences, game theory is used to model tactical situations (games), in which an individual's success in making choices depends on the choices of others. Game theory provides a way to understand various kinds of confrontation and offers an explanation of why cooperation may be the ideal response in some situations. Individuals and groups can avoid some traps in game theory by cooperating instead of allowing destructive competition.

Game theory applied to the OR suite

All parties working in the OR generally share common goals (such as maximizing the health of the patient), although conflicting goals may occur. In the OR, iterative prisoner dilemmas can be observed – a series of games in which participants can choose to cooperate or defect with another participant [25].

Understanding the types of interactions (games) helps the participants better predict outcome and adapt their own behavior to optimize that outcome. Types of games seen in the OR suite include the following [26,27].

- Zero–sum (win–lose) game – for example, OR time is often allocated across surgeons from a fixed amount of staffed OR time: if surgeon A is allotted more time, this amount of time must be deducted from one or more of his or her colleagues.
- Nonzero–sum games – for example, cooperative interaction and synergies between surgeons, anesthesiologists, OR nursing staff, and the hospital administration can improve efficiency and throughput, and hence productivity.

Numerous examples exist of selfish actions in the OR suite:

- anesthesiologists being inflexible in the required preoperative evaluations, unreasonably limiting their work hours, unnecessarily canceling or

delaying cases, obstructing the OR schedule and inconveniencing patients, or taking a passive role in the turnover and flow of cases;
- surgeons by making unreasonable demands on access, providing inaccurate information about the case (e.g., duration, medical information, urgency, etc.), demanding immediate compliance with their wishes, and defecting through disruptive behavior or gaming to get their cases done at night;
- hospital administration not providing adequate space or support personnel (e.g., concentrating on short-term budget issues).

A poorly running OR is comparable to "mutual defection." This can be illustrated by comments from staff such as "Why should I do this-or-that when so-and-so won't do his job?" In such a situation, it is not clear whether the players cooperate until one player defects and then defect forever or whether they have deduced that in a finite series of games the one strategy that minimizes unfair gain by others is for both players to defect. For salaried employees, working quickly in an OR is "rewarded" with additional cases but no increase in compensation. Once observed, they may appear to be people not working as efficiently.

In cooperative games, a good leader gathers the best players to win the game and makes OR nurses understand that it is their job to help the surgical team – for example by helping to make sure there are no retained sponges [28]. Understanding game theory helps a leader recognize the interdependence of all players in the game, the need to become allocentric, and the need to think ahead, considering all possible consequences.

Challenges of OR leadership

Organizational structures of OR leadership

Hospitals have always been in search of the optimal OR leadership structure. For example, in the literature of the 1950s, a textbook contained descriptions of the ideal OR structure and recommended that "the administration of the surgical department shall be under the direction of a competent registered nurse who has executive ability and who is specially trained in operating-room management" [29]. In 1983, an article about OR management delineated eight managerial measures to improve OR management efficiency and effectiveness. One of these measures was the identification of a clear line of authority and appointment of an individual with far-reaching responsibilities, including

policy making, running the daily schedule, and disciplining people [30]. The article pointed out that not only would this person have to be a senior physician with institutional authority but also be recognized as being in charge.

There is no perfect organizational structure. The organizational structure of an OR suite must be individually tailored to its internal and external needs.

Small organizations often feature a flat hierarchy and do not require many formal organizational structures. These organizations benefit from close relationships between the people working in the OR suite. This allows quick and informal problem solving. An OR charge nurse or nursing director as the sole formal leader may be sufficient in small OR suites, as ad hoc problem-solving groups form spontaneously and dissolve naturally.

Large organizations with several surgical subspecialties require a more complex organizational and leadership structure because cooperation and coordination of tasks between departments is a challenging task. The OR suites of large medical centers often feature several complementary leadership structures (Table 1.4).

Outside the United States, OR management is a relatively young science and leadership literature a relatively new phenomenon. In Germany, OR management appeared in the scientific literature in 1999 for the first time. The fact that this topic produced interest there much later than it did in the United States may be explained by the introduction of the German Diagnosis Related Groups reimbursement, a prospective payment system (PPS) for inpatient hospital services in 2003. In the United States, PPS was introduced in the 1980s. With the introduction of government-mandated health-care cost-containment measures as PPS, hospital revenues declined and hospital and physician executives started to find new ways to increase OR efficiency (see Chapter 6).

The appearance of the OR management in the hospital, medical management literature, and scientific literature parallels the introduction of PPS. In the German OR management literature, a team-oriented (or transformational) leadership style has been discouraged for OR suites with more than 20 people working in them, because it is believed that only a transactional leadership style with a formal distance between the OR manager and the "team" allows the former to pursue the agreed-upon targets [34]. In a 2002 survey from Switzerland, 49% of responding hospitals indicated

Table 1.4 Leadership positions and structures for the surgical suite

Physician OR leadership position (e.g., OR Medical Director)	May be a facilitator, mediator, and negotiator position to balance the priorities of each group in the OR (surgeons, anesthesiologists, nurses, hospital administrators, etc.).
Alternatively, the OR Medical Director may be positioned to be a distinct authority	A position frequently recommended by the German OR management literature ("OR manager") [31,32]. This may be explained by the fact that in Germany, as in many other European countries, most physicians are employed by the hospital. Wherever there are many independent, powerful physicians (especially surgeons), a tall or centralized organization with a top decision-making leader may be an ineffective leadership structure.
Standing OR Committee with strategic and oversight responsibilities (e.g., "OR oversight committee," "OR board").	This committee may consist of the chairs of surgical services and/or departments, the chief of the anesthesia department and nurse managers of the perioperative area, and representatives of the hospital administration. The role of this committee is to provide fair and balanced OR governance [33].
Additional smaller OR management teams may be formed with operational responsibilities (e.g., OR executive committee).	A typical formation includes a senior surgeon and anesthesiologist (who may be the medical co-directors of the OR suite), the director of surgical services, and a senior hospital executive.
Administrative Executive Physician	This position may be labeled Chief Medical Officer (CMO) or Vice President of Medical Affairs (VPMA), and refers to a position often used as third-party mediator to facilitate finding solutions between two conflicting parties (e.g., between two different surgical departments or between the hospital administration and anesthesia department).

that their OR suite did not have a formal OR director [35]. Fifty-two percent of the OR leadership respondents had responsibility for strategic planning, 11% for finances, 89% for day-to-day operations, and 63% for human resources.

Lonely at the top

Leaders are often alone with their thoughts because they need to keep an emotional distance and avoid a conflict of interests in their professional environment [34]. Leaders are able to develop a relationship with people based on respect, not on friendship [36]. In addition, leaders are often surrounded by people with completely opposite opinions on a certain topic for valid reasons. Decision making in uncertainty is a task that exacerbates the leader's loneliness. Making decisions unpopular with some stakeholders and being attacked for those decisions may increase isolation for the leader.

One of the interesting observations by leaders is to see how streams of information dry up when a person becomes the head of an organization or a group. People are less comfortable speaking freely with a leader and communicate more formally, as if they were talking to the institution rather than to the leader. For the leader, the risk then is that the ability to figure out what is really going on decreases. A leader in the surgical suite needs to work hard to get people to share their views, and must proactively develop positive relationships so that colleagues feel comfortable providing their honest opinions.

Culture and informal organization

Understanding the organizational culture of the OR suite is key to successful and effective leadership. For example, change management and implementing patient safety initiatives are hard to accomplish without knowing the values, assumptions, preferences, unwritten rules, and behaviors of a workplace. If leaders do not become conscious of the culture in which they are embedded, those cultures will manage them [37]. The leadership needs to perceive the functional and dysfunctional elements of the existing culture and to manage cultural evolution and change in such a way that the group can thrive.

Organizational culture is the essence of the informal organization [38]. In addition to the formal relationships shown on organizational charts, in every OR suite information relationships exist and there may be an informal network, coalitions of people, and even hierarchy. For example, a powerful surgeon may be able to exert his or her influence on the scheduling process and circumvent official scheduling rules. These informal affiliations shape the organization's culture, and they can either facilitate or impede change. An important aspect of perioperative leadership is understanding and accepting these relationships, managing the informal chain of command, and even leveraging these affiliations.

People alignment and change

Tensions between the different professional groups working in the OR have probably existed since the first surgeries were performed. A nursing report from Australia in the early twentieth century noted that the "disaccord between nurses and physicians often led to troubles in the OR because the physicians would never announce the beginning of surgeries in a timely fashion, but would then suddenly appear in the OR where they would have to wait for the nurses to be finished with their preparatory work" [39].

A core issue for leaders of the OR suite is that the goals of the various professions are not well aligned with those of the hospital and the OR suite. This dilemma is known in economics as the "principal-agent problem," where difficulties arise under conditions of incomplete and asymmetric information when a principal hires and motivates an agent to act on his or her behalf [40]. One of various mechanisms that may be used to try to align the interests of the agent in solidarity with those of the principal is performance measurement. In the OR environment, well-designed reporting systems must report relevant performance measures (key performance indicators). This feedback is provided to those owning the critical processes and should be gauged relative to the OR suite's goals and its most important stakeholders. The OR environment with conflicting goals requires strong leadership to enforce hospital and OR suite strategies.

In US hospitals, the shift toward employment of physicians continues to grow, becoming the dominant alignment model. There will be less emphasis on solitary leaders and more on teams of leaders. There will be broadened leadership communities inside and outside the organization [21].

How can a leader assess his or her individual impact on culture and perimeter of control in the organization? Covey and Gulledge encouraged leaders to work within their smaller circle of influence, in which they can make a difference, rather than spending time in their circle of concern, in which they have little ability to contribute [41]. Effective leaders recognize two primary types of change: from the outside in (structural) and from the inside out (cultural/behavioral). A focus on cultural change is core to sustaining structural change.

However, for leaders it is difficult to simultaneously tackle all "soft" issues (such as culture and motivation) that are relevant for transforming organizations. Sirkin *et al.* have found that focusing on these issues alone may not bring about change because companies also need to consider the "hard" factors, such as the time it takes to complete a change initiative, the number of people required to execute it, etc. [42]. There is a consistent correlation between the outcomes of change programs (success versus failure) and the following four variables.

D – The *duration* of time until the change program is completed if it has a short life span; if not short, the amount of time between milestones.

I – The project team's performance *integrity*; that is, the capabilities of project teams.

C – *commitment* to change the senior executives and staff.

E – The *effort* over and above the usual work that the change initiative demands of employees.

The "DICE" framework comprises a set of simple questions that help executives score their projects on each of the four factors. Companies can use DICE assessments to force conversations about projects, to gauge whether projects are on track or in trouble, and to manage project portfolios.

Social capital

Waisel described social capital as an overall indicator of the quality of the relationships within a community and applied it to the OR suite [25]. Increasing social capital improves communication and trust, which in turn improve most cooperative undertakings. In the OR suite, the social capital benefits of expectations of trust, robust norms, and better communication help to achieve community goals.

The norm should be that medical professionals seek flawless behavior, particularly with regard to interacting with others and respecting operational guidelines. Other than small teams, large groups of people are less likely to have developed personal histories of successful interactions. In the absence of a personal history of trust, the expectation of trust from social capital permits individuals entering into negotiations to assume that they will be treated in a fair, appropriate, and civil manner. Functional operational guidelines help to develop trust in the organization. Improved behavior and successful interactions increase trust and communication, which in turn improves the OR working environment and increases the success of cooperative ventures, such as having more efficient operating rooms.

Importance of building trust on survival of coalitions

Dialogue promotes understanding between parties in conflict and the resulting relationship promotes trust between diverse entities [43]. This trust is based on the fact that there is respect for one another's opinion and that team members are willing to listen and share viewpoints openly. If and when leaders promote an environment in which they are comfortable taking on the challenging dialogues (i.e., productive conflict), they can effectively lead change and build respect in the perioperative setting. This leads to a stronger team and better adherence to patient safety measures. A common example is of OR nurses speaking up before a wrong-site surgery, preventing disaster.

The impact of leadership on patient safety and quality initiatives

Many have stated that the magic ingredient to success in patient safety is leadership [2]. Communication and leadership failure are two of the most frequent causes of adverse events [44]. Previous studies have identified that the nontechnical skills of teamwork, communication, and situation awareness are the most important for working safely and effectively in a surgical environment and for minimizing technical errors [45,46].

How is a leader able to move the team to the next level of safety culture? Before a change can be successfully implemented, the leader must first assess and understand the culture. Only a deep awareness of the organization's culture allows the leader to set off effective change.

In the UK in 1997, the concept of "clinical governance" was introduced into the National Health Service (NHS), relating to a comprehensive framework to improve the quality of care. Clinical governance is defined as a framework through which NHS organizations are accountable for continuously improving the quality of their services and safeguarding high standards of care by creating an environment in which excellence in clinical care can flourish. Leadership, teamwork, effective communication, and ownership and systems awareness are the foundations of clinical governance [47].

Successful centers are more likely to have a shared sense of purpose, leaders with a hands-on leadership style, and clear accountability structures [48,49].

Leaders may have a direct impact on the behaviors of the employees, by joining in the execution of the strategy and clarifying the expected results and aligning the rewards system. The leader must insure the right person for the right role, and with execution as part of the expected behavior, it becomes part of the culture [50].

There is evidence that preventability of harm to patient and sustainable transformation to a higher state of reliability is directly related to governance board engagement and administrative execution [51]. Risk-adjusted mortality rates have been shown to be significantly lower for hospitals whose governing boards have a quality committee than for those who don't. Hospital boards seem to be more successful when they set specific aims to reduce harm and make a public commitment to measurable quality improvement [52].

There exists evidence that greater engagement of hospital leadership at the board and executive level is associated with better quality outcomes, as measured by the CareScience Quality Index – a single quality measure embracing risk-adjusted adverse outcome rates for mortality, morbidity, and complications [53].

One of the major patient safety organizations in the United States, the National Quality Forum (NQF) studies on seven dimensions of culture revealed the following findings [21]:

- communication – high-performing organizations have very clear communication channels within their structures and systems and excellent links with outside organizations;
- underlying values – leaders drive values, values drive behaviors, and the collective behaviors of the individuals in an organization define the corporate cultures and drive performance;
- leadership – the success of high-performing organizations revolves completely around leaders at every level and the structures and systems they put in place enable expressions of the group values;
- teamwork – high-performing organizations are invested in the knowledge and skill development to build a great team;

- unity and trust – unity around a constancy of purpose cannot happen without trust;
- reliability – high-performing organizations have formally or informally adopted the characteristics of high-reliability organizations (e.g., Six Sigma);
- energy state – cultures that are transforming or constantly improving have a capacity for extra effort over and above that needed to deliver basic care.

However, more than ten years after the Institute of Medicine (IOM) report "To Err Is Human," the efforts undertaken for improving health-care quality and patient safety haven't yet achieved a breakthrough. Katz-Navon *et al.* have identified conflicting messages of health-care organizations about the relative value of productivity and safety as possibly one essential issue [54]. While the usual official mission of a health-care organization includes high quality and patient safety, maintaining these tenets often entails working at a slower pace and exerting extra effort, conflicting with the organization's other goals – optimizing productivity and economic efficiency.

For example, despite national efforts to prevent wrong-site surgeries, they have become more prevalent. These "never events" are becoming more common because of growing time pressures, and they require changing hospital culture and ensuring that physicians collaborate and follow standardized protocols. For senior hospital leaders this is a major challenge to insure that the time and resources needed to improve broken processes are made available [55].

Summary

Being a leader in a medical environment may be different from being a chief executive officer of a corporation, as the optimal combination of leadership styles may be different. For example, in a physician group, the chief needs to be wary of an authoritative style, as the OR environment and medical group is a collegial place in which numerous people have a collective responsibility and ownership for the organization. The successful OR manager has the difficult task of being professional and steady-mannered while taking public criticism openly and accepting personal weaknesses in a very dynamic environment.

Appendix A. Characteristics of leadership

Integrity: core to building trust

- Promptly takes ownership of difficult situations
- Perceived as direct, truthful
- Can present the unvarnished truth in an appropriate and helpful manner
- Keeps confidences
- Not afraid to fail
- Admits mistakes
- Doesn't misrepresent for personal gain

Vision and purpose

- Communicates a competing and inspired vision or sense of core purpose
- Dissatisfied with the status quo
- Talks beyond today and about possibilities
- Shoulders blame rather than searches for excuses
- Optimistic
- Creates milestones and symbols to rally support
- Makes the vision sharable by everyone
- Inspires and motivates entire units

Political savvy

- Can maneuver through complex political situations
- Sensitive to how people and organizations function
- Anticipates where difficulties/barriers are and plans approach accordingly
- Views politics as a part of organizational life and works to adjust

Decision making

- Makes good decisions based upon a mixture of analysis, wisdom, experience, and judgment
- Most solutions and suggestions turn out to be correct and accurate when judged over time
- Sought out by others for advice and solutions
- Resists being hypnotized by complexity

Negotiating

- Understands no one conflict resolution type is best but that several are needed depending on situation
- Settles differences
- Can win concessions without damaging relationships
- Can be both direct and forceful as well as diplomatic
- Gains trust quickly of parties to the negotiations
- Has a good sense of timing

Motivating others

- Creates a climate in which people want to do their best
- Possesses knowledge and skills to recognize and develop talent
- Motivates many kinds of direct reports and team or project members
- Pushes tasks and decisions down
- Ready to drive continuous process improvement
- Empowers others
- Invites input and shares ownership and visibility
- Makes each individual feel their work is important
- People like working for and with them

References

1. Merriam Webster Online Dictionary. 2011. www.merriam-webster.com/ (last accessed June 30, 2011).

2. C. R. Denham. May I have the envelope please? *J Patient Saf* 2008; **4**: 119–23.

3. J. Hoyle. *Leadership Styles*. Thousand Oaks, CA: Sage Reference, 2006.

4. D. Goleman. Leadership that gets results. *Harv Bus Rev* 2000; **78**: 78–90.

5. W. L. Gardner, B. J. Avolio, F. O. Walumbwa. *Authentic Leadership Theory and Practice: Origins, Effects and Development*. Oxford: Elsevier JAI, 2005.

6. D. Goleman, R. Boyatizis, A. McKee. *Primal Leadership. Realizing the Power of Emotional Intelligence*. Boston: Harvard Business Press, 2002.

7. L. A. Hill. Where will we find tomorrow's leaders? *Harv Bus Rev* 2008; **86**: 123–9.

8. D. McGregor. *The Human Side of Enterprise*. New York: McGraw-Hill, 1960.

9. D. McGregor, J. Cutcher-Gershenfeld. *The Human Side of Enterprise*, annotated edn. New York: McGraw-Hill, 2006.

10. D. Goleman. What makes a leader? *Clin Lab Manage Rev* 1999; **13**: 123–31.

11. C. D. Naylor. Leadership in academic medicine: reflections from administrative exile. *Clin Med* 2006; **6**: 488–92.

12. L. R. Hearld, J. A. Alexander, I. Fraser, *et al*. Review: How do hospital organizational structure and processes affect quality of care? A critical review of research methods. *Med Care Res Rev* 2008; **65**: 259–99.

13. M. J. Gilmartin, T. A. D'Aunno. Leadership Research in Healthcare: A Review and Roadmap. *Acad Manag Ann* 2007; **1**: 387–438.

14. C. Vance, E. Larson. Leadership research in business and health care. *J Nurs Scholarsh* 2002; **34**: 165–71.

15. S. Xirasagar, M. E. Samuels, T. F. Curtin. Management training of physician executives, their leadership style, and care management performance: An empirical study. *Am J Manag Care* 2006; **12**: 101–8.

16. C. Carruthers, J. Swettenham. Physician leadership: Neccessary and in need of nurturing – now. *Healthc Q* 2011; **14**: 6–8.

17. A. M. Desai, R. A. Trillo, Jr., A. Macario. Should I get a Master of Business Administration? The anesthesiologist with education training: training options and professional opportunities. *Curr Opin Anaesthesiol* 2009; **22**: 191–8.

18. R. Aggarwal, S. Undre, K. Moorthy, *et al*. The simulated operating theatre: comprehensive training for surgical teams. *Qual Saf Health Care* 2004; **13 Suppl 1**: i27–32.

19. R. Cullen, S. Nicholls, A. Halligan. Reviewing a service – discovering the unwritten rules. *Clin Perform Qual Health Care* 2000; **8**: 233–9.

20. T. A. Judge, J. E. Bono, R. Ilies, *et al*. Personality and leadership: A qualitative and quantitative review. *J Appl Psychol* 2002; **87**: 765–80.

21. C. R. Denham. Values genetics: Who are the real smartest guys in the room? *J Patient Saf* 2007; **3**: 214–26.

22. R. E. Freeman. *Strategic Management: A stakeholder Approach*. Boston: Pitman, 1984.

23. R. K. Mitchell, B. R. Agle, D. J. Wood. Toward a theory of stakeholder identification and salience: Defining the principle of who and what really counts. *Academy Manage Rev* 1997; **22**: 853–86.

24. L. Fisher. *Rock, Paper, Scissors: Game Theory in Everyday Life*. London: Hay House, 2008.

25. D. B. Waisel. Developing social capital in the operating room: The use of population-based techniques. *Anesthesiology* 2005; **103**: 1305–10.

26. A. P. Marco. Game theoretic approaches to operating room management. *Am Surg* 2002; **68**: 454–62.

27. A. P. Marco. Game theory in the operating room environment. *Am Surg* 2001; **67**: 92–6.

28. S. B. Dowd, A. Root. The hospital manager and game theory: Chess master, poker player, or cooperative game player? *Health Care Manag (Frederick)* 2003; **22**: 305–10.

29. M. T. MacEachern. *Hospital Organization and Management*. Berwyn, IL: Physicians' Record Co., 1957.

30. W. F. Hejna, C. M. Gutmann. The management of surgical facilities in hospitals. *Health Care Manage Rev* 1983; **8**: 51–5.

31. A. Baumgart, G. Schupfer, A. Welker, *et al*. Status quo and current trends of operating room management in Germany. *Curr Opin Anaesthesiol* 2010; **23**: 193–200.

32. G. Schüpfer, M. Bauer. Wer ist zum OP-Manager geeignet? *Anaesthesist* 2011; **60**: 251–6.

33. P. Patterson. Is your OR's governing structure up to today's intense demands? *OR Manager* 2008; **24**: 1, 6–7.

34. M. Bauer, J. Hinz, A. Klockgether-Radke. Göttinger Leitfaden für OP-Manager. *Anaesthesist* 2010; **59**: 69–79.

35. T. J. Sieber, D. L. Leibundgut. Operating room management and strategies in Switzerland: Results of a survey. *Eur J Anaesthesiol* 2002; **19**: 415–23.

36. S. Birk. The 10 most common myths about leadership. *Healthc Exec* 2010; **25**: 30–2, 34–6, 38.

37. E. H. Schein. *Organizational Culture and Leadership*. San Francisco: Jossey-Bass, 2010.

38. D. J. Teece. Firm organization, industrial structure, and technological innovation. *J Econ Behav Organ* 1996; **31**: 193–224.

39. E. P. Evans. Nursing in Australia. *Int Nurs Rev* 1938; **12**: 261.

40. K. M. Eisenhardt. Agency Theory: An Assessment and Review. *Acad Manage Rev* 1989; **14**: 57–74.

41. S. R. Covey, K. A. Gulledge. Principle-centered leadership and change. *J Qual Particip* 1994; **17**: 10.

42. H. L. Sirkin, P. Keenan, A. Jackson. The hard side of change management. *Harv Bus Rev* 2005; **83**: 108–18, 58.

43. M. M. Chadwick. Creating order out of chaos: a leadership approach. *AORN J* 2010; **91**: 154–70.

44. The Joint Commission. Improving America's Hospitals: The Joint Commission's Report on Quality and Safety 2007. The Joint Commission, 2007, pp. 45–8.

45. M. Leonard, S. Graham, D. Bonacum. The human factor: the critical importance of effective teamwork and communication in providing safe care. *Qual Saf Health Care* 2004; **13 Suppl 1**: i85–90.

46. S. Yule, R. Flin, S. Paterson-Brown, *et al*. Non-technical skills for surgeons in the operating room: A review of the literature. *Surgery* 2006; **139**: 140–9.

47. M. E. Braine. Clinical governance: Applying theory to practice. *Nurs Stand* 2006; **20**: 56–65; quiz 6.

48. A. S. Frankel, M. W. Leonard, C. R. Denham. Fair and just culture, team behavior, and leadership engagement: The tools to achieve high reliability. *Health Serv Res* 2006; **41**: 1690–709.

49. M. A. Keroack, B. J. Youngberg, J. L. Cerese, *et al*. Organizational factors associated with high performance in quality and safety in academic medical centers. *Acad Med* 2007; **82**: 1178–86.

50. J. Collins. Level 5 leadership. The triumph of humility and fierce resolve. *Harv Bus Rev* 2001; **79**: 66–76, 175.

51. H. J. Jiang, C. Lockee, K. Bass, *et al*. Board engagement in quality: findings of a survey of hospital and system leaders. *J Healthc Manag* 2008; **53**: 121–34; discussion 35.

52. J. Conway. Getting boards on board: engaging governing boards in quality and safety. *Jt Comm J Qual Patient Saf* 2008; **34**: 214–20.

53. T. Vaughn, M. Koepke, E. Kroch, *et al*. Engagement of Leadership in Quality Improvement Initiatives: Executive Quality Improvement Survey Results. *J Patient Saf* 2006; **2**: 2–9.

54. T. Katz-Navon, E. Naveh, Z. Stern. The moderate success of quality of care improvement efforts: Three observations on the situation. *Int J Qual Health Care* 2007; **19**: 4–7.

55. R. L. Kane, G. Mosser. The challenge of explaining why quality improvement has not done better. *Int J Qual Health Care* 2007; **19**: 8–10.

The path to a successful operating room environment

Ross Musumeci MD, MBA
Alan D. Kaye MD, PhD
Charles J. Fox III MD
Richard D. Urman MD, MBA

A closer look at the OR Manager/Director   15

Psychology in the OR   16

Emotional intelligence   16

Emotional pathways   17

The components of emotional intelligence   17

Measuring emotional intelligence   18

Resonant and dissonant leadership   19

The importance of emotional intelligence and resonant leadership   19

Improving emotional intelligence   20

Psychology in the OR: transactional analysis   20

One example, structural analysis   20

Team training   22

Summary   23

The operating room typically has a fast paced, high stress environment with complex professional interactions. Clinical competence is a basic requirement for work in the operating room, but to excel it is necessary to manage those interactions successfully. A firm understanding of human behavior and important leadership skills make this task much easier. There are over a dozen subgroups of workers who must act as a cohesive team to achieve optimal performance and provide excellent patient care (Figure 2.1).

A closer look at the OR Manager/Director

There are at least four distinct stakeholders in the OR: hospital administration, nursing, anesthesiology, and surgery. Each of these stakeholders has their own interests that may not coincide, and the OR Manager/Director must be able to balance the needs of these different groups in order to maximize productivity and minimize conflict. The key characteristics of an effective OR Manager/Director are listed in Table 2.1.

A more detailed job description of the OR Manager/Director can be found on the website of the American Association of Clinical Directors (AACD) at www. aacdhq.org.

Anesthesiologists who have the characteristics listed in Table 2.1 are particularly qualified to fill the OR Manager/Director position because they typically have a constant presence in the OR without the need for office hours, and they usually have a clear understanding of OR processes. Hospital administrators may prefer anesthesiologists or nurses for the OR Manager/Director position, because their economic interests are often directly aligned with those of the hospital.

A successful OR Manager/Director must have the support of the hospital Chief Executive Officer (CEO) and the chairpersons of the departments of surgery, nursing, and anesthesiology. It is necessary for all departments to give up some of their own authority and control so that the OR Manager/Director can run the OR in a manner that benefits everyone. The OR Manager/Director must also have the support of their own specialty group, because the position will require time that could otherwise be spent on their own specialty group activities. For this reason, and also to emphasize the neutrality of the OR Manager/Director position among all departments, the OR Manager/Director and/or the manager/director's practice should be compensated by the hospital.

Operating Room Leadership and Management, ed. Kaye A.D., Fox C.J. and Urman R.D. Published by Cambridge University Press. © Cambridge University Press 2012.

Table 2.1 Characteristics of an effective OR Manager/Director

Strong problem-solving and organizational skills

Even-tempered

Ability to commit significant amount of nonclinical time

Strong clinician garnering respect of other clinicians

Strong interpersonal and negotiation skills

Ability to understand business/financial concerns of institution and physicians

Understanding of perioperative processes

Understanding of scheduling systems and information technology

Good understanding of organizational dynamics; ability to understand divergent needs and concerns of different stakeholders and bring them together

Commitment to overall performance of OR suite rather than individual department

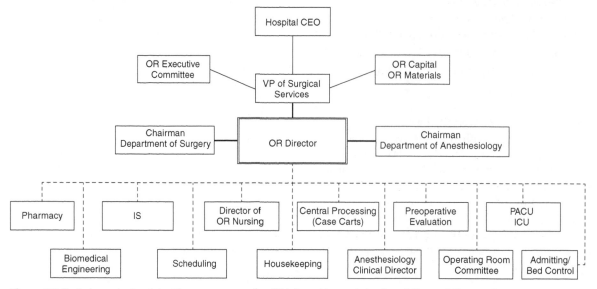

Figure 2.1 Typical organizational chart for management of an OR (taken with permission from: R. Urman, S. Eappen. Operating room management: Core principles. In: C. A. Vacanti, P. K. Sikka, R. D. Urman, M. Dershwitz, B. S. Segal. *Essential Clinical Anesthesia*, 1st edn, Cambridge University Press, 2011).

Psychology in the OR

An understanding of fundamental psychology is extremely valuable in any professional setting, but this is particularly true in the stressful and emotionally charged environment of the OR. Understanding psychological insights quickly can significantly improve the quality of communication. Indeed, for leaders in the OR, recruiting staff members who possess strong psychological insights can make a significant contribution to the success of the group. Moreover, members of surgical, nursing, and anesthesia teams who are effective leaders typically possess these valuable abilities.

Interpersonal difficulties are common in the OR, and those that achieve the greatest success and respect in that setting are able to communicate effectively and overcome situational problems.

Emotional intelligence

One aspect of psychology that is particularly relevant to the practice of medicine, and the OR environment in particular, is emotional intelligence (EI). It is a set of skills that enables a person to recognize their own and others' emotions, and to use that information in ways that improve their interpersonal interactions. Emotional intelligence is a topic that is relatively unknown in medicine, but it is well known in the business community. This section will discuss the components of EI, ways to measure it, its relevance to practice management, and its application to the practice of medicine in general. This subject presents readers with a huge opportunity for self-improvement on both a personal and professional level. The only requirements are an open mind and a motivation.

Weschsler first referred to the collection of skills that comprise EI when he noted the difference between "intrapersonal and interpersonal" intelligence in the 1940s. However, the term "emotional intelligence" was coined by Leuner in 1966. The first models of EI were introduced in the late 1980s and early 1990s by Greenspan and Salovey & Meyer. The concept was fully popularized in the business community through a series of articles and books published by Daniel Goleman starting in the late 1990s. Dr. Goleman presented the topic in a simple fashion and made a compelling argument for the importance of EI as a leadership skill. Subsequently, many others have published on the topic with variations in the style and structure that they use to present the topic.

As it is a relatively new concept, it is no surprise that there is some controversy surrounding the nature of EI and the validity of it as a psychological construct. Arguments exist about whether it is an ability that is learned, a trait that is inherited, or some combination of the two. Some psychologists argue that tests for measuring EI are collectively quantifying other individual abilities for which proven testing already exists, and that EI adds nothing new. Dr. Goleman has also attracted his share of critics who say that he uses proprietary data that are unavailable for outside review to support his claims of the value of EI as a leadership skill.

Despite all the controversy, there is evidence supporting the worth of EI in professional interactions, with increasing value at higher levels of leadership. The popularity of Dr. Goleman's writing over the past decade indicates that his way of presenting the concept of EI has struck a chord among those in the business world. Leadership is a somewhat nebulous concept that is difficult to define accurately, and identifying the core elements necessary for high-quality leadership is even harder. Whether EI is a new concept or not, it appears that the way it has recently been presented has made its utility as a leadership skill more obvious and easier

to understand, thereby making it more accessible for those of us who are not psychologists.

Emotional pathways

If we dramatically simplify the human emotional reaction to outside stimuli, there are two main pathways through which we respond. There is a relatively fast and unconscious pathway that travels through the amygdala, and a slower, more deliberative pathway that travels through the prefrontal cortex. It is the faster pathway through the amygdala that Goleman refers to as the "low road," which is responsible for some of the more interesting and problematic emotional responses humans have.

It is this pathway that is responsible for the phenomenon of "emotional contagion." If a human subject is asked to look at pictures of the face of another individual with emotional expressions, the subject will eventually begin to take on the emotional state, and even the physiologic response of the person in the pictures. This happens without any conscious action on the part of the subject and happens without their knowledge. It is as if the individual "feels" rather than sees the emotion in the pictures. Scientists now understand that the human limbic system functions as an "open loop," meaning that human emotions are responsive to the emotions of others around them. If two individuals that are monitored engage in a conversation, their moods and their vital signs tend to converge to a similar state within a period of 15 min. An understanding of this phenomenon helps to explain why people who work together over long periods of time seem to take on similar emotional states. It follows that the leaders of an anesthesia department, or a medical group, must be particularly careful about the emotional state they project, as everyone usually watches "the boss."

If reactions through this unconscious, faster pathway are to be managed for better outcomes in our interpersonal interactions, it is necessary to anticipate how we are likely to behave in difficult situations. It makes sense that a little self-education on how to anticipate and be proactive in managing our own emotional responses might be useful, as the logic provided by the slow-moving prefrontal cortex is going to arrive too late to prevent the low road from reacting!

The components of emotional intelligence

The components of emotional intelligence differ slightly depending on which author one reads, but the differences are minor. Goleman divides the four components of emotional intelligence into the categories of "personal competence" and "social competence." Under each category, the components include awareness and management.

- Personal competence
  1. Self-awareness
  2. Self-management
- Social competence
  3. Social awareness
  4. Relationship management

The names of all of the components of EI make their descriptions self-evident, but there is more to them than the names imply. Self-awareness means that one needs to be able to read one's own emotions, and many of us are probably already fairly good at that. However, if one makes an effort to pay attention to one's own emotional state, there is probably more that can be learned. More important than knowing how we feel at any given time is learning how those feelings affect our behavior. Learning how feelings affect our behavior is much less obvious to the individual than it is to the observers around them. For example, learning that you are particularly prone to having a short temper when you become stressed or easily distracted from details when you are angered would be valuable information the next time you find yourself experiencing those emotions.

Individuals with high levels of self-awareness are confident. They have already made an accurate and realistic self-assessment, so they know their strengths and weaknesses, and they are able to use their assessment to guide their decisions. They know where they are headed and why. Because they are well grounded, they do not feel compelled to act impulsively, but instead are reflective and thoughtful. When they do act, it is with conviction and genuineness.

Self-management involves the ability to maintain control over your emotions, and requires that you have already attained an adequate level of self-awareness, because you cannot control what you cannot perceive. Similarly, you cannot hope to control the emotions of others until you can control your own, making self-management an essential skill for leadership. Individuals that are skilled in self-management tend to be honest and transparent, and act only in ways that are consistent with their own values rather than following the crowd. They are driven to an inner standard of excellence and are able to maintain discipline and

motivation in pursuing it. Because their inner emotional turmoil is minimized, they are able to cope with external uncertainties more effectively. This makes them adaptable, optimistic and ready to seize opportunities when they present themselves.

Social awareness includes empathy, or the ability to sense others' emotions and to understand their perspective. This is true both at an individual and an organizational level. Individuals skilled in social awareness are able to sense the emotional currents, the politics, and the decision-making networks within an organization. They are able to sense the requirements for effective communication in a given situation and to determine what is needed to motivate people.

Relationship management requires an individual to use their social awareness to guide communication in a positive way. Leaders with good relationship management skills are able to guide followers with a compelling vision. To do this, they utilize a range of tactics for persuasion. They take an interest in developing others as a means of both improving the health of the organization and developing a sense of support and community among the group. They also realize the importance of workplace relationships, and understand that nothing important is completed alone. They seek common ground, and work on building a network. Their communication and persuasion skills allow them to act as change catalysts or conflict managers, and they are effective at teamwork and collaboration.

Measuring emotional intelligence

Several tests are available for measuring emotional intelligence, and quantifying EI may be useful in certain circumstances. Some of the better-known tests for EI are:

- the Mayer–Salovey–Caruso Emotional Intelligence Test (MSCEIT);
- the Emotional Competency Inventory (ECI);
- the Emotional and Social Competency Inventory (ESCI);
- the Bar-On Emotional Quotient Inventory (EQ-i);
- the Trait Emotional Intelligence Questionnaire (TEIQue).

There are also testing services that are available online for both self-evaluation and 360-degree evaluations. A full discussion of the characteristics and individual merits of the available tests is beyond the scope of this chapter.

Resonant and dissonant leadership

Leaders with high levels of EI are able to provide "resonant" leadership. The term "resonance" refers to the reinforcement of sound through synchronous vibration, and individuals in a resonant group "vibrate" with the leader's enthusiastic energy. Resonant leaders are attuned to group emotions and are able to communicate in a way that connects with those they seek to persuade. They can sense the mood of a crowd and modify their communication style to suit the immediate needs of their audience. They speak enthusiastically and authentically and drive group emotions in a positive direction.

Dissonant leadership represents the other end of the spectrum. Dissonance refers to an unpleasant sound due to a lack of harmony. Individuals in a dissonant group are out of sync, and beset with negative emotions, which distract them from important tasks in the workplace. Dissonant leaders are out of touch with group emotions, and as a result tend to drive group emotions in a negative direction.

The importance of emotional intelligence and resonant leadership

Daniel Goleman has investigated the characteristics that distinguish truly successful leaders from others. He found that individuals with high levels of intelligence and training do not always make the best leaders. They may have a wealth of good ideas, but without the ability to motivate others to execute them, the ideas themselves are worth little. Goleman found that while adequate training and intelligence are entry level requirements for leadership, it is an individual's emotional intelligence that determines whether they excel, and the importance of emotional intelligence increases at higher levels of leadership.

A quote from the first lines of Goleman's book, *Primal Leadership*, explains why this might be so: "Great leaders move us. They ignite our passions and inspire the best in us. When we try to explain why they are so effective, we speak of strategy, vision or powerful ideas. But the reality is so much more primal: Great leadership works through the emotions."

Intelligence, training, and a well-reasoned argument are not always enough to inspire people to follow. The way to achieve an action on something is to get people emotionally involved and inspired. They must be motivated, not just convinced.

This is true in the OR. Anesthesiologists, nurses, and surgeons work in a high-pressure environment that demands self-control and teamwork. Furthermore, anesthesiologists, nurses, and surgeons work alongside hospital administrators and others, all of whom have motivations that do not fully coincide. The organizational dynamics of the hospital are complex. In this setting, a resonant leader can have a significant impact on the workplace environment. Resonant leaders are skilled in conflict resolution and persuasion, and are able to successfully navigate the complex political landscape of the OR. They are inspirational leaders whose optimism and motivation serve to increase teamwork and efficiency. They have a positive impact on the job satisfaction of department employees and may also be able to improve the group's relationship with hospital administration and the security of their hospital contract. Anyone who has spent time in more than one anesthesia, nursing, or surgery department can readily attest to the fact that there are significant differences in the workplace environment between departments and that those differences can have a big impact on how much they enjoy their work. Such differences are largely due to the effect that the group's leader has on department employees.

Traditional medical school training does not include EI, which is somewhat curious given the high level of EI that medical practice requires. This is especially true for anesthesiologists, who have approximately 5–10 min to reassure their nervous patients during the preoperative interview. A study in the *Journal of the American Medical Association* that examined differences between physicians with fewer or more than two lifetime malpractice claims showed that the physicians with fewer claims spent more time with their patients, used more humor in their patient interactions, and spent more time eliciting their patients' questions and concerns. This supports the contention that EI-related skills are important in reducing the likelihood of malpractice claims. In the author's personal experience, it is also true that anesthesiologists who have previously established good relationships with nurses and surgeons are more likely to be perceived positively and supported by them in the event of a bad outcome and a subsequent malpractice case. Within the anesthesia practice, good relationships among partners are invaluable to the long-term health of the group. Groups comprised of individuals with higher levels of EI are less likely to have significant conflict that goes unresolved.

A meta-analysis of EI published in the *Journal of the Royal Society of Medicine* examined available data on the subject in 2007 [1]. They found that EI is a valid construct that is worthy of further research, and that it is a valuable predictor of performance in the workplace. It correlates well with academic success, and is a better predictor of job performance and satisfaction than traditional personality measures. However, there are few studies specifically related to EI and health care. Most of the existing studies contain unsubstantiated claims of its importance, and make the assumption that it is a quality that can be altered or changed. Although there is evidence of the value of EI in the business world, the same is not yet been demonstrated in health care, and the positive impact of resonant leadership that is discussed in this chapter is extrapolated from results in the business world, not proven through rigorous, scientific study. Areas that are cited by the study for future research include medical student selection and training, its impact on quality of care, and its impact on the job satisfaction and burnout rate of health-care workers.

Improving emotional intelligence

The first step for those who are interested in improving their EI is to recognize the potential benefits. Habits and behaviors that have been ingrained for many years are not readily amenable to change, so a significant degree of motivation is necessary to succeed. Unless the potential benefits of improved EI are understood and internalized, it is unlikely that one will have sufficient motivation for this undertaking. It is also important to realize that attention to EI skills is an ongoing effort, not a time-limited process.

Further reading and self-education are also advisable. Although the basic concepts of EI are amenable to this brief description, there is much more to the topic that should be well understood before embarking on an attempt at improvement. The books on this subject are filled with illustrative stories that help to solidify the concepts of EI, and to clarify what is needed to improve.

There are differing opinions on specific means for improving EI skills, and on whether it is even possible to do so. The process is complex, but the basic steps are straightforward. An initial self-assessment should determine areas of strength and potential areas for improvement. Testing may be helpful. Using your self-assessment, a comparison with the existing reality, and the desired future provides a roadmap for change. It

is an iterative process of self-observation and attempts at behavior modification in which individuals debrief themselves after an encounter in which they are either satisfied or unsatisfied and then make a plan for their next encounter.

Although this topic may seem straightforward, many find it to be compelling. We deal with human emotions every day, and they become such a routine part of our daily lives that we take them for granted. The construct of EI brings them back into focus and emphasizes their importance in our professional lives. The process of paying closer attention to how we interact with others almost invariably provides information that is actionable and potentially valuable.

Psychology in the OR: transactional analysis

Transactional analysis is a method to rapidly analyze and understand behavior. In short, it allows one to focus on elements of one's personality that are flawed, allowing one to respond better to others without conflict. In *Born to Win*, the defining book on transactional analysis, a description of "winners" is presented: winners are not helpless, they are authentic. They are not isolated, and they work for the greater good of the situation. Their timing is right with responses appropriate to the situation, making the other person involved feel dignified and worthwhile [2].

Transactional analysis provides a method to achieve awareness and self-responsibility on a daily basis. It involves four types of analysis. Structural analysis is the analysis of individual personality; transactional analysis is the analysis of what people do and say to each other; game analysis is the analysis of ulterior transactions leading to a payoff; and script analysis is the analysis of specific life dramas that a person compulsively plays out [2].

One example, structural analysis

Structural analysis involves gaining an understanding of another person's thoughts, feelings, and behaviors [2]. A multitude of factors, which can originate from previous experiences in a person's lifetime, can dictate how that person communicates. The thoughts, feelings, and behaviors of an individual are identified as "ego states," which are described as "parent," "adult," and "child."

Parent ego state reflects behaviors and attitudes incorporated from external sources, usually one's parents [2]. An example of the parent ego state in the OR

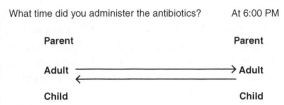

Figure 2.2 An example of a complementary transaction.

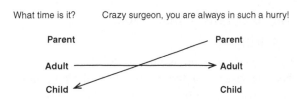

Figure 2.3 An example of a crossed transaction.

is someone criticizing a hairstyle, the color of the OR, nurturing feelings, or critically commenting on the fact that someone was injured because they were out late. Anytime one behaves like their parents, they are in the parent ego [2].

The adult ego state reflects objective information gathering, rational thinking, and problem solving. The adult ego state calculates and responds in a dispassionate manner, much like a computer [2]. For example, asking someone what 8 plus 3 equals, the adult ego would respond after calculation with the answer 11. If the surgeon asks the anesthesia provider what the blood pressure is at the moment, communicating the current blood pressure would be an adult ego state response.

The child ego state reflects all the natural impulses from childhood. An example in an OR is an anesthesiologist saying that surgeon X scares them, or that they wish they could take time off to have fun. Anytime you act or feel as when you were a child, including joy, laughter, rebellion, and sorrow, you are in a child ego state [2].

Complementary transactions

In a complementary transaction, an inquiry from one particular ego state is met with a response from the same ego state [3]. Complementary transactions can occur between any of the ego states. Figure 2.2 gives an example of a complementary transaction.

Crossed transactions

A crossed transaction occurs when an inquiry from one particular ego state is met with a response from a different ego state. The results of a crossed transaction can rapidly escalate into an argument, friction, withdrawal between two people, hostility, emotional pain, and other destructive consequences. Figure 2.3 gives an example of a crossed transaction.

The successful OR worker must master the art of communication and identify pathological interactions in others. The ability to understand pathological forms

of communication in others gives you the opportunity to make accommodations for them and rescue an otherwise failed interaction.

Transactional analysis is one tool available to improve communications and to attempt to insure a well-functioning workplace. As might be expected, pathological behaviors can be clearly and rapidly identified and proper responses taught to any individual. The many concepts described within transactional analysis include practical lessons well suited for the OR.

Below is a summary of items to consider when trying to improve self-awareness and management of emotions, or to develop effective communication skills.

To develop high self-awareness:

- reflect on the encounter *when you are calm* and engage in an inner dialogue;
- seek input from others and be honest with yourself;
- make accurate appraisals of what is going on;
- get in touch with your feelings;
- pay attention to your actions/observe their impact;
- learn what your intentions/goals are each day.

To manage your emotions:

- take charge of your thoughts;
- don't overgeneralize;
- stay away from destructive labeling/avoid mind reading;
- don't have rules about how others should act;
- don't inflate the significance of an event.

To develop effective communication skills:

- use sensitivity;
- use self-disclosure;
- acknowledge ownership of your statements;
- use assertiveness;
- use dynamic listening.

The role of the human resource department

A hospital's human resource (HR) department has become crucial to the success of today's hospital. Health-care institutions are under enormous pressure to control costs and improve quality, and for most institutions this involves reducing personnel. This reduction in human capital has forced new responsibilities on the doctors, nurses, technicians, and administrators working in the hospital setting. Effectively managing this scenario requires managers to take a more active role in developing very accurate job descriptions and protecting these "multitaskers" from burnout by creating a work culture that is enjoyable and fair. The HR department plays an important role by ensuring a safe and fair workplace environment, by managing employee benefits in a way that makes employees feel valued, and by delicately handling a difficult situation in the event that an employee's contract must be terminated. Their success or failure can profoundly affect the hospital's culture and patient outcomes.

Successful hospitals create a culture of accountability. The current national culture, which shuns personal responsibility, makes it more difficult for hospitals to do this. The HR department, in many instances, must educate its workers on accountability and explain how this will improve patient outcome and personal satisfaction. OR Committees have limited means to deal with dysfunctional workers who happen to play important roles as nurses, anesthesiologists, or surgeons. Educational seminars on team training and EI training (discussed earlier in this chapter) involve case presentations and "role-playing." Team training involves active participation and illustrates the importance of every job if excellent patient outcomes are to be achieved.

The diversity of our nation has changed dramatically in the last 20 years and will continue to evolve. Because of this, hospitals must remain diverse and culturally sensitive by reflecting the community in which they reside. Hospital HR departments should insist on culturally diverse employment for all segments working within the hospital. Excellent patient outcomes can only be achieved if cultural beliefs and needs are understood. According to Anderson *et al.*, there are six HUMANE steps that health-care institutions can take to become culturally competent: **h**ire a diverse workforce [4]; **u**nderstand the community in which the hospital exists [5]; **m**ake cultural competency a business priority [6]; **a**dopt cultural and communication capabilities that reflect the community [7]; **n**urture the community's culture by engaging leaders and staff in outreach programs [8]; and constantly **e**valuate and continue to develop programs that encourage community involvement [9].

Disruptive behavior is a major issue for hospital HR departments. Although disruption can occur within any segment of the hospital workforce, the majority of recent work deals with the disruptive physician. Recent changes in health care have resulted in a loss of physician autonomy, which has caused an increase in frustration and disruptive behavior. Most recent research links workforce safety and patient outcomes with teamwork. The physician acts as the leader of the team, so the effectiveness of their communication with team members directly affects many aspects of patient care.

Disruptive behavior by one team member can negatively impact a whole department. Hospital policy and medical staff by-laws must exist and clearly state a course of action to deal with these individuals. An aggressive, zero-tolerance stance toward disruptive behavior is advisable for a productive and patient-centered work environment. From an educational standpoint, case studies vignettes and workshops on improving communication skills between team members are important ways to reinforce or instruct team members on how to conduct themselves properly.

Team training

In 1999, *To Err is Human* revealed that approximately 98 000 deaths occur annually as a result of medical errors. This resulted in a public outcry for patient safety. The federal government, through the Agency for Healthcare Research and Quality (AHRQ) and the Department of Defense (DoD), has served as the leader in this movement. They have implemented a team approach to patient safety and initially put their program in place, through the DoD, within military treatment facilities and casualty combat care arenas. The initial results show promising results, so the Joint Commission and the Accreditation for Graduate Medical Education moved quickly to laud the importance of teamwork in patient safety.

The program, initiated by the DoD and the AHRQ, is called the TeamSTEPPS program. Success in the military arena and subsequent requests from healthcare institutions for a similar program has accelerated the push for the establishment of a national program through the AHRQ. Currently, the AHRQ is developing the infrastructure necessary for national implementation of a TeamSTEPPS program. The program consists of three phases.

Phase I, the assessment phase, evaluates the organizational readiness of your institution and identifies potential leaders that will make up the institutional change team. This stage also identifies barriers to this change and whether sufficient resources are in place to support the proposed change. The AHRQ offers an assessment tool that aids health-care organizations in a site appraisal. It provides direct feedback on: assessing awareness about safety issues; evaluating specific patient safety interventions; tracking change in patient safety over time; setting internal and external benchmarks; and fulfilling regulatory requirements or directives.

Phase II involves the planning, training, and implementation of the TeamSTEPPS program. In this phase, the change team must complete a 2½-day train-the-trainer program. Provided in this session is the TeamSTEPPS curriculum, which includes case studies, scenarios, multimedia, and simulation. Each department involved in the change will take part in a 4-h session aimed at developing a plan tailored to fit their unique situation. Peer and instructor feedback helps the participants fully understand the mission and crystallize learning objectives. Once the learning objectives are understood, the plan can be adapted easily to numerous situations.

The goal of Phase III is to sustain and spread the advances achieved through teamwork performance, clinical practices, and outcomes. During this phase, participants integrate teamwork skills and tools into their daily practice and monitor the ongoing effectiveness of the TeamSTEPPS intervention. They develop an approach for continuous improvement and spread the intervention throughout the organization. This ongoing process is managed by the change team and involves continual training of the core curriculum through refresher courses and new employee orientation.

Summary

The nature of the OR environment makes an understanding of psychological concepts extremely valuable. The high level of stress that exists in the OR tends to magnify existing, undesirable personality traits, and to make effective communication more difficult. Without effective communication, it is challenging to navigate successfully the complex organizational dynamics and politics that exist in the OR. Developing a better understanding of the nature of human interactions, and improving one's skills in this area, is not easy but is worth the time and effort. Multiple conceptual frameworks exist, and the user should choose one that resonates with them, because motivation is the key to success. Emotional intelligence, transactional analysis, and other available models provide a framework for readers to take routine skills of personal interaction that they take for granted, and turn them into potent tools that can enhance their professional performance. Attention to this area of performance, along with the assistance of a good HR department to insure a healthy workplace environment, can have a profoundly positive impact on teamwork, job satisfaction, and patient care.

References

1. Y. F. Birks, I. S. Watt. Emotional intelligence and patient-centred care. *J R Soc Med* 2007; **100**: 368–74.

2. M. James, D. Jongeward. *Born to Win*. Boston: Addison-Wesley Publishing Company, 1971, pp. 2–20.

3. FS Perls. *Gestalt Therapy Verbatim*. Boulder, CO: Real People Press, 1969, pp. 121.

4. D. Goleman. What Makes a Leader? *Harv Bus Rev* 1998; **Nov–Dec**.

5. D. Goleman, R. Boyatzis, A. McKee A. *Primal Leadership, Learning to Lead With Emotional Intelligence*. Boston: Harvard Business Press, 2002.

6. H. Weisinger H. *Emotional Intelligence at Work*. San Francisco: Jossey-Bass Inc., 1998.

7. D. L. Van Rooy, C. Viswesvaran. Emotional intelligence: A meta-analytic investigation of predictive validity and nomological net. *J Vocat Behav* 2004; **65**: 71–95.

8. W. Levinson, D. L. Roter, J. P. Mullooly, V. T. Dull, R. M. Frankel. Physician-patient communication. The relationship with malpractice claims among primary care physicians and surgeons. *JAMA*.1997; **277**: 553–9.

9. Goleman D. *Social Intelligence, The New Science of Human Relationships*. New York: Bantam Books, 2006.

Suggested reading

A. Alonso, D. Baker, R. Day, *et al*. Reducing medical error in the military health system: How can team training help? *Hum Resour Manage Rev* 2006; **16**: 396–415.

American Organization of Nurse Executives. 2006. AONE guiding principles for excellence in nurse/physician relationships. http://net.acpe.org/services/AONE/Index. html (last accessed January 21, 2012).

L. M. Anderson, S. C. Scrimshaw, M. T. Fullilove, J. E. Fielding, J. Normand; Task Force on Community Preventive Services. *Am J Prev Med* 2003; **24**(3 Suppl): 68–79 (Review).

D. P. Baker, J. M. Beaubien, A. K. Holtzman. *DoD Medical Team Training Programs: An Independent Case Study Analysis*. Washington, DC: American Institutes for Research; 2003.

S. R. Covey. *The 7 Habits of Highly Effective People*, 3rd edn. New York: Free Press; 2004.

L. T. Kohn, J. M. Corrigan, M. S. Donaldson. *To Err is Human*. Washington, DC: National Academies Press; 1999.

J. Longo. Jan. 31, 2010. Combating disruptive behaviors: Strategies to promote a healthy work environment. *OJIN: The Online Journal of Issues in Nursing* Vol. 15, No. 1, Manuscript 5.

G. Porto, R. Lauve. 2006. Disruptive clinician behavior: A persistent threat to patient safety. Patient Safety & Quality Healthcare. www.psqh.com/julaug06/disruptive. html (last accessed January 21, 2012).

E. M. Rogers. *Diffusion of Innovations*, 5th edn. New York: Free Press; 2003.

Strategic planning

3

Michael R. Williams DO, MD, MBA

Introduction   25
Development of purpose   26

Strategic planning   27
Summary   31

Introduction

In his book, *Sensemaking in Organizations*, Karl Weick describes the story of a small Hungarian military unit on maneuvers in the Alps of Switzerland [1]. It seems that the young lieutenant in charge dispatched a small group of men into the icy wilderness for a reconnaissance mission. After two days, the group had not returned, and the lieutenant feared he had sent these men to their death in an ill-fated mission. However, later that day the men suddenly appeared, marching back into camp unharmed. When he asked them how they found their way back to camp they simply explained when they thought all was lost one of the men found a crumpled map in his pack. They reviewed the map, checked their provisions, and devised a plan to return back to the base camp to join their fellow soldiers. As they were explaining this the lieutenant asked to see the map and only then did anyone realize that the map was a map of the Pyrenees and not the Alps!

This story exemplifies the fact that you can have the wrong map, yet still get to your destination if you have a purpose and are willing to try. Most organizations become lost because they invest a great deal of time and effort on developing a map, but do little to understand their purpose. Other organizations begin with a defined purpose, but never take the time to design and build a map, providing a pathway to achieve the purpose. The union of purpose and planning leads to a strategic purpose for the organization. Design, implementation, and execution of strategic action plans ultimately leads to an organization that provides strategic performance. Organizations that achieve focused strategic performance year after year become highly successful, high-performing organizations. They are built upon a clear purpose, great planning, active execution of the plan, accountability for the goals and targets at all levels, and finally follow-through by leadership.

The focal subject of this book is the development and enhancement of operating room (OR) leadership and management. In every imaginable modern healthcare structure the OR exists as a subunit of a larger organization, whether a hospital, ambulatory surgery center, office-based surgical suite, or even a military field unit surgical suite. They all exist within a much larger organizational structure. It will be important for operating leadership to understand how the strategic planning and purpose of the OR must support the strategic planning and purpose of the larger organization it serves. This chapter will focus on the steps required to assess purposeful planning for the larger organization. However, the OR's strategic planning process can follow the same steps, as described below. These steps include discussions of the organization's mission, vision, and values statements. These are key corporate documents, which create the foundational structure for a corporate purpose, and in turn build the necessary foundation needed to begin a strategic planning process. Collectively, these define the reason to exist and the behaviors by which those in the organization's community agree to live to achieve the defined purpose. Once purpose is better defined with some clarity, a map must be developed in order to clearly delineate the pathway to follow to achieve the purpose. We will call the map the "strategic plan." Strategic planning

Operating Room Leadership and Management, ed. Kaye A.D., Fox C.J. and Urman R.D. Published by Cambridge University Press. © Cambridge University Press 2012.

has an inherent process that will be described in more detail below.

Development of purpose

To fully develop the reason this organization has to exist, and the value it adds, three statements should be developed. These statements, which by their very formation will aid in clarification of the purpose, are the "mission statement," "vision statement," and the "statement of values."

Mission statement

The mission statement is probably the most important piece of the organization's overall development of purpose. Great leaders in history have not been remembered and respected because of their charisma or their image, but rather because of the mission they pursued and believed in could be easily understood and agreed with by their followers and admirers. For this reason, the mission statement must be objective and easily understood so that everyone is clear on how his or her individual role drives the overall mission. Peter Drucker, considered by many to be the father of modern management, once stated "One of our most common mistakes is to make the mission statement into a kind of hero sandwich of good intentions. It has to be simple and clear" [2].

A well-written mission statement should have at least three parts. First, be aware of needs that exist in your market area or your area of expertise. Do these needs translate into opportunities for the organization? If so, can the organization perform these and perform them well in a way that makes a difference? Second, take a look at what the organization truly believes in. If there are strong beliefs, these can often be transformed into strong actions that have real meaning. The third important aspect speaks to team and organizational commitment to the stated mission. Do those who must deliver on the stated mission truly believe in it? If the entire community can commit to the tenets of the mission statement it has a much higher chance of being successful. Drucker discusses the story of the Ford Edsel car, which failed miserably on the market. As Drucker describes it, the Edsel did not fail as a result of poor planning or engineering. In fact, it is considered one of the best-engineered and researched automobiles in history. However, no one at Ford truly believed in it or fully committed to it [3]. Although an organization can set audacious goals, the goals must have the commitment of the entire populace of the organization. In conclusion, before writing the mission statement, be sure you understand the needs of the industry, market, and customers served; next, validate that the organization has the competencies and capacities to deliver on these needs; and finally, check the team commitment to this mission.

The first mistake many groups make when building an organizational mission statement is being too verbose. Lengthy mission statements quickly lose meaning and clarity. In order to be effective, a mission statement must be easy to read and understand, while being meaningful to all members of the organization's stakeholder group. It must be concrete and direct in message. It must answer the question "How do we intend to be the absolute best in this industry in delivering our specific mission?" [4].

The mission statement should balance what we know to be possible and within our limits with the stretch goals that appear to be unobtainable. Planners must always consider the organization's strengths, weaknesses, resources, and people skills among other qualities. According to Drucker, "It should be a precise statement of purpose, not a slogan, and should fit on a T-shirt" [5]. The words it contains must be carefully selected for clarity and meaning. The power of the statement will be found in its brevity and simplicity. Finally, the most senior leaders should be writing the mission statement in the organization – the people who are ultimately responsible for achieving it. Once the mission statement is developed the vision and values statements can be constructed. From that point forward, all of the organization's decisions must be linked to the mission.

Vision statement

Many people confuse vision statements with mission statements and often mix the distinct purpose of each statement. These two statements are very different in content and purpose, yet must work to support each other in parallel. Therefore, it is important to have one of each before beginning a strategic planning process. Like the mission statement, the vision statement must be concise, clear, and vivid in language. It should be inspiring and challenging, and it should avoid use of complicated concepts.

Most vision statements reveal a compelling idea of what ultimate desired outcome might be achievable in 5–10 years or longer. The idea is to create a mental picture that stirs emotions, inspires the team, and calls everyone to action. Vision statements are not built around goals, but rather describe the ultimate outcome of the organization's goals and do not come with any expectation of measurability. They simply describe the best possible outcome and do not provide any form of a measurement of success. This is the function of the organization's goals and objectives. They must inspire, motivate, and stimulate a "what if" form of creativity. Vision statements, like mission statements, should be developed by the most senior leaders. These leaders will create the inspiring vision as the best possible outcome achievable via the mission statement, goals, and objectives.

Although knowledge from the mission statement, goals, and objectives allows one to see things as they are, imagination stimulated by the vision statement allows one to see what is possible. It is important to open up all the possibilities in the visioning process in order to release a tremendous source of creativity, passion, and energy. Two examples of corporate vision statements include those of Toyota and Amazon. Toyota's Global Vision Statement is *"Toyota will lead the way to the future of mobility, enriching lives around the world with the safest and most responsible ways of moving people. Through our commitment to quality, constant innovation and respect for the planet, we aim to exceed expectations and be rewarded with a smile. We will meet challenging goals by engaging the talent and passion of people, who believe there is always a better way"* [6]. In comparison, Amazon's corporate vision statement is *"Our vision is to be earth's most consumer centric company; to build a place where people can come to find and discover anything they might want to buy online"* [7]. Be creative, audacious, brief, and inspiring. Take a long forward view and the power of the vision statement will be unleashed.

Values statement

The potential power of the statement of values for the organization is often greatly underestimated. Organizational values must be direct reflections of the character values believed and lived each day by the organizational membership. When writing the values statement the leaders must allow the frontline staff to open their inner selves, expressing what they truly believe in a very honest, open manner. Values provide the compass when we are lost, the principles we must depend upon, and the behaviors that define how the organizational culture will act in good times and bad [8]. In short, values reflect our personal and organizational "line in the sand" and are our defined "guardrails" along our journey.

Values should align with the mission and vision statements. They should be empowering, and help to provide clarity for each individual in the organization or department. Properly constructed value statements should easily drive employee engagement and a commitment to the mission of the organization or department. In writing the values it is important to be clear and direct. The language used should be very simple. The stated list of values is unique in that it should be constructed with input from everyone in the organization. Leaders must avoid dictating values. Rather, leaders should clearly express the values they personally believe in, and then work to become knowledgeable of the values the organizational community believes in. The combination of these two lists will begin to build a values statement that the entire organization can believe in and honor with their daily actions.

Strategic planning

Properly executed strategic planning is often the first step in any organization's journey to become a high-performing organization. This process draws the map that the organization will follow to achieve its stated mission. This is a process that must be performed by the organization's highest-level leaders, with oversight by the organization's governing body. Poor planning leads to poor performance. The planning must be carried out with a serious focus on gaining answers to many questions. What is occurring in our industry currently and what trends are expected over the next three to five years? What is our understanding of our competitors and their capabilities? What are our capabilities? What can we execute better than anyone else?

The following information will discuss the process in more specific detail.

Timeline

Many organizations have a strategic planning process in place that works well for their annual calendar. However, for those that do not we will present a suggested timeline example for a calendar-year-based organization to follow. The OR leadership will need to understand and honor the planning timeline followed by the larger organization. However, the OR leadership will be responsible for developing a more focused plan that is specific with regard to OR goals, objectives, measures, and targets, while assuring that the OR plan directly supports the organizational plan. Timing for the OR plan will need to begin after completion of the

Table 3.1 An example of a calendar-year-based planning cycle

February 2013	Begin strategic planning process for 2014
May 2013	Present draft of leadership plan to governing body
June – August 2013	Move draft leadership plan to final form
August 2013	Present final leadership plan to governing body
September 2013	Begin taking plan to support departments
October 2013	Develop departmental action plans
November 2013	Finalize full organizational plan
January 2014	Full organizational plan becomes actionable

larger organizational plan. However, it will be clear that there is much information gathering needed before beginning the focused planning process.

For a calendar-year-based organization, the final approved strategic plan must be ready to become actionable by January 1 of each year. The specific time-line chosen is dependent upon factors unique to each organization. These include the size of the planning team, capabilities of the team, access to necessary data, frequency of planning meetings, and the hierarchy of who must give input to the developing plan.

A sample calendar-year-based planning cycle is shown in Table 3.1.

SWOT analysis

The SWOT (strengths, weaknesses, opportunities, and threats) analysis should be one of the earliest actions completed so that the leadership can assess the current positioning of the organization.

The entire planning team should participate in this self-analysis. Input should be sought from many stakeholders. Once the information is gathered it can be edited, clarified, simplified, and then prioritized. The four parts of the assessment – the departmental or organizational strengths, weaknesses, opportunities, and threats – are equally important, and with adequate input from different perspectives inside the organization, the SWOT analysis will achieve its full potential.

The SWOT analysis always begins with an assessment of the organization's strengths. "Strengths" refers

to the capabilities of an organization, an operation, or a department. The assessment should focus on an understood ability to make improvements in or perform certain activities or functions. If they are lacking or become diminished, the organization or department will suffer in some way.

Next is an assessment of the organizational and/or departmental weaknesses. This assessment is a close, focused look at the existing shortage in capabilities, lack of competencies, and lack of resources within the organization. The weaknesses part of the assessment can be very insightful. However, in many organizations where honesty is not a part of the culture, the weaknesses portion of the assessment may be understated.

The opportunities section requires a more forward-looking view of the organizational and departmental potential, both in the external and internal environments. This section of the assessment requires consideration of industry trends, customer needs, stakeholder needs, team member skill development, and possible competitive advantages that should be given attention in the future in order to gain a competitive advantage.

Finally, the threats include those factors that alone, or in combination, could cause the business to fail, lose market share, or become weaker at the least. Threats have the potential to cause permanent damage to the organization, or at least stop the forward progress of the organization. Threats should be considered as permanent injuries, not temporary "bumps in the road."

Competitive analysis

The basic origin of the word "strategy" comes from a military application for planning a specific action in order to obtain a certain goal. Even with the non-military use of the word "strategy," there is an implied need for the understanding of the organization's competitors, and the need to position the organization in the competitive environment before building a plan to obtain the set goals. Competitive analysis becomes an integral requirement of any strategic planning process. The strategy of an organization or department should focus on the unique qualities and abilities that separate the organization from all its competitors. What sets this organization apart? What makes it unique? The SWOT analysis should help with this understanding. The competitive analysis can take many forms; however, the best is "Porter's five competitive forces that shape strategy" [9].

The five forces include the "threat of entry," the "power of the buyers," the "threat of substitute products or services," the "power of the suppliers," and the "rivalry among existing competitors." In addition to an understanding of each of the five competitive forces, an understanding of industry analysis is also very important. The scope of this chapter does not allow for a full in-depth discussion of these forces: a brief discussion of each is described below; for further understanding the reader is directed to the book *On Competition* by Michael E. Porter [10].

The threat of entry focuses on the issues created by a new competitor entering the organization's market with new capabilities, new capacities, different pricing structure, lower costs, and an immediate ability to take away market share and affect the profitability of the organization. In the case of threat of entry, it is important for the organization/department to be aware of their industry on a national, state, and local level. Leadership should always be aware of growing industry trends that might attract the attention of possible new entrants to the market. For an OR, this might be a new ambulatory surgery center, a new surgeon opening an office-based surgical suite, or an industry trend that is moving certain procedures from the OR to the physician's office.

The power of buyers represents the power of the customer and can create competitive forces by forcing down prices, demanding higher quality, and/or demanding other new services. Buyers can gain large amounts of power in industries where the prominent products are relatively standardized and undifferentiated. This allows the buyers to leverage one organization against the other. Nongovernmental, commercially insured buyers of health-care services are now more price sensitive than previously as insurance deductibles and copays are much larger. Governmentally insured (i.e., Medicaid, Medicare, etc.) buyers who have small to nonexistent deductibles remain much less sensitive to pricing. An example of this might be the impact that low-priced, cash-based imaging centers have had on hospital-based imaging departments. To clearly understand the competitive power of buyers the organization/department must clearly understand the needs and wants of their customers as well as the ability of the customer population to shop around for services.

The threat of substitutes is of concern when new services, technologies, or procedures are being created that will remove the need for these same services and procedures to be performed in the OR. Substitutes could occur downstream or upstream of the OR. For example, for many years ORs performed large numbers of gastric ulcer operations. Several years ago acid-blocking medications were created that reduced the incidence of gastric ulcers, which in turn greatly reduced the need for these surgeries. Substitutes can cause permanent negative impact on the profitability of the organization and OR, especially if the substitute attacks a high-frequency procedure for the OR. Another example is the impact cardiac stents and cardiac angioplasty has had on the number of open-heart procedures performed.

The power of suppliers focuses on the competitive threat of all those sources of resources required for the organization or OR to function. In the case of the OR, suppliers include surgeons who bring the patients, primary-care physicians and mid-level providers who refer patients to surgeons, and equipment and supply vendors who provide the necessary supplies for the surgeries to occur. Vendor suppliers can gain power and pricing strength when the number of vendors is concentrated and there are no substitutes for what they provide. Vendors can also increase prices and power when their supplies are in high demand, when the vendors do not depend upon the organization or industry for much of their revenue, when the cost of switching to other vendors is high, and when products among vendors are well differentiated. Referring physicians can gain power as suppliers by limiting the flow of patients to the OR and the organization.

Rivalry among existing competitors is the most obvious source for competitive threats and is usually the one organizations focus on the most. This focus on known competitors can be accurate or can create a distraction from the other sources of competitive threats when the existing competitors do not present much competition.

It is important to be aware of this rivalry when certain situations exist, including when there are numerous competitors in the same market of the same size and power offering the same list of services, when barriers to exit from the industry are high, and when the overall industry growth rate is slow. This rivalry of existing competitors is most destructive when it leads to pricing competition, and can greatly impact profitability. This is especially harmful when fixed costs of the organization are high and pricing decreases start to drive margins closer to the total cost levels.

Industry analysis is heavily based upon the understanding of Porter's five competitive forces. The five forces reveal the drivers of the industry competition, the attractiveness of an industry at a given time, and allow better understanding of the positioning of the organization in the industry. This focus on competitive forces and gaining a better understanding of the industry allows the organization to direct energy on driving improved economic value. The organizational strategic plan can then be designed with a much better understanding of where the competitive strengths and weaknesses exist. Better focus on decision making should be the result of this effort.

Goals, objectives, measures, actions, and targets

When the organization begins the actual process of strategic planning, it is important that a leadership team focused on the planning process be identified. This team can begin communication with members of the governing body to gain alignment on the organizational goals before initiating the planning process. For the strategic plan to be effective and easier to execute, the number of goals should be limited to one for each of the major focus areas of the organization or department, and no more than five to six in total. Most healthcare organizations will have focus areas such as people, growth, finance, community, quality, and service. A common mistake is to have too many goals, making it difficult for the resources of the organization to be focused and applied where needed.

Once the goals are clearly stated, one to two objectives per goal are agreed to. The objectives must describe brief action statements that will lead to accomplishment of the stated goal they support. Goals drive the overall strategic direction of the organization and become extremely important. Planning groups and members of the governing body should give ample time to clearly state the organizational goals. Goals and objectives must be clear, "high level" in focus, and achievable. The objectives must be clearly measurable with achievable targets. Also, supporting departments such as the OR must be able to develop their action plans consistent with the organizational objectives and goals.

Each stated objective must be measurable in a way that is available in the organization's data, easily understood, and in units of measure that clearly signify their importance to the organization. Therefore, when measures are established for each objective, it is important that team members, at all levels, are able to easily interpret what the individual measure indicates and what the directional trends in the measures indicate. As departments begin to develop their individual supporting strategic documents, it is important that they have their own measures that provide direction and accountability for the department staff. Action plans are developed for each objective at all levels of the organization. These action plans must be specific, easy to place into action, and flexible as progress with the strategic plan moves forward or action plans become irrelevant.

Targets for each measurable objective need to be achievable and clearly driven by the action plan. Targets should be established at levels that require effort to reach, but are not unobtainable. Unobtainable targets quickly become irrelevant to the organizational teams. Targets must be kept real and attainable, but not so low that they are too easy to reach.

Monitoring

Every well-designed strategic plan will become actionable and measurable with carefully conceived targets to attain. In order to hold the organizational team accountable for performance on the strategic plan, there must be a way to monitor incremental achievements as the strategic plan year progresses. Active monitoring of the plan allows the organizational team to "keep score" as progress on the plan is made or not made throughout the year.

The best monitoring tool is the Balanced Scorecard, developed by Dr. Robert Kaplan and Dr. David Norton in the early 1990s [11]. The balanced scorecard provides several advantages for monitoring the strategic plan. First, it provides a single-page summary of current status on the key issues/targets of the strategic plan. Second, it provides focus and clarity for any teams within the organization/department that might be working on different aspects of the strategic plan at the same time. Third, it allows for fixed periodic measured results to be published, which allows mid year course corrections as needed with the strategic plan. Last, it has been shown to enhance other improvement programs in existence in the organization, such as activity-based costing, Six Sigma, Lean, etc. Other attributes of the balanced scorecard include the ability to better balance financial and nonfinancial measures, balance long- and short-term measures, and balance lead indicators with lag indicators so that you can look at outcomes of decisions as well as predictors of certain interventions. This discussion only serves as a brief introduction to the balanced scorecard as a tool.

Summary

Proper strategic planning is one of the most important processes an organization can use to drive higher levels of performance. It is also a process that requires a willingness to work through multiple steps in the process and understanding that the more effort the team makes to understand strategic plan the better the end product. Strategic planning forces the organizational leadership to revisit the organization's mission, vision, and values. Also, an annual strategic assessment, in the form of a SWOT analysis, is healthy at least on an annual basis if not more often. Focused energies on the organization's strategic initiatives will produce better performance with clear measures and open sources of reporting and scoring by using the chosen monitoring tool. Highly successful organizations are focused, strategic organizations that master the art of planning with purpose. Also, they complete the execution loop of strategy execution, accountability of clear measures, and follow-through with ongoing monitoring of the organization's results. These are the organizations that succeed year after year.

References

1. K. E. Weick. *Sensemaking in Organizations*. London: Sage Publications, 1995, pp. 54–5.

2. P. F. Drucker. *Managing the Nonprofit Organization*. New York: Harper, 1990, p. 5.

3. P. F. Drucker. *Managing the Nonprofit Organization*. New York: Harper, 1990, p. 7.

4. J. Welch, S. Welch. *Winning*. New York: HarperCollins, 2005, p. 14.

5. E. H. Edersheim. *The Definitive Drucker*. New York: McGraw-Hill, 2007, p. 170.

6. The Toyota Global Vision 2011. www.toyota-global.com/company/vision_philosophy (last accessed April 29, 2012).

7. The Amazon.com Vision Statement 2011. Amazon.com FAQ's. http://phx.corporate-ir.net/phoenix.zhtml?c=97664&p=irol-faq (last accessed April 29, 2012).

8. J. Kouzes, B. Posner. *The Leadership Challenge*, 4th edn. San Francisco: John Wiley & Sons, 2007, p. 52.

9. M. E. Porter. *On Competition,* updated and expanded *edition*. Boston: Harvard Business School Publishing, 2008, pp. 3–24.

10. M. E. Porter. *On Competition,* updated and expanded edition. Boston: Harvard Business School Publishing, 2008.

11. R. Kaplan, D. Norton. *The Balanced Scorecard: Translating Strategy into Action*. Boston: Harvard Business Press, 1996.

Chapter 4

Decision making
The art and the science

Michael R. Williams DO, MD, MBA

In any moment of decision the best thing you can do is the right thing, the next best thing is the wrong thing, and the worst thing you can do is nothing.

Theodore Roosevelt

Introduction   32
Building the decision team   32
Framing the decision   33
Develop and evaluate possible alternatives   34

Evaluation of alternatives and use of analytical tools   34
Role of bias in decision making   36
Make the decision and begin implementation   37
Summary   37

Introduction

Decisions are a part of our daily life. We are confronted with choices every day and in most cases must make decisions with limited information. Many of these daily decisions have a minor impact on our lives; however, some of them carry great impact. This impact may be focused only on our individual lives or may also impact the lives of many other people. How we make decisions is extremely important; however, most of us do not consider or take time to understand the best ways to make decisions. The question is often "Why did that individual or those people make such a bad decision?" When we are not included in the decision process, we often feel frustration and waning support for the decision. The leadership of the operating room (OR) or surgical services department of every hospital is faced with decisions on a daily basis. Sometimes such decisions have focused impact on certain stakeholder groups, such as physicians, surgical technicians, anesthesia personnel, nursing staff, and patients and their families. At other times such decisions impact the lives of only a few individuals. This chapter will focus on helping leaders better

understand how to avoid making poor choices, how to structure a decision-making process that will engage the talents and perspectives of the entire team, frame the decision in the proper context, evaluate all appropriate alternatives using different analytical tools, be aware of possible decision biases, and finally move to make the decision and implement it.

Building the decision team

The first step of a successful decision-making process is the building of an informed, thoughtful, and focused team. Arguably, this step could be considered the most important in the process. The right team will move the decision process a great distance toward the goal of making the best decision. This step in the overall process must be approached by the leader with a clear understanding of both how a team functions, and those qualities important to have on a high-performing team. In Patrick Lencioni's book, *The Five Dysfunctions of a Team*, he clearly describes those qualities [1]. The five dysfunctions that must be avoided are: the "absence of trust," "fear of conflict," "lack of commitment," "lack of accountability," and "inattention to results." Trust

Operating Room Leadership and Management, ed. Kaye A.D., Fox C.J. and Urman R.D. Published by Cambridge University Press. © Cambridge University Press 2012.

forms the foundation needed for the other team functions to work.

Begin by gathering individuals who trust each other. If this is not possible, trust must be established as quickly as possible in order to move through the decision-making process quickly. The absence of trust allows the team to move forward with a foundational flaw and leads to future failure. The higher the level of trust, the faster the team can move on the work ahead of it. Everyone must be willing to share mistakes and weaknesses in order to show they can be vulnerable to others on the team.

Without trust it will become impossible to avoid the second dysfunction: fear of conflict. When fear of conflict exists, team members remain guarded in discussion and are incapable of engaging in an open exchange of ideas. This results in the suppression of their true feelings on most issues and therefore prevents the team from adequately exploring all alternatives presented in the decision-making process. When the team has lack of trust and fear of conflict they begin to feel as if the team meetings are not worth the time needed and begin to demonstrate a lack of commitment to the team's assigned work.

Lack of commitment to the team is the third dysfunction. In meetings these individuals never air their true feelings on the matters being considered. They never buy in to the process or the final decision, yet they often act as if they are in full agreement with the team at meetings, only to express lack of support for the team and the decision when outside the team. This lack of commitment leads to the fourth dysfunction: the avoidance of accountability.

When individuals are not trusting, fear conflict, and/or lack commitment to the team, they begin to hesitate to hold team members accountable to the work of the team. Because they do not believe in the team or its work, they will choose to avoid accountability. When accountability is absent, the focus on results and the measurement of results ultimately cause the team to fail, and decisions they make will fail or at least never reach their full potential.

The final dysfunction, inattention to results, allows individual team members to focus on their personal needs and interests. This focus on individual needs always overshadows any concern or focus on the needs or work of the team. Therefore, most decisions made by such a team will fail, and ultimately the team will fail.

The team should be constructed with a focus on avoiding these dysfunctions and looking to build a team with the desirable qualities enhanced. Other important considerations include finding people with full authority to allocate necessary resources to the final decision and the authority to implement the final decision. Key stakeholder groups should be represented either directly or indirectly. Both proponents and opponents of the decision at the start of the process should be included. These different perspectives add value and a rich quality to the discussion and final decision. Outside opinions should also be sought as necessary from consultants with an expertise in the areas being evaluated for the decision [2]. Keep the size of the team manageable and consider the meeting environment and location of meetings so that open discussion and trust can be fostered and developed. Last, consider any positional hierarchy on the team so that meetings can be held in an open environment. Even the setting of the meeting can give way to a sense that only one or two individuals will make the decision: for example, a table in a boardroom with only one chair at the head of the table. There will need to be a team leader; however, the role of the leader should be focused on facilitation of open discussion, and not decision making, in the team meetings.

Framing the decision

Framing is the second step in the decision-making process and is equally important to the first step of assembling the team. If framed incorrectly, the right decision may not even be considered, much less reached as the final outcome. However, proper framing will set the direction of discussions and can often speed the process on the proper path. Framing is the responsibility of the team leader, as he or she will also facilitate the discussions and insure that the focus stays inside the proper frame. Alan Rowe describes frames as "the prisms through which we view the world ... they determine both what we see and how we interpret it" [3].

Avoid framing with current assumptions only or intuitive guesses by team members as to the meaning of the decision. When set, the frame will guide all future team discussions, options considered, alternatives developed, and certainly final decisions made. The team leader must be vigilant for team members attempting to frame the decision from an individual perspective. Those individuals who understand framing will also know the power of the frame in leading to the final decision. Indeed, as Jeffrey Pfeffer states in *Managing with Power,* "Establishing the framework within which issues will be viewed and decided is often tantamount to determining the result" [4].

The leader should make sure to encourage and direct the framing to remain focused on the course that most benefits the organization. Don't allow the team to automatically accept an initial framing. Ask for many different team opinions and perspectives before making any decisions. Look for personal and individual biases. Also, uncover and challenge any assumptions that might exist under a dominant member's presence and opinions. Lastly, ask the leader to place him or herself in the perspective of other members to clearly look at different angles to the frame [5]. This deliberate attempt to find the best frame for the benefit of the organization and the team sets the frame and moves the process forward. The team will appreciate the sincere attempt by the leader not to dominate the framing of the issue. At the end of the process, the decision will have better support by the entire team and will be more easily implemented across the entire OR. Finally, do not hesitate to adjust the frame or reframe the decision if issues or alternatives develop that significantly change the direction of the decision from the organization's perspective.

Develop and evaluate possible alternatives

All good decision makers should seek multiple possible alternatives before making a decision. Finding, selecting, and evaluating alternatives will allow the best possible decision to be found and chosen by the team. The team should seek to avoid a simple yes or no decision, which is what occurs in the absence of alternative choices. The team leader must encourage a search for varied alternatives that look from several different perspectives and angles represented by the members of the team. If the leader does not seek alternatives, the risk will exist that the team will develop a single focus, leading to a single, untested decision. This atmosphere prevents innovative thought and appropriate vetting of the eventual decision.

In order to encourage development and discussion of alternatives, the leader should encourage outside opinions at the team meetings, look at other like companies in order to benchmark how they have addressed similar questions, ask team members to step out of their traditional job roles and think from a different perspective, ask probing questions, allow views and discussions different from that of their own, revisit

abandoned alternatives from time to time in order to reevaluate their relevancy, and consider hybrid alternatives as well [6].

Also, the team leader must establish some rules for the group to follow in order to encourage the development of alternative thoughts. Such rules should allow for and encourage active listening, equal respect for all team members, acknowledgement of failures without judgment, and tolerance of conflicting views. The leader must keep the discussion focused on the issues and alternatives and not on the individuals presenting their thoughts, while keeping the atmosphere in the room as light and unthreatening as possible.

According to David Matheson and Jim Matheson in *The Smart Organization,* the best alternatives have certain characteristics, given below.

- They are broadly constructed and not only a simple variation of another alternative or concept. They should offer a broad range of options.
- They are true alternatives and not just "straw men" presented to make another choice appear superior and reasonable. False choices must be avoided.
- They are feasible choices given the organization's resources, capabilities, and capacities. It is important to remain realistic regarding what the organization can do. The team can build a feasibility test that each alternative must be able to pass. It is important not to waste the team's valuable time on alternatives that can never become a reality for the organization.
- They are sufficiently numerous to represent a true choice. However, be mindful that each selected alternative must be fully evaluated, so be selective in the process [7].

The next step in the decision-making process is to take each alternative and analyze it using a varied set of analytical tools. These are discussed below.

Evaluation of alternatives and use of analytical tools

Most likely, each alternative will need to be fully evaluated from a variety of perspectives using different analytical tools. It is important for the team to enumerate those variables important to the final decision and therefore create a screen or filter by which each alternative can be evaluated. Such variables might include *time* to implement, *benefits* to the organization if chosen and implemented, the *ethics* of the decision and whether there are any ethical or *legal issues*, what are the required *resources* to complete implementation, *how feasible* is the alternative and what are the possible obstacles to implementation. Additional variables could include the *overall risk* of the alternative, the *financial impact* of the alternative at maturity, what *intangibles* might be affected by the alternative, and lastly the *costs* to implement and use the alternative on a long-term basis.

As the decision team filters each alternative for all the variables listed above they will need to be aware of the further analysis necessary for each choice. Analytical tools are available to assess the financial impact of each possible choice, the probability of a particular alternative succeeding or failing, the development of further details that exist inside each alternative and how each alternative performs in a "trade off" against other alternatives, and prioritization of each choice as to how it best addresses the key objectives of the overall decision.

From a financial analysis perspective there are several commonly used analytical tools. These include the return on investment (ROI), net present value (NPV), internal rate of return (IRR), breakeven analysis, and sensitivity analysis. These will be described below as to their individual benefits and the process involved in completing each. Other tools such as the prioritization matrix and the decision tree will also be discussed below. Any discussion of advanced decision support computer software or related enterprise-level software is beyond the intended scope of this chapter.

The ROI is a calculation of the percentage return from the chosen investment that can then be compared to other investment returns that might be expected from alternative investments using the same capital dollars. The net return of an investment is simply the subtraction of the total costs of the project from the total cash benefits. Then the ROI is calculated by dividing the net return by the total investment amount. For example, let's assume that an item of imaging equipment is being evaluated with an upfront cost of $400 000 and with an expected annual return of $100 000 per year over 5 years. The total return would be $500 000 and the net return would be $500 000 minus the total cost of $400 000 ($500 000 – $400 000 = $100 000). The net investment return of $100 000 is then divided by the total investment cost of $400 000 ($100 000/$400 000 = 0.25), resulting in a healthy ROI of 25%.

The NPV takes into consideration the fact of using today's dollars and adjusting future values for the time value of money and the fact that future dollars are never worth more than present dollars. When cash flows can be predicted, the best predictive financial tool to use is the calculation of the NPV. The NPV takes into consideration the future cash flows, the ongoing cost of capital or risk, and the initial investment cost to start the project. In the end, the NPV gives an accurate assessment of the present value of the decision today while using future dollars in the calculation. It can be a complicated calculation; however, most financial calculators and computer spreadsheet programs can perform the actual calculations, and they will not be discussed here. It is most important for the decision team to estimate future cash flows from the possible investment and alternate investments being evaluated. It is also important for the team to determine the discount rate or the rate of return if the same dollars were placed into an alternative investment with similar risk. The future cash flows are then discounted by the discount rate and the sum of these discounted cash flows results in a total present value. Total investment costs of the project are then subtracted from the total present value to give the NPV. This NPV can then be compared to similar NPV calculations of other investment alternatives under consideration. A possible example of the use of this might be if a surgical department was considering expanding to include a new service line not currently provided.

The IRR is similar to the NPV calculation. It is defined as the discount rate that will cause the NPV to be equal to zero. Then, when comparing alternative decisions, the one with the higher IRR will be the best from a financial return perspective. In most cases, the IRR of a given decision alternative should be higher than the risk-free treasury bond rate and higher than the organization's hurdle rate or internal discount rate.

The breakeven analysis is useful when evaluating an investment that will allow new revenue generation or enhanced revenue from an existing service. An example might be the addition of a specific spinal surgical procedure to an existing spine program in a hospital not currently performing these procedures. The breakeven analysis would help the team determine how many of these procedures at a given unit value would need to be completed in order to reach a break-even state with the total investment costs of the program. The variables to be considered would include the unit contribution amount, unit variable costs, and total fixed costs. The unit contribution amount is the "contribution margin" of each procedure – that is, the

Alternative	Lower costs (4)	Higher revenues (3)	Short implementation (2)	Patient satisfaction (1)	Total score
A	$5 \times 4 = 20$	$1 \times 3 = 3$	$10 \times 2 = 20$	$10 \times 1 = 10$	53
B	$8 \times 4 = 32$	$1 \times 3 = 3$	$8 \times 2 = 16$	$6 \times 1 = 6$	57

Figure 4.1 A prioritization matrix.

procedural revenue minus the variable cost of each procedure. The total fixed costs are then divided by the unit contribution of one procedure with the resulting quotient being equal to the number of units needed for a break-even volume. This is the total number of these procedures needed to cover the fixed costs of this alternative. The team must then decide if this volume is achievable – and if so, over what time frame – and what resources exist or are needed to support such an endeavor.

Sensitivity analysis is a tool that allows the decision team to take the previously calculated NPV amount and then assess the probability of specific variables required in the alternative actually occurring. After the probability of a single variable is changed, the NPV can be recalculated using a computer spreadsheet. This analysis allows individual items to be changed to determine the overall impact on the program's financial outcome.

For a more complete review of these financial analytical tools with examples of the needed calculations, consult any business finance text or similar searches on the web. As to other types of nonfinancial analysis, consider the prioritization matrix and the decision tree. These will both be discussed in more detail below.

The prioritization matrix is a useful tool to analyze the nonfinancial value of a particular alternative. With this tool, the team must develop a clear list of expected objectives that would be achieved if the program alternative were successful. Each objective is then prioritized and weighted accordingly. Also, each alternative being analyzed is assigned a probability (using a scale of 1 to 10, with 10 being the best) of achieving each selected objective. A total score is then calculated and the alternative with the highest score is the better choice (see Figure 4.1).

In Figure 4.1, alternative B would be the better alternative given this set of probabilities and weighted objectives.

The decision tree tool builds a "roadmap" of possible decisions inside a single alternative with assigned probabilities to each decision pathway. To provide the most accurate assessment of the given alternative using the decision tree, the decision team must ask each member, and outsiders as needed, for individual estimates of probabilities in order to develop a final probability set for each decision node. For completeness' sake, each member of the team should also estimate financial values with each probability if possible. Decision trees work best when the team can accurately predict probabilities and financial outcomes of the separate parts of the given alternative (see Figure 4.2) [8].

For a more detailed discussion on using and constructing more complex decision tree tools, refer to the web as well as statistical texts and decision theory business texts.

Role of bias in decision making

Despite best efforts on the part of decision team members, it is normal for specific types of decision biases to enter into the decision-making process. It is best for all members of the team to be frequently reminded by the team leader and other members how they can be aware of and guard against the several forms of cognitive decision biases.

The first form of bias is the "overconfidence bias." People by nature are overconfident in their personal decisions and judgments; they are also overly optimistic in these decisions and judgments. The combination of overconfidence and optimism can lead to faulty decisions. The second form of bias is the "sunk-cost effect." The sunk-cost effect describes how humans will invariably commit to decisions in which they have already invested a large amount of time, money, or other personal resources. These previous investments of resources in one alternative investment prevent individuals from making a clear alternative decision that might be better. Third is the "recency effect," also known as an example of the "availability bias." This bias is in effect when those making the decision place too much emphasis on

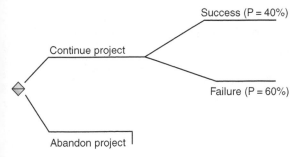

Figure 4.2 A decision tree – basic form.

information that is readily available when faced with the decision. They focus on recent events they think are similar to the decision facing them. The fourth bias is the "confirmation bias," which causes humans to gather information that confirms their existing views about a decision, and causes them to devalue any information that does not support their preconceived ideas about the decision. Fifth is the "anchoring bias," whereby the decision evaluation is begun from an arbitrary reference point, which if improperly placed, or anchored, will skew the final decision to a faulty conclusion. There are several other cognitive biases; however, those mentioned above are the most common. So how can the decision team diminish the effects of these biases? Mainly by keeping a high level of awareness in the team so that they can recognize if these start to appear in the decision process. Also by looking for forms of measurable feedback once the decision is made in order to retrospectively review how the decision was made and if any bias impacted the final decision.

Make the decision and begin implementation

After the team has agreed on an amount of time to complete its assessment of the decision and alternatives, the leader must move the team to a close. Even with disagreement between team members, the team leader must move to get the decision finalized. First, he or she must keep the team's focus on the previously agreed upon common goal. Also, the team might agree to briefly revisit and reexamine all alternatives and related summary assumptions. If the process begins to drag on, the leader will need to set a clear time deadline. The leader may need to remind the entire team that if a consensus decision cannot be reached, a majority vote will carry the final decision. Both deciding too early and too late in the process can be problematic; therefore a vote may be needed to reach the deadline. After the decision is made, the team should agree to come out of the final meeting in unity behind the final decision despite the voting results.

Next the decision will need to be explained to those in the organization who will be affected by it or expected to carry out the implementation. Explain how the process worked and why the final alternative was chosen. Clearly describe the implementation process and timeline while recognizing all those who participated in the decision process. Lastly, ask for feedback and allow the post-decision process to be a time of learning for the future. This also allows others to be heard and valued even though they were not directly involved in the process.

Summary

High-reliability organizations allow the formation of a well-tested process for decision making. There is a proven process described that, when followed, will allow the best decision team to be selected, a clear process to be defined, and alternative decisions to be developed and analyzed individually and in comparison with each other. Also, the team will engage in open discussion, the avoidance of cognitive biases, and ultimately reach the best alternative of those considered. Finally, the decision will be reached, and clearly communicated, and then the implementation process will begin. Those organizations that are best at decision making will always use every opportunity to learn from each decision made, in order to improve in the future. Whether in the surgical suite or in the organization as a whole, those leaders who have a better understanding of decision making will always be in the best position to lead others in easy and difficult times alike.

Decision making is a leadership skill that is worthy of the time required to develop it further. Few leaders are fully competent at it or work to become competent at it.

References

1. P. Lencioni. *The Five Dysfunctions of a Team*. San Francisco: Josey-Bass, 2002, pp. 188–9.

2. R. Luecke. *Decision Making, Five Steps to Better Results*. Boston: Harvard Business Press, 2006, p. 13.

3. A. J. Rowe. *Creative Intelligence*. Upper Saddle River, NJ: Prentice Hall, 2004, p. 68.

4. J. Pfeffer. *Managing with Power*. Boston: Harvard Business Press, 1992, pp. 63–4.

5. R. Luecke, *Decision Making: Five Steps to Better Results*. Boston: Harvard Business Press, 2006, pp. 27–8.

6. R. Luecke, *Decision Making: Five Steps to Better Results*. Boston: Harvard Business Press, 2006, pp. 57–8.

7. D. Matheson, J. Matheson. *The Smart Organization*. Boston: Harvard Business Press, 1998, pp. 42–3.

8. R. Luecke. *Decision Making: Five Steps to Better Results*. Boston: Harvard Business Press, 2006, pp. 54–5.

Chapter

Health care and economic realities

Robert Lynch MD

Hospital revenue and the impact of operative
services   40
Hospital expenses and
the impact of operative
services   41

Risk profile of the OR in an academic
environment   42
OR efficiency   42
Graduate medical education   43
Summary   44

Every discussion about the US system of health care could start with a statement about the profound pace of change. The twentieth century alone saw an explosion in technological advances, from modern sterile techniques, modern anesthesia, antibiotics, blood and blood product replacement, and organ transplantation to mechanical substitutes or assistive devices for the kidneys, heart, and lungs. The first decade of the twenty-first century has seen an explosion in microsurgical techniques and robotic surgery, and the incorporation of molecular biology into all aspects of medicine. The latter portends a future of highly personalized medicine, with both diagnosis and therapy driven out of medicine's ability to unlock the genetic foundation of health and disease.

At the same time, our advances have created new problems. Antibiotics have become increasingly ineffective, just as we are realizing that hospitals and other health-care institutions are major contributors to the problem. In just over a century, the industrialized world replaced epidemic illnesses, childbirth, and malnutrition as major causes of mortality and morbidity with the complications of our newly won longevity and the lifestyles afforded us by our industrial accomplishments. Perhaps most challenging is that the above mentioned technological march combined with aging populations has produced a cost spiral that exceeds the rate of economic growth and is therefore unsustainable. Even in industrialized countries with "low" per capita health-care spending, the rate of increase will eventually overwhelm their ability to pay for it.

At the time of writing, the US health-care system is attempting to incorporate the massive changes required by the Affordable Care Act (ACA). The ACA is in part a response to the rising cost pressures noted above. It does many things, but in short, the effect of the ACA to providers is to expand coverage while reducing payments for a unit of service. At the same time, it accelerates the linking of payments to performance. This means linking payments to improved outcomes, reduced complications, and patient satisfaction.

Hospitals are in the middle of all these issues and pressures. With some exceptions, hospital utilization is expected to decline as the result of better outpatient management strategies and pressure from both private and government payers. At the same time hospitals are the main entry point for new technologies that are adding costs faster than reimbursement is increasing. Patients in hospitals today are sicker than ever, and their care is more complicated. This adds to the challenges of functioning in a pay-for-performance world that will not subsidize complications.

The ACA puts economic pressure on insurers, suppliers, and providers. All will attempt to turn to hospitals to offset this impact. In the case of physicians, there will be an increasing trend toward hospital employment or subsidization. This will be driven by physicians trying to preserve incomes. It will also be driven by pay-for-performance, with both hospitals and physicians working to coordinate patient care between the hospital and the office. Employment is the most effective vehicle to foster this coordination. On balance, employing physicians is a net expense for hospitals.

For hospitals to survive economically in this environment, they must execute strategies that leverage those aspects of their business that have the highest margins. Every hospital has business that for a number of reasons is unprofitable. What makes the enterprise viable is making sure that profitable business is sufficient to subsidize all aspects of the hospital. In an academic medical center this is doubly true, as such centers frequently end up subsidizing the academic mission. In reality, most medical schools cannot survive without hospital subsidies. Hence at an academic medical center the ability to leverage profitable business is necessary not only for its own health but also for that of its affiliated school.

As a general rule, the highest margin aspect of hospital-based care is procedural. Nowhere is this truer than in the operating room (OR). At the same time the cost and risk aspects of the OR constantly threaten to tip the economic balance. When this is complicated by a teaching hospital's academic mission, which adds cost and reduces efficiency, one realizes the challenges of sustaining quality care and academics in an economically sustainable manner.

In the end the hospital OR is the focal point of all the challenges facing health care. It is where the rising cost of technology and declining reimbursement meet sicker (riskier) patients. It is where the expectations of good outcomes are the most evident and the complexity of modern medicine requires perfect execution to achieve them. It is also a major focal point for the educational mission of an academic medical center. Academic medical centers not only tend to treat more complex patients using the latest technology, but also have multiple layers of trainees from students to fellows that must have a meaningful educational experience. This must happen despite the inherent conflict that education creates, with the pressures on improving operating efficiency and quality.

Hospital revenue and the impact of operative services

Hospital operating profit margins have hovered around an average of roughly 2–4% between 2005 and early 2010. The range of profitability is wide, however, with a significant number of hospitals losing money in any given fiscal year. Despite the relatively level average margins, the percentage of hospitals with negative margins grew from 20% in 2005 to 38% in 2010 [1]. This trend is disturbing, as the ACA is predicted to put pressure on revenues. Unless hospitals adapt, this trend will lead to closures and/or consolidations.

The major variables that influence a hospital's total margin are its payer mix, case mix, and cost structure. Payer mix, for example, is a significant variable. Looking at Medicare alone, in not-for-profit hospitals the median profit margin in 2008 was zero. In essence, half the hospitals reported lost money on Medicare [2]. Medicare generally pays less than commercial health maintenance organization (HMO) and preferred provider organization (PPO) payers, and more than Medicaid. Hospitals that are highly profitable tend to have more commercial business and are in a strong position to negotiate favorable rates. The ACA is expected to lead to a decline in traditional employer-sponsored commercial coverage and an increase in Medicaid. It will be impossible for every hospital to improve its payer mix and case mix in this environment, although some will be successful. All hospitals will be aggressively addressing cost through increased efficiencies.

Most of a hospital's revenue comes from inpatient care. Typically half a hospital's admissions come through the emergency department. The other half is heavily biased toward elective admissions, particularly operative care and major procedures. Although there is a wide range, our hospital is fairly typical, with surgical patients generating almost 40% of our revenues. The total includes major hospital-based outpatient services, such as cancer chemotherapy and radiation therapy.

It is very difficult to influence payer mix and case mix in the emergency department, but hospitals do have some influence over both in the OR. This is why hospitals aggressively recruit surgical specialists whether they are subsidized or not. Winning physician loyalty through improved access, throughput, and quality (including patient satisfaction) is essentially a universal strategy. These also have a synergistic effect on cost.

Whether a physician should be employed or subsidized is a complex legal and business discussion, but surgical specialties are frequently candidates for such relationships. In academic medical centers, the faculty are typically not full-time clinicians with academic responsibilities taking up the rest of their time. For many faculty members, their clinical practice will not cover all their salaries and benefits, necessitating some subsidy of their academic time from within the medical school. From a strategic perspective, it is important for the academic medical center to coordinate on the recruitment of those disciplines that help it increase its margins. Given the magnitude of surgical revenues, this will typically mean specialists that drive OR volume.

In summary, revenue from surgical patients represents a plurality of a hospital's income. In a time where the average hospital is operating at low margins, the health of their OR business is key to making or losing money. This is going to be increasingly true as more patients shift to government payers. Hospitals strive to improve operating functions, not only for efficiency, but also to recruit and retain productive surgeons. Subsidies and employment for physicians are becoming increasingly important. In academic settings, academic medical centers and their affiliated medical schools frequently collaborate on such key recruits.

Anesthesia services drive much of what goes into improving access, throughput, and quality. When functioning well they can help drive surgical volume and its related revenues. This is much more challenging in an academic environment, but it can be addressed. Residents by definition are not able to function at the level of an attending anesthesiologist and can negatively impact throughput and cost. Conversely residents are increasingly driving both business and quality improvements as a formal part of their training. Anesthesia services must be partners in improving operations and growing the business line if hospitals are to succeed in the future. This is particularly true at academic medical centers.

Hospital expenses and the impact of operative services

Hospitals are a high-volume low-margin business. Average profit margins of 2–4% mean that on average costs come close to approximating revenues. Clearly managing costs is critical to the financial health of any hospital. Although procedural-based areas such as the OR constitute a disproportionate share of a hospital's revenues, they also constitute a disproportionate share of the costs.

Labor typically makes up 50–60% of a hospital's operating expenses. Per-patient-served labor costs are even higher in the OR. Aside from call coverage, ORs are staffed proportionally to utilization (with some adjustment for complexity). In essence, total hours of utilization are correlated with labor costs. What dictates efficiency is how many cases can be done per staffed hour. The staffed hours include all time from opening to closing a room. Therefore delays in first starts, extended turnaround time, last-minute cancellations, and cases that run longer than usual all contribute to staffed hours while adding nothing to revenue. To maximize efficiency and cost-effectiveness, these variables must be managed. This can be challenging in an academic setting, where trainees do not function with maximum efficiency and the variety of cases and the variability of academic schedules makes it challenging to develop the kind of routines and practices that maximize efficiency.

Supplies typically make up 15% of a hospital's operating expenses. Supply costs in the OR are a disproportionately large share of the hospital total. Technology and intensity drive OR supply costs. Every hospital deals with the constant pressure to adopt new devices, which almost universally come with a higher price tag. Newer devices also do not tend to be part of the bulk-purchase contracts that hospitals negotiate with vendors. Teaching hospitals magnify this, as surgical caseload is skewed toward complex and high-risk cases and faculty tend to be very interested in new technologies. Trainees also add to costs if for no other reason than that there are extra hands and bodies involved. Anecdotes about extra breakage and wastage probably have some truth, but they are hard to quantify.

Capital, particularly for medical equipment, is an almost universal issue. Although funded and accounted for differently, it is a major part of the true expense of running a clinical enterprise. Physicians are frequently unaware of the major capital needs just to provide and maintain the physical plant. Clinical equipment ultimately competes for such funding. Conversely new medical equipment may be supported by a potential for a return on investment in the form of new clinical volume/revenue. The nature of the OR is that it is particularly capital intensive. It is driven by new technologies and very aggressive marketing to physicians. In an academic setting, this is particularly true, as faculty tend to be aware of new technologies and strive to offer cutting-edge care that is the hallmark of a teaching hospital. Teaching hospitals also tend to have a broad clinical portfolio, which demands an equally broad capital investment.

An academic anesthesia program has the ability to influence all three of these costs. Ideally the members of the program take the lead in driving efficient OR utilization, participate in supply contract selection, help enforce contract adherence, and take the lead in equipment prioritization and selection and utilization.

Risk profile of the OR in an academic environment

In the United States medical malpractice is frequently cited as a significant driver in the cost of health care. The actual costs for liability coverage for hospitals, however, are closer to 2% of all expenses. What is debated and hard to quantify is the cost of "defensive medicine." Regardless of the financial impact, the real issue is whether the defensive behaviors are wasteful (e.g., unnecessary imaging studies) or whether they improve practice (e.g., adoption of strategies to reduce central-line infections).

The Department of Justice (DOJ) analyzed claims data in seven states that require public reporting of claims [3]. Three of the states reported only on claims against physicians, whereas the rest reported on all providers. Over half of all claims reported were for injuries claimed during inpatient hospital care. About half of all claims are filed against surgeons. These data support the assumption that the OR is a high-risk environment in terms of generating claims.

Claims probably understate the magnitude of the problem. In 2010, 9894 paid claims against physicians were reported to the National Practitioner Data Bank [4]. If the DOJ ratio applies, then about 5000 claims were for care provided in a hospital. To put this in context, the AHA reports there are just over 5800 hospitals in the United States.

The Institute of Medicine put the issue in perspective. In its seminal report *To Err is Human*, it pointed out that between 44 000 and 98 000 people die each year as a result of preventable errors [5]. They noted that such errors were likely to occur in operating rooms, intensive care units, and emergency rooms. Since the report was published, much has been done to improve patient safety, particularly focusing on operative care. Led by the government, payers have begun to withhold payment for the treatment of preventable complications, and hospitals have adopted policies of not charging for such treatments.

While it represents voluntary reporting, the Joint Commission (JC) publishes sentinel event trends. In 2010 three of the top four sentinel event categories were related to the OR. Clearly when looking at the most significant outcomes, the OR is a high-risk environment. The JC data also demonstrate that the health-care system can improve. For over a decade, the number 1 sentinel event was wrong patient/wrong site/wrong procedure. Owing to a system-wide effort to improve patient and procedure identification, this category fell to number 3 in 2010.

Clearly the OR is a high-risk environment and is a source of a significant number of errors and unexpected outcomes. This represents not only a malpractice liability issue but also a significant financial risk. More importantly, it is a failure of our health-care system to live up to our mandate to do no harm. Academic medicine has recognized the importance of these issues and has adopted patient safety into all levels of training. Specific to the OR, anesthesia services are in the best position to drive the changes needed. This must be a collaborative effort, as even something as simple as preventing a wrong site procedure requires the participation of the entire operative team. From a position of training, presence, and authority, the anesthesiologist is in the best position to drive the changes needed. Hospital administrations have begun to recognize this and are empowering their anesthesia services as leads in quality improvement. Anesthesiologists and residents are frequently serving on hospital-wide quality improvement and risk-reduction committees and teams.

OR efficiency

As noted earlier, OR efficiency is a major determinate of costs and, by extension, profitability. It is also a significant driver of physician loyalty and satisfaction. From a strictly business perspective, hospitals want surgeons to use their facilities. In the context of fee-for-service medicine, surgeons have the same economic pressures that hospitals do. It is in both the surgeon's and the hospital's best interests to make efficient use of the OR. In reality, OR efficiency and physician satisfaction are tightly linked.

In a perfect world all cases would start on time; patients would always be fully cleared for surgery in advance; cases would run as long as scheduled; complications would not happen; equipment and supplies would always be available and would never break; turnaround time would be consistently short; surgeons would always have the time slot they wanted to operate; and emergency cases would never displace scheduled cases. The above list may seem obvious or even whimsical, but it illustrates the fact that there are a finite number of things that drive efficiency and satisfaction. Furthermore, all of them can be influenced. It is beyond the scope of this chapter to delve into all the strategies that can influence these issues. All hospitals do work to improve them, but with varying degrees of success.

An efficient OR has obvious economic benefits, as it is maximizing the use of facilities. This produces the largest return for the fixed expenses and maximizes the effectiveness of the semi-variable and variable expenses. Chief financial officers and managers spend a lot of energy pushing their organizations toward these goals. As an efficient OR also supports the surgeon's practice, it improves their satisfaction. Hospitals have realized that physicians have some degree of discretion as to where they operate, whether on a case-by-case basis or driving their overall recruitment and retention at a hospital. All things being equal, a surgeon will prefer to operate where their needs for efficiency are met and they are most satisfied. Over time, an efficient OR can grow surgical volume as a result.

Although the surgeon is a "customer" of the OR that hospitals strive to satisfy, he or she can contribute to the very problems that hinder their practice. The OR is a very real example of a place in which the customer must participate in improvement efforts. Surgeons, however, vary in terms of their OR issues and their willingness and ability to participate in such activities. To involve surgeons effectively requires leadership from hospital-based anesthesiologists. They alone are in the best position not only to lead a team approach but also to deal with surgeons on a peer-to-peer basis. Hospitals must make sure their anesthesiologists understand all the issues involved and that they are empowered to take a leadership role in addressing them.

Graduate medical education is increasingly preparing trainees not only to be functional clinicians but also to take a leadership role in the business of medicine. This includes not only quality and patient safety initiatives, but also process improvement issues. The OR is a rich environment for positively influencing both. Academic anesthesia departments can take an even greater role in terms of improving OR functions and patient safety. Perhaps more importantly, they can develop the next generation of clinician/managers who will be needed in the future.

Graduate medical education

Graduate medical education (GME) in the United States is primarily based in hospitals. This is a direct result of the decision to fund GME through the Centers for Medicare & Medicaid Services (CMS). As a result, hospitals receive funding proportionate to the number of residents, fellows, beds, and services provided to CMS beneficiaries. Funding supports direct costs (salaries and benefits of trainees), indirect costs (increased overhead of supporting trainees in the hospital), and capital. Reimbursements from nongovernmental payers are sometimes negotiated at higher rates at teaching hospitals.

Although hospitals are generally paid more for having GME programs, they are not necessarily reimbursed fully for the increased costs of supporting postgraduate education. Direct salary and benefit costs for trainees are fully reimbursed, only if the proportion of care provided to government beneficiaries is high enough. Indirect costs are hard to quantify, and there is less consistency in how they impact hospitals. A number of factors influence such costs. It has long been established that teaching programs utilize more resources for a given diagnosis-related group. This mainly stems from overutilization of ancillary services, but it can be influenced by a number of things.

With new limits on resident work hours and duties, hospitals have had to increase support. This ranges from nurse practitioners and personal assistants to assist in patient care to adding additional ancillary support staff. Specifically for anesthesia, this means additional certified registered nurse anesthetists (CRNAs) and technicians. Resident supervision can mean limits on admissions and patient load, leading to additional teams or nonteaching hospitalists. Both are typically subsidized by the hospital.

For anesthesia, 1:2 resident supervision requirements can require more attending physicians. To the extent that hospitals subsidize staff, this can be a significant impact. With increased emphasis on quality of life, call rooms and meals have been improved and formal teaching and work space provided or upgraded. Depending on specific hospital circumstances, this can impact capital and operating budgets.

There is a trend toward hospitals subsidizing their anesthesia services. This has complex causes, ranging from undersupply, declining professional reimbursement, and competition with ambulatory surgery centers. Between 1997 and 2007 the percentage of hospitals paying a subsidy increased from 15% to 75%. The size of the actual subsidies showed a proportionate increase as well. In teaching programs, faculty typically are allotted "academic time" for the purposes of teaching or research. This limits the amount of time a given member of staff is available for strictly clinical duties. In the case of anesthesia, this can mean subsidizing more total staff than would be justified based on strictly patient-care demands. This is exacerbated by the staffing ratios for resident supervision noted earlier.

From a strictly financial standpoint, teaching hospitals have higher revenues per patient than nonteaching hospitals. Conversely they also have higher expenses. What this means to a specific hospital's bottom line is a complex interplay of multiple factors influencing both revenues and expenses.

Academic medical centers do not exist solely for financial reasons, and nor should their value be measured in strictly financial terms. Teaching hospitals are the major venue for educating our health-care workforce at all levels. Likewise academic medical centers are a major site for clinical research, and they indirectly support basic research at their affiliated medical schools. These factors are also true for academic anesthesia programs.

Although one could argue that these benefit society at large, there is also an argument that they benefit the teaching hospital as well. Teaching hospitals tend to function as quaternary/tertiary referral centers. They have a disproportionate share of Level I trauma centers, complex surgical programs, transplant programs, and highly specialized disease management programs. To sustain all these programs and attract the physicians necessary to run them is incredibly difficult without the financial structure and the environment of an academic medical center. Lastly, at a time when future physician supply is again projected to be inadequate, teaching hospitals are in an excellent position to recruit young physicians from their own training programs and to attract established faculty from outside their community.

Surgical and procedural specialties play particularly important roles in supporting academic medical centers. Having well-functioning ORs and an engaged supportive anesthesia program is critical to their success. The financial and administrative challenges of supporting GME in anesthesia can conflict with these goals. These conflicts can be managed, and the positive benefits of well-run education programs can be leveraged as a result.

Summary

For hospitals to survive in our changing health-care environment they must grow revenues despite downward pressures on reimbursements. They must focus on expanding business in areas that have more favorable reimbursement to subsidize areas that are less well reimbursed. For academic medical centers, this also means that they must also be able to subsidize the academic mission and their affiliated school. This puts tremendous pressure on those high-margin areas to execute well and to develop new business. Although many areas can be the focus for most hospitals, operative services will be a significant part of their strategies. This means minimizing risk, adverse events, and costs while maximizing efficiency and physician and patient satisfaction. Teaching hospitals must do these things while integrating the academic mission into their operations.

Anesthesia services are a critical component of successful operative and invasive programs. In many ways, anesthesiologists are in the best position to manage many of the complex variables that determine the success of such programs and services. Academic anesthesia programs have an especially important role, driven by the imperative to incorporate quality improvement/risk reduction and management into GME. From a hospital's perspective GME presents both financial and operating risks and opportunities. Hospital administration must partner with departmental leadership to achieve the mutual goals of successful clinical and academic programs.

References

1. Thompson Reuters. *Hospital Operating Trends Quarterly*. Ann Arbor, MI: Thompson Reuters, 2010. Available online at: http://healthcare.thomsonreuters.com/thought-leadership/assets/HospOperatingTrendsQuarterly_Dec_2010.pdf (last accessed May 10, 2012).

2. J. Carlson. On the margins of Medicare. *Modern Healthcare* 2012. Available online at: www.modernhealthcare.com/article/20120102/MAGAZINE/301029885# (last accessed May 10, 2012).

3. T. Cohen, K. Hughes. *Medical Malpractice Insurance Claims in Seven States, 2000–2004.* Bureau of Justice Statistics, Special report 2007. Available online at: http://bjs.ojp.usdoj.gov/index.cfm?ty=pbdetail&iid=783 (last accessed May 10, 2012).

4. Kaiser Family Foundation, statehealthfacts.org. Available online at: www.statehealthfacts.org/ (last accessed May 10, 2012).

5. Committee on Quality of Health Care in America, Institute of Medicine, L. T. Kohn, J. M. Corrigan, M. S. Donaldson. *To Err is Human: Building a Safer Health System.* National Academy Press, 1st edn. 2000.

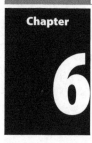

Chapter 6

Influence of staffing and scheduling on operating room productivity

Franklin Dexter MD, PhD
Richard H. Epstein MD, CPHIMS

Definitions 46
Operating room efficiency on the day of surgery 50
Tactical versus operational OR management decisions 52

Planning service-specific staffing and scheduling cases based on increasing OR efficiency 54
Impact of reducing times on productivity 61
Summary 63

This chapter focuses on the determinants of operating room (OR) labor productivity and costs. It is intended to help readers understand how evidence-based management can be applied when planning staffing for their facilities (i.e., hospitals, day surgery centers, etc.). Both productivity and the cost of OR staffing are inextricably linked to the choices of how many ORs to open at the start of the day and how to schedule cases into those locations.

Definitions

Staff scheduling and assignment

"Staff scheduling" is the process of deciding which nurses, anesthesia providers, and other personnel work each shift on each day. Staff scheduling for a future date is usually performed before the surgical cases to be performed on that date have been scheduled. For example, the OR nurses create their work schedule 2 months in advance: Ms. Jamison and Mr. Green are scheduled to work 08:00 h to 16:00 h on March 8.

"Staffed hours" are hours that the OR nurses and the anesthesia group schedule their providers to cover when not on call (e.g., 07:00 h to 15:00 h) and "staff assignment" is the process of deciding who will take care of patients in a given location on a specific day. Most assignments are typically made on the weekday prior to the date of surgery. For example, tomorrow,

Dr. Waters will be supervising two certified registered nurse anesthetists (CRNAs) in ORs 9 and 10.

Elective, urgent, and emergent cases

We are not aware of any one best answer as to what constitutes an elective, urgent, or emergent case [1]. Still, differentiating among such cases is necessary to plan staffing. The following is a set of reasonable definitions that provide for different operational decisions.

An "elective case" can be defined as one for which the patients can wait at least 3 days for surgery without sustaining additional morbidity [2]. The choice of 3 days corresponds to patients waiting from Friday to Monday. At a facility with patients scheduled for elective surgery on Saturdays, 2 days would be used as the threshold. For example, shoulder arthroplasty and breast biopsy cases are elective.

An "emergent case" can be defined as one for which the patient is likely to sustain additional morbidity and/or mortality unless surgical care is started in less time than needed for a team to be called in from home. In this context, "likely" to have a worse outcome means based on scientific studies, such as published observational studies. By using this evidence-based definition, the appropriateness of the relevant staffing decision can be made by reviewing data on previous emergent cases [2]. For example, cesarean sections because of a

Operating Room Leadership and Management, ed. Kaye A.D., Fox C.J. and Urman R.D. Published by Cambridge University Press. © Cambridge University Press 2012.

prolapsed umbilical cord or placental abruption are emergent.

An "urgent case" is defined as one for which the safe waiting time lies between that of an emergency and an elective case [2]. Almost all non-elective cases are urgent cases. For example, appendectomy is an urgent case. The procedure is not an emergency, because the patient can wait long enough for an OR team to come to the hospital from home. A cadaveric renal transplant would also be urgent, rather than emergent, for the same reason.

From a practical viewpoint, sufficient staff need to be present in-house to deal with emergent cases, whereas providing staff who take call from home to cover urgent cases that cannot be covered by the in-house call team is a viable approach. The cost differential between having sufficient staff in-house to handle urgent cases versus having them taking call from home can be considerable [2,3].

Definitions related to service-specific staffing

"Surgical service" refers to a group of surgeons who share allocated OR time (i.e., service-specific staffing). An individual surgeon, a group, a specialty, or a department can function as a surgical service, depending on how OR time is allocated. "Service" simply refers to the unit of OR allocation. For example, two ORs are allocated to the urological surgeons practicing at a hospital, any of whom can schedule cases in these rooms daily. Then, "Urology" is a service. As another example, two general surgeons are partners in General Surgical Associates (GSA), one of two independent general surgery groups that practice at a hospital. If these two general surgeons are together allocated OR time, then they represent a service, "GSA." A third example is a busy orthopedic surgeon, Dr. Bones, who is personally allocated 8 h of OR time every Tuesday. Then, from the perspective of allocating OR time and scheduling cases on Tuesdays, "Dr. Bones" represents a surgical service, even though there may also be an "Ortho" service. The service-specific staffing is that one OR for 8 h every Tuesday.

Even when a surgical suite does not have a formal organizational plan for allocating ORs (i.e., "block schedule"), there can be service-specific staffing (i.e., OR allocations). In this regard, "services" need not be specific clinical subspecialties in the medical staff organizational structure. Rather, they reflect the activities of individuals or groups of surgeons who use the OR facilities and thus require organized staffing to support those activities. In some circumstances, several disparate subspecialties (e.g., "Oral surgery" and "Plastic surgery") may share allocated OR time and thus function as a service.

For example, an eight-OR surgical suite has the official policy that all of its cases are scheduled on a first-scheduled, first-served basis. However, in reality, cases of the same specialty are usually scheduled into the same ORs, as this simplifies the distribution of resources (e.g., surgical equipment, video towers) and assignment of nursing and anesthesia teams who specialize in the area of surgical practice. Some nurses preferentially care for patients undergoing neurosurgery and otolaryngology cases, some mostly gynecology or general surgery, and so forth. In this case, the services correspond to the specialty teams.

"Allocated operating room time" is the interval of OR time with a specified start and end time on a specified day of the week that is assigned by the facility to a surgical service for scheduling cases (Figure 6.1). Some facilities have OR time that is staffed and available for cases, but not allocated to a specific service. Such OR time has been allocated to a "pseudo-service," variably named the "Open," "Unblocked," "First-scheduled, First-served," or "Other" service.

For example, urology is allocated OR time in two rooms from 07:00 h to 16:00 h on Monday to Friday. This does not mean that the department's surgeons are limited to scheduling cases only if they can be completed by 16:00 h. Instead, it means that staffing has been *planned* for the department's surgeons between 07:00 h and 16:00 h. The definition applies whether or not at that hospital it happens that the department's surgeons actually finish by 16:00 h. If the urology service's cases run past 16:00 h, and if nursing and anesthesia teams were to plan their staff scheduling to match the allocated OR time, then they would need to work beyond the end of regularly scheduled hours.

The "operating room time" of a case is defined as the interval from when a patient enters an OR until that patient leaves the OR (i.e., "wheels-in" to "wheels-out"). This definition is used often, because these events are unequivocal and thus have good interrater reliability. The use of anesthesia information management systems to provide such data automatically can make OR management easier [4].

"Turnover time" is the time from when one patient exits an OR until the next patient on that day's OR schedule enters the same OR [5,6]. Separating turnover time from the OR time of a case permits the two to be

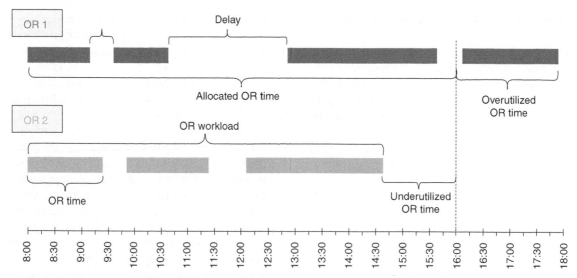

Figure 6.1 An example of an OR schedule.

studied statistically as separate processes (see Impact of reducing surgical and turnover times, below). Cleanup and setup times characteristically are recorded separately from OR times, but then combined. In part, this is because it is hard to define when cleanup has ceased and setup has begun for the next case, and these activities may overlap. Turnover times include cleanup times and setup times, but should exclude planned or unplanned delays between cases (e.g., when a to-follow surgeon is given a scheduled 12:30 h start time and the prior case in the OR ended at 11:00 h, or if the second of three cases in an OR cancels and the third patient is not available) (Figure 6.1). Hospital surgical suites may consider times between cases that are longer than a defined interval (e.g., 90 min) to represent delays, not turnovers, when computing turnover times to focus statistics on the latter cleanup and setup times [5]. This is because it is difficult to determine retrospectively the cause of such outliers, and these are usually unrelated to the process of room setup and cleanup. It is common for hospital analysts to ignore this distinction, resulting in invalid estimates of the actual turnover time and its variance.

For example, staffing is planned from 07:00 h to 15:00 h. A patient arrives at the holding area at 07:45 h, her IV is placed at 07:50 h, she enters the OR at 07:59 h, the trachea is intubated at 08:12 h, the operative site is prepared at 8:15 h, and the incision is made at 08:23 h. The patient leaves the OR at 10:59 h. From the perspective of OR scheduling, the case starts at 07:59 h. The OR time of the case is 3 h.

In another example, a surgeon is scheduled to perform a hepatic resection. However, soon after incision, the patient is found, unexpectedly, to have widespread peritoneal metastases and the incision is closed without performing the planned procedure. The patient exits from the OR 2.5 h earlier than planned. Including a planned 0.5-h turnover, the second case of the day could start 3 h earlier than planned. However, the second case of the day in that OR will be performed by a different surgeon. He is unavailable, caring for patients in his outpatient office. The result is a delay of 3 h. That delay should not contribute to the calculation of turnover times.

"Operating room workload" for a service is its total hours of cases including turnover times (Figure 6.1). This excludes the urgent cases for that service if separate OR time is allocated for urgent cases performed by all services. Turnover times are applied, by convention, to the service performing the prior case in the OR. Thus there is no turnover time for the last case of the day in that OR.

"Underutilized operating room time" = [allocated OR time] – [OR workload], or zero if this value is negative (Figure 6.1) [7]. This means that underutilized OR time equals the allocated OR time minus the OR workload, provided the allocated OR time is larger than the OR workload. Otherwise, the underutilized OR time is 0 h. Thus, underutilized OR time represents the time for which staffing was planned, but no work was performed.

"Adjusted utilization" = 100% × (1 – [underutilized OR time] ÷ [allocated OR time]) [6]. For example, staffing is planned from 08:00 h to 16:00 h. An OR's last case of the day ends at 14:00 h. The OR workload is 6 h. There are 2 h of underutilized OR time. The adjusted utilization is 75%, where 75% = 100% × (1 − 2 h ÷ 8 h) [6]. The maximum value of "adjusted utilization" is 100%.

"Overutilized operating room time" = [OR workload] − [allocated OR time], or zero if this value is negative (Figure 6.1) [7]. Thus, overutilized OR time represents the time during which work was performed but staffing was not planned in advance. For example, an OR is staffed from 08:30 h to 18:00 h. The last case of the day in the OR ends at 20:00 h. Then, there are 2 h of overutilized OR time. The adjusted utilization ignores overutilized OR time, which is one of the reasons why utilization is not a useful metric for facilities that typically do not finish the OR schedule prior to the end of allocated OR time.

"Inefficiency of use of operating room time" = [(cost per hour of underutilized OR time) × (hours of underutilized OR time)] + [(cost per hour of overutilized OR time) × (hours of overutilized OR time)] [7–9]. The cost of an hour of overutilized OR time is always more expensive than the cost of an hour of underutilized OR time.

"Operating room efficiency" is the value that is maximized when the inefficiency of use of OR time has been minimized [7]. "Efficiency" is characteristically thought of as the ratio of an output to the necessary input. For example, in a factory producing widgets, efficiency can be the number of widgets produced divided by the labor cost of producing those widgets. Thus, efficiency could be increased by producing more widgets with the same number of workers, or the same number of widgets with fewer workers. In the OR setting, when surgeons and patients are provided open access to OR time on any future workday, the output (e.g., number of cases performed) is a constant (see Tactical versus operational OR management decisions, below). One cannot "manufacture" more cases on the day of surgery. Maximizing "efficiency" then is achieved by minimizing the input. That occurs when service-specific staffing and case scheduling are so good that there are both 0 h of underutilized OR time and 0 h of overutilized OR time. In practice, this is an unachievable goal, because of variance in surgical times for identically scheduled cases. Thus, optimizing OR efficiency requires a managerial objective to minimize the total cost of the underutilized and overutilized OR time.

For example, vascular surgery is allocated two ORs every Friday. Why was this decision made? If the department's surgeons were allocated three ORs, then much of the OR time would be underutilized, which would reduce OR efficiency. If the department had been allocated one OR, then the surgeons would have been working late to finish their cases, resulting in much overutilized OR time, which would also reduce OR efficiency. The choice of two ORs provided the best balance.

In our experience, this example provides what most facilities consider the objective of OR allocation: providing the right amount of OR time to get the cases done (i.e., not too much nor too little). That is the essence of operational OR management decision making. This objective *must* be differentiated from the longer-term tactical stage of OR allocation, wherein an increase or reduction in allocated OR time is expected to result in a change in OR workload [10].

The example also shows why good operational decisions cannot be made based on OR utilization. True, OR allocation would not be three ORs, based on either OR efficiency or OR utilization, because there would be many hours of underutilized OR time. However, the choice of one or two ORs would not be clear based on OR utilization, because the resulting hours of overutilized OR time are not included in the calculation of utilization (which, by definition, cannot be higher than 100%). In contrast, decision making based on OR efficiency considers both the expected underutilized and overutilized OR time. At facilities in which there is substantial overutilized OR time, basing allocations on utilization statistics will have a large negative impact on OR efficiency.

For example, Dr. Sato is an orthopedic surgeon in a solo practice. She is allocated OR 1 on Mondays and Wednesdays for 10 h, from 07:00 h to 17:00 h. Dr. Ho is another orthopedic surgeon in a solo practice. He is allocated OR 1 on Tuesdays and Thursdays for 10 h, also from 07:00 h to 17:00 h. Both Drs. Sato and Ho consistently perform slightly fewer than 10 h of cases in their allocated OR time, virtually never more. Both perform spinal surgery cases. However, Dr. Sato tends to perform one more case of the same type as Dr. Ho within the allocated OR time because Dr. Sato operates much more quickly than Dr. Ho. The OR efficiency is identical and unaffected by how quickly Dr. Sato operates (see continuation of the example at the end of this section).

Managerial cost accounting

"Labor cost" equals the sum of two products: staffed hours multiplied by the cost per hour of staffed hours and hours worked late multiplied by the cost per hour of hours worked late. More complicated managerial accounting models generally are not needed for the purposes of OR allocation and case scheduling. Labor cost can generally be estimated as the sum of the allocated OR time multiplied by the cost per hour of staffed hours and the hours of overutilized OR time multiplied by the cost per hour of overutilized OR time.

"Operating room productivity" equals the OR workload divided by the labor costs. For example, the only anesthesia service that a group provides at an outpatient surgery facility is OR anesthesia. Staffing is planned for five ORs from 07:00 h to 17:00 h. There is virtually never any overutilized OR time. Then, each increase in OR workload (i.e., the cases performed) results in an increase in OR and anesthesia group productivity.

For example, a hospital has substantial underutilized OR time and substantial overutilized OR time. Recent increases in elective OR workload have resulted in cases finishing in the early evenings, resulting in increased overutilized OR time. The increase in OR workload could be reducing OR productivity. That would be happening if the cost per hour of overutilized OR time is much higher than the cost per hour of regularly staffed hours. Although it may seem good to make operational OR management decisions based on increasing OR productivity, we recommend against the approach. Instead, make operational OR management decisions to maximize OR efficiency. Usually the decisions will be the same, but not always.

We recommend decision making based on OR efficiency for two reasons [1,11]. First, whereas decisions based on OR efficiency are invariant to the perspective of the cost assessment, decisions based on labor cost are not. There is no one best answer as to whose labor costs should be used to make decisions. For example, although from the perspective of the anesthesia group, the ideal would be to make the decisions based on its labor costs, other reasonable options include the labor cost of the hospital or society. Second, labor costs vary depending on staff scheduling and staff assignment, whereas OR efficiency does not. If labor costs were used, distributed decision making would no longer be consistent, depending on the perspective of who makes the decision. For example, if one CRNA works overtime to cover for another CRNA who has called in sick, that would affect decisions based on labor costs but would not affect decisions based on OR efficiency.

"Revenue" is the money received from third parties in return for having provided care for a specific patient.

"Variable costs" are costs that increase proportionately with the volume of patients receiving care [12].

For example, the amount of anesthetic medication used will vary with the number of patients who receive anesthesia care. Hence, pharmacy costs are variable costs.

"Fixed costs" are those costs that are not related to the volume of patients receiving care. For example, the surgical tables cost the same regardless of how often they are used. Surgical tables are a fixed cost.

For example, a new eight-OR ambulatory surgery center has virtually no overutilized OR time but considerable underutilized OR time. On a short-term basis, labor costs can be viewed as fixed. Even if OR workload increased moderately, all the cases would still be completed within the allocated OR time. The number of OR nurses needed to staff the ORs would be unchanged. However, on a longer-term basis, labor costs could be reduced by closing an OR if the OR workload does not increase sufficiently.

"Contribution margin" is equal to revenue minus the variable costs for providing care to those patients. These include revenue and variable costs associated both with the current case and those related to subsequent care owing to complications. For example, consider the calculation of contribution margin for a colon resection in which the wound becomes infected. Revenue and variable costs need to be included as a result of the original surgery as well as the full hospitalization, including three trips back to the OR to wash out the wound.

"Profit" is equal to revenue minus the sum of fixed and variable costs. This is the same as contribution margin minus fixed costs. For example, let us return to the orthopedic surgeons, Drs. Sato and Ho, who were described previously. Dr. Sato performs one extra spinal surgery case in the same number of hours of OR time than does Dr. Ho. For the anesthesia group, Dr. Sato is more profitable than is Dr. Ho, because the anesthesia group gets more revenue for the same fixed costs of staffing the OR. However, the implants that Dr. Sato chooses cost 80% of the revenue whereas those that Dr. Ho chooses cost 50% of the revenue. Thus, for the hospital, Dr. Sato is less profitable than Dr. Ho [13]. Both still have a positive contribution margin, but only slightly so for Dr. Sato.

Operating room efficiency on the day of surgery

Operating room efficiency is maximized by choosing staffing and scheduling cases to minimize the inefficiency of use of OR time, the latter being [(cost per hour of underutilized OR time) × (hours of underutilized OR time)] + [(cost per hour of overutilized OR time) × (hours of overutilized OR time)]. If one considers the cost of 1 h of overutilized time to 1 h of underutilized time to be the fixed ratio, R, (typically 1.5 to 2.0), the value to be minimized can be expressed in terms of hours: (hours of underutilized OR time) + R × (hours of overutilized OR time). This relationship is further simplified on the day of surgery.

At most surgical facilities, OR nurses are full-time hourly or salaried employees. Thus, on the day of surgery, the increment in nursing labor cost from 1 h of underutilized OR time is negligible relative to the cost from 1 h of overutilized OR time. Finishing cases early, but still before the end of staffed hours, reduces labor costs negligibly versus the labor cost that would result from a reduction in overutilized OR time. The same applies to CRNAs and/or anesthesiologists who are employees of the surgical facility or corresponding anesthesia group.

Few anesthesiologists and CRNAs in private practice can earn enough money to cover the cost of their salary plus benefits unless they are scheduled to care for whatever patients may need urgent surgery along with patients having elective, scheduled surgery. Thus, the incremental revenue lost on the day of surgery by having 1 h of underutilized OR time is negligible relative to the indirect/intangible costs from working late unexpectedly (i.e., the opportunity cost of being idle is effectively zero) [14,15].

Consequently, on the day of surgery, the cost per hour of underutilized OR time is negligible relative to the cost per hour of overutilized OR time [1,16]. Thus, on the day of surgery, minimizing the inefficiency of use of OR time (see Definitions, above) requires only that management minimize the hours of overutilized OR time, as the cost per hour of this time is a constant [1,16]. As explained below, "minimizing" on the day of surgery includes case and staff assignment decisions, as all cases are performed unless patient safety would be affected.

Case scheduling to maximize OR efficiency minimizes hours of overutilized OR time, as previously reported for surgical suites [17]. The following two scenarios illustrate the implications of the results.

For example, an anesthesiologist is assigned to an OR staffed from 07:00 h to 15:00 h, but with one expected hour of overutilized OR time. The anesthesiologist works quickly. She places every intravenous catheter and arterial cannula on the first attempt and performs a fiberoptic intubation in 10 min. Because of her rapid work, the cases finish at 15:00 h, preventing 1 h of overutilized OR time. Thus, the anesthesiologist has increased OR efficiency [16].

A different anesthesiologist is assigned to another OR staffed from 07:00 h to 15:00 h, but with 7 h of scheduled cases. The anesthesiologist works equally quickly, resulting in cases finishing at 14:00 h instead of at 15:00 h. Because overutilized OR time was not reduced, the anesthesiologist did *not* increase OR efficiency [16].

These scenarios show that "working fast" is *not* synonymous with increasing OR efficiency. The last scenario of the preceding section showed that working fast is not synonymous with maximizing profit, either. Analogously, "working slowly" is *not* synonymous with decreasing OR efficiency. Sometimes, "working fast" may increase OR efficiency, and "working slowly" may decrease OR efficiency. But this will be entirely dependent on the circumstances.

For example, a different anesthesiologist is supervising resident physicians in two ORs. Staffing is planned from 08:00 h to 16:00 h. The anesthesiologist needs to decide which of the two ORs to start first. One OR is scheduled with two cases from 8:00 h to 18:00 h, the other with five cases from 08:00 h to 15:00 h. To maximize OR efficiency, the anesthesiologist should first start the OR expected to have 2 h of overutilized OR time [16].

By following this simple principle, individual and collective decision making can be closely linked to enhancing OR efficiency. Without understanding the principles of OR efficiency, the anesthesiologist is likely to have made the opposite decision because there are more cases in the other OR.

The same principles and use of scenarios can be applied to housekeepers, OR nurses, managers, postanesthesia care unit nurses, etc. [4,9]. In essence, all decision making on the day of surgery that has "improving efficiency" as the goal revolves around this concept of reducing overutilized time. Again, working faster per se does *not* increase OR efficiency; rather, OR efficiency is increased only when working faster reduces overutilized time.

For example, staffing is planned from 07:00 h to 15:00 h. Recently the hospital hired a new OR nurse. On Monday, she assisted in OR 12, resulting in cases finishing at 14:00 h instead of 15:00 h. On Tuesday, she assisted in OR 14, resulting in cases finishing at 16:00 h instead of 17:00 h. She increased OR efficiency more on Tuesday than Monday, because reducing 1 h of overutilized OR time increases OR efficiency more than does reducing 1 h of underutilized OR time.

Tactical versus operational OR management decisions

Consider a common OR management problem: staffing is planned from 07:00 h to 15:00 h. A surgeon has been allocated 8 h of OR time every Wednesday for years, and the hospital has an "official" policy that elective cases may only be scheduled into allocated time. The surgeon has always underestimated the OR times of his cases in order to bypass this constraint. He has never finished before 18:00 h and usually ends between 19:00 h and 20:00 h.

The anesthesiologists and OR nurses may complain about working late every Monday because the surgeon is being allowed to "overbook" his schedule. They may lobby to have a committee meet to rectify the situation. Simultaneously, the administrators may discuss the surgeons' lack of respect for rules and hospital resources. Nevertheless, physicians who refer their patients to the surgeon reward him by continuing to send him work because their patients are pleased with his expeditious service.

The fundamental issue is the surgeon's frequent misrepresentation of the estimated OR times of his cases, in order to get them onto the OR schedule [18]. The merits of the tactical issue (i.e., whether this is overall good or bad practice) have little relevance to OR productivity. The relevant operational decision is clear: managers should change staffing to match the reality of the existing workload. Doing so neither increases nor reduces OR capacity or convenience for the surgeon and his or her patients. What it does is to reduce labor costs by reducing the hours worked late in lieu of staffed hours. From the surgeon's perspective, the only thing that will change is that he can provide more realistic estimated operating times, as there will no longer be a need to "adjust" the times in order to get the cases running past the end of the regular workday on the schedule. From the perspective of the anesthesiologists and the OR nurses, complaints about working "late" will disappear, as the regular hours in the surgeon's OR now extend to 12 h, and staff working in that OR can expect to work for this period of time.

For example, when an anesthesiologist was hired, the job description said that work hours were 07:00 h to 17:00 h, and he accepted a salary based on this assumption. Yet, every Wednesday for the past 5 years, the anesthesiologist has finished working between 19:00 h and 20:00 h. Staffing is subsequently changed to be to 20:00 h because that is the reality of the existing OR workload. Planning the staffing to 20:00 h does not change the workload. Rather, it results in the work being planned long in advance.

In the two preceding scenarios, the surgeon and patient are choosing the day of surgery. Cases are not being turned away, provided they can be done safely, even if they will likely be performed in overutilized OR time [19]. Subject to that priority, OR time can be allocated based on maximizing OR efficiency. To describe operational reality, mathematics needs to be based on the surgeon and patient having open access to OR time on the workday of their choosing.

For example, all ORs are allocated at a hospital for 8 h. The adjusted utilizations range from 75 to 85% among the surgical services. Thus, there is essentially only underutilized OR time. At this hospital, allocating OR time based on OR efficiency would give precisely the same result as allocating OR time based on adjusted utilization. This is because virtually no OR ever finishes late. A zero has been substituted for the hours of overutilized OR time in the equation for the inefficiency of use of OR time (see Operating room efficiency on the day of surgery, above). The surgeons can be considered to have open access to OR time on the workday of their choosing, and they have chosen to perform cases only when they can be completed within allocated hours.

The two preceding scenarios demonstrate that service-specific staffing can be considered for any facility when decisions are made based on OR efficiency and on surgeon and patient open access to OR time on any future workday. The next scenario shows that the assumption of fixed hours applies only to a minority of surgical suites [8].

For example, an ambulatory surgical center has a policy that OR time is allocated based on OR utilization. Staffing is planned from 07:00 h to 15:00 h. This policy is enforced strictly. A surgeon asks to book a case to start at 13:00 h, with an expected (realistic) OR time for the case of 2.5 h. He is told "No," that would be unacceptable, because the case will probably end at 15:30 h.

The preceding scenario will seem unreal to most clinicians in the United States. That is the point. Only scheduling cases if they can reasonably be expected to finish by the end of allocated OR time is not the reality of short-term operational decision making at many facilities. Although considering a facility to have fixed hours of OR time is an accurate and practical model from a tactical perspective, it is not realistic for day-to-day decision making for all surgeons at a surgical suite [1,19–21].

We return to the first scenario of this section, which describes persistent overutilized OR time. Should the surgeon be encouraged to continue to schedule cases beyond the hours that have been allocated? That is a reasonable tactical question, which includes consideration of the financial impact of the surgeon's cases versus the long-term effects on hiring and retention of OR nurses and anesthesia providers [10]. The tactical decision can, and probably should, be considered from multiple perspectives, including societal. However, the operational decision making focuses on the reality of the existing workload. Operational decisions, specifically service-specific staffing, are what most managers can control.

Truly not having fixed hours of OR time, despite an official policy against overbooking elective cases, is particularly common in hospitals at which surgeons mischaracterize cases as "urgent" to get them onto the OR schedule.

For example, an academic department is allocated three ORs from 08:00 h to 16:00 h on all weekdays. No elective case is scheduled unless it will fit into the 8 h based on mean historical OR time data from the OR information system. The service schedules 20% of its OR hours as urgent cases. Many of these patients probably could have waited safely for several days for surgery. Thus, these were elective cases. The surgeons called the cases "urgent" to achieve open access to OR time and thus bypass the policy against overbooking. The OR efficiency would have been greater had more OR time been allocated originally. This would have allowed the cases to be performed in allocated, rather than in overutilized, OR time.

Suppose that on a long-term (tactical) basis, the behavior of the academic surgeons is considered so bad that penalties are applied. Then there would be very little overutilized OR time. The methods described in this chapter would be valid and appropriate, but not necessarily a useful improvement. Consequently, there is reason to consider whether the behavior of the above surgeons is inherently bad.

From the societal, hospital, and surgeons' perspective, probably the behavior is good, or at least not bad enough to penalize the surgeons. They are serving as their patients' advocates, assuring timely surgery. Most patients only have two preoperative visits with the surgeon, making surgeon flexibility to schedule initial consultations very important to growth in surgical practices [22]. Further, in some health-care systems, including that in the United States, the more cases that the surgeons perform, the higher are hospital and physician contribution margins.

Hospitals receiving fee-for-service reimbursement achieve an overall positive contribution margin for the elective cases of almost all surgeons [10,20,23] because a large percentage of OR costs are fixed (e.g., surgical robots, video equipment for minimally invasive surgical suites, and anesthesia machines). If professional revenues for the anesthesia providers and surgeons were also considered in the calculation of contribution margin, then every surgeon would provide an overall positive contribution margin for their elective cases. The implication, then, is that if a case can be performed safely, it is economically irrational not to perform the case [10,20,24].

The rationale for providing surgeons with open access to OR time, provided a case can be performed safely, makes particular sense for hospitals with intensive care units (ICUs) that are often full. For patients needing such care, the ICU is a frequent bottleneck that results in delays or cancellations of surgical cases. There are two ways to approach this problem, other than simply providing and staffing more ICU beds.

One strategy to reduce the risk of delays or cancellations is to adjust the days that services are scheduled to perform surgery [25,26]. Although such techniques can be implemented practically [25,26], the incremental benefit to hospitals may be small. If most surgeons schedule patients for ICU admission on the same days of the week, usually the cause of case cancellations is visible to the surgeons. The surgeons generally suffer more, financially, from case cancellations and delays than do hospitals and anesthesiologists. In this situation, the hands-on facilitation of a local OR manager or an expert in managing organizational conflict can help, with tabular and graphical summaries of the impact of decisions on cancellations [26]. Such interventions are valuable and important [27]. However, they are not commonly decisions made by anesthesia group managers or OR nursing directors, although they can facilitate such processes.

The second of the two strategies is to provide surgeons with flexibility in the days when they have OR time. Cases should get onto the OR schedule to assure that the expensive bottleneck (the ICU) is always full. For example, although 90% of patients may have ICU lengths of stay <2 days following coronary artery bypass graft (CABG), there can be marked variability in length of stay [26,28]. Consequently, predictions can be inaccurate for the number of open ICU beds available daily as a result of patient transfers from the unit. When the bottleneck to doing surgery is downstream from ORs and the service time for that downstream process is highly variable, then flexibility in scheduling the OR cases is needed to maximize throughput. This does present some inconvenience to surgeons and patients, in that they do not know with certainty the date when the procedure will be performed until very close to the day of surgery, but it is preferable to having the case cancelled on the day of surgery owing to inadequate ICU resources.

The same logic applies to expensive capital equipment (e.g., intraoperative magnetic resonance imaging), which, like the ICUs, is a fixed cost that is best kept as fully utilized as possible. In the future, more ORs will include more technologically advanced equipment, resulting in even higher capital costs. The percentage of hospital costs for surgery that are attributed to labor is likely to decrease as capital costs increase to support these and other expensive technologies. To maximize use of that equipment, surgeons should have open access to OR time to do a case on whatever future workday they are available, provided the case can be performed safely using existing equipment. For example, if two surgical services have allocated time on the same day of the week and are vying for the one operative robot, providing the services with the ability to book elective cases on days other than on the date of their surgical block will increase the utilization of this expensive resource.

The caveat of allowing open access to OR time "provided the case can be performed safely" is of strikingly large importance. Safety includes access not only to specialized surgical equipment, but also to limited ICU beds, hospital ward beds, postanesthesia care unit beds, nonfatigued staff, etc. What can be done safely limits how much work can be done in a surgical suite on any given day [1,9,10,26,29]. Characteristically, tactical decision making limits what can be done safely. Then, operational decision making functions within these boundaries.

Based on these arguments, realistic operational decision making needs to function within a structure that allows the surgeon and patient to choose the day of surgery. The reason this is so important is that surgeons are not the individuals primarily responsible for

OR efficiency through their filling of the OR time allocated to them. Rather, the parties primarily responsible for OR efficiency are the nursing and anesthesia group managers who choose the OR allocations to match staffing to the surgeons' workloads. The latter refers almost entirely to the durations of the hours in each OR into which cases are scheduled, numbers of ORs usually only being numbers of flexible rooms to facilitate turnovers and urgent cases, etc.

For example, for 1 week each year, most of the otolaryngologists are away at a conference. There is substantial underutilized OR time, resulting in poor OR efficiency. This is an example of poor OR management. The managers should have increased OR efficiency by adjusting staffing to match the surgeons' and patients' hours (e.g., by encouraging months in advance for some nurses and anesthesia providers specializing in this area of care to use some of their accrued vacation).

Planning service-specific staffing and scheduling cases based on increasing OR efficiency

Allocating OR time (i.e., planning service-specific staffing) and scheduling cases based on OR efficiency can increase OR productivity by reducing labor costs.

Performing calculations using complete enumeration

In practice, OR allocations that are calculated based on OR efficiency are done by service and day of the week. That is because day of the week is the best predictor of a service's workload [8,30]. Calculating an OR allocation means determining how many ORs should be staffed daily for each service and, for each of these ORs, how many hours of staffing should be planned (e.g., 8, 10, or 13 h) [8,30]. Calculations of optimal allocations can be done by complete enumeration. Specifically, all possible staffing solutions are considered, starting with 0 h and progressively increasing staffed hours until additional increases in the staffed hours cause the efficiency of use of OR time to decrease for that service [30]. If shifts of 8, 10, and 13 h are considered, then the successive choices are 0, 8, 10, 13, 16, 18 h, etc. Increasing the staffed hours causes the efficiency of use of OR time to increase progressively to a maximum, after which it decreases [8]. The complete enumeration can be constructed such that every series of cases performed by the same surgeon on the same day would be performed in its original sequence and take the same amount of OR time. The only change is in the start times.

For example, a surgeon is currently allocated 8 h of OR time individually on Tuesdays. The surgeon historically has done 9 h of cases every Tuesday. The hospital calculates that the expense of 1 h of overutilized time is twice that of 1 h of underutilized time, and inefficiency is expressed in terms of the number of equivalent underutilized hours. Candidate allocations are 0, 8, 10, and 13 h. The inefficiency of use of OR time for each potential allocation is determined from the cost of the underutilized and overutilized hours that would have resulted. A 0-h allocation (A) would have resulted in 9 h of overutilized time, with an inefficiency of use of OR time proportional to 18 h. An 8-hour allocation (B) would have resulted in 1 h of overutilized time, with an inefficiency proportional to 2 h. A 10-h allocation (C) would have resulted in 1 underutilized hour with an inefficiency proportional to 1 h. Finally, a 13-h allocation (D) would have resulted in 4 h of underutilized time with an inefficiency proportional to 4 h. As the most efficient solution (i.e., smallest value of the inefficiency of use of OR time) was allocation C, the surgeon should have been allocated 10 h of OR time in order to maximize the efficiency of use of OR time.

There is a unique solution to the choice of the OR allocation that will maximize OR efficiency if OR allocations can be of any duration (e.g., 9.27 h) [8] but not necessarily when fixed choices (e.g., 8, 10, 13 h) are considered. When two choices provide nearly the same inefficiency of use of OR time, the OR workload can be reviewed to consider which most closely matches how the surgeons in the service have historically been using their OR time.

For example, the cardiac surgeons perform an average of 14 h of cases each Tuesday, with a range of 12 to 15 h. Forecasted OR efficiency would be nearly identical whether 13 h of OR time were allocated in one OR or 8 h in each of two ORs. The cardiac surgeons have had two ORs (i.e., reliable first case of the day start times) for the past 6 years. They have consistently scheduled cases into those ORs such that there is only underutilized OR time, not overutilized OR time. Two ORs would be the most reasonable choice. In this example, planning OR allocation based on OR efficiency versus adjusted utilization results in the same decisions.

Maximizing OR efficiency is the same as minimizing the sum of underutilized hours and overutilized hours multiplied by the relative cost of overutilized to underutilized OR hours (see Definitions, above) [8].

Thus, only the relative cost of overutilized to underutilized OR hours needs to be known, not the costs per se [8]. A commonly used [30] value for this ratio of costs is 1.75. This includes the direct costs of overtime at "time and a half" (1.50) and an increment (0.25) for indirect (intangible) costs of employee dissatisfaction, resignation, and recruitment and training [30]. Because of the marked effect of limiting consideration to common staff schedules (e.g., 8 or 13 h), the resulting inefficiency in use of OR time is characteristically highly insensitive to local experts' uncertainty in the choice of the value of this parameter [31].

For example, on three Wednesdays, a service performed 12, 7, and 15 h of cases, including turnover times. There are 8-h shifts, with overtime scheduled by rotation using a late list. The relative cost of overutilized to underutilized hours is considered 1.75. If the service were allocated 8 h of OR time each Wednesday, then the cost of the inefficiency of use of OR time would be proportional to 20.25 h, where 20 h = (0 underutilized + 1 underutilized + 0 underutilized + 1.75 × [4 overutilized + 0 overutilized + 7 overutilized]). If the allocation were two 8-h ORs each Wednesday, the cost would be proportional to 14 h, where 14 h = (4 underutilized + 9 underutilized + 1 underutilized). If the allocation were three 8-h ORs each Wednesday, the cost would be proportional to 38 h, where 38 h = (12 underutilized + 17 underutilized + 9 underutilized). Therefore, the service should be allocated two 8-h ORs to maximize OR efficiency.

There is only one answer to the question, "How close are current OR allocations to those that would maximize OR efficiency?" In contrast, there is no one answer to the question, "How close are current OR allocations to those that are optimal based on OR utilization?" The reason is that there is then the subsequent question of how to determine the optimal OR utilization. The best OR utilization varies among services because it is sensitive to many parameters, such as staffed hours, turnover times, day-to-day variability in OR workload, statistical distribution of OR times of cases, and so forth [19,32]. Years of data can be required to estimate these parameter values sufficiently accurately to use them to decide on the OR utilization to use as the service's goal [33]. Allocating OR time based on OR efficiency simultaneously takes into account all of these issues. When a manager says "We allocate OR time based on OR efficiency," that is close to a sufficient statement to describe precisely what happens in practice because the choice of the relative cost of overutilized to underutilized OR time is invariably close to 1.75 and insensitive to any differences. In contrast, when a manager says "We allocate OR time based on OR utilization," that alone says virtually nothing about what happens in practice at the surgical suite.

Calculated staffing (OR allocations) differ from those in current practice

OR managers' efforts to reduce labor costs must focus predominantly on OR allocation and case scheduling, because almost all of anesthesia providers' costs are labor costs. The viability of a surgical facility depends on the economics of the anesthesia providers. For 11 of 12 facilities studied, allocating OR time based on OR efficiency achieved significantly lower labor costs than the plans that were being used by the local managers [30,34,35]. For ten of the 11 facilities, the statistical method approach resulted in plans that reduced labor costs by at least 10% [30,34,35]. The percentage increases in OR efficiency were, by definition, even more.

A common anecdote reveals how poorly many facilities plan service-specific staffing. Often OR nurses and anesthesia providers report that every OR finishes at least an hour or two late every day. To consider the irrationality [36] of the situation, suppose that the relative cost of overutilized to underutilized OR time were 2.0. Then, it would be twice as expensive to finish late versus early. Thus, with appropriate OR allocations, the odds for each service and OR to finish early should be approximately two chances in three. That is, if staffing decisions were made rationally, a given OR would finish early on 2 of every 3 days.

In practice, percentage reductions in labor costs are not proportional to the number of ORs [30,34]. Even at facilities for which each allocation is for one room, but either for 8 h or 10 h, savings are found [37]. Surgical suites at which many hours of OR time are allocated to services do not have the largest percentage improvements from applying the operations research to OR management.

The explanation for this observation is that the principal challenge faced by managers is not the number of ORs to be allocated to services, but how to manage variability in OR workload from week to week. The fact that the OR allocation decision is stochastic is the conceptual problem in the practicing managers' decisions. The poor decisions are caused by psychological biases that are observed for such decisions in other industries [36]. Implementation of improved decisions is not achieved by education, but rather by automating reliance on decision-support software [36].

For example, consider a service with OR workload averaging 6.5 h every Friday [38]. Because there are no overutilized hours, allocation based on OR efficiency is identical to allocation based on OR utilization [37]. Once this principle is understood by managers, analysis is unneeded in the future. One analysis is sufficient. In contrast, suppose that the same facility has three of its eight ORs as unblocked, open, first-come, first-served "other" time. The surgical suite staffs in 8-, 10-, and 13-h shifts. Then, those three ORs could be allocated as 8/8/8, 8/8/10, 8/10/10, 10/10/10, 8/8/13, 8/13/13/, 13/13/13, 8/10/13, 10/10/13, and 10/13/13. Intuition will not help with this complex decision. The value of education is by increasing trust in relying on the statistical results [39,40].

Urgent cases

Some hospitals have one or more ORs allocated for urgent cases during the regular workday. Typically, the appropriate number of ORs is chosen for such urgent cases by considering them to be performed by a pseudo-service, the "Urgent" service. Then, the methods above are applied. At facilities not planning an OR for urgent cases, when calculating OR allocations for elective cases, each urgent case should be attributed to its surgical service.

The relative cost of overutilized to underutilized OR time may be appropriately higher for the urgent service than the other elective services, because the choice affects not just how often staff work late, but also patient waiting time for urgent surgery. However, urgent cases often cannot start immediately (e.g., because the surgeon is not available), such that overutilized OR time would occur regardless of calculations. In practice, the use of the same relative cost for overutilized to underutilized OR time as above (e.g., a factor of 1.75) can provide answers that clinicians consider reasonable.

Amount of data required for calculations

To assess the amount of data required to produce acceptable results, a long series of data from a surgical suite was divided into training and testing datasets, with different training periods [11]. The complete enumeration was applied to the training data, and the expected labor costs that would have occurred during the subsequent testing period were calculated.

Each increase in the number of months of data up to 9 months resulted in a statistically significant reduction in expected labor costs. There were large incremental benefits in using at least 7 months of data. For the studied hospital, there was no advantage to using more than 1 year of data.

The minimum amount of data needed for calculating OR allocations based on OR efficiency can be particularly important to managers at facilities purchasing a new OR information system, anesthesia information system, or anesthesia billing system. The minimum period of data indicates the time from installation of the system to when management changes based on resulting data can be implemented. Application of the statistical methods using as little as 30 workdays of system data provided better OR allocations to reduce labor costs than OR allocations established by the practicing managers with years of data [11].

Sources of data

Data for analysis can come from an OR information system, an electronic anesthesia information management system, or anesthesia billing data [41]. Data from an OR information system have the advantage of virtually always having necessary data fields completed. Anesthesia billing data have the advantage of accuracy, because billing errors can be costly or even lead to challenges of fraudulent behavior. When using anesthesia billing data, if the OR in which the case was performed is not available from the data, then the anesthesia provider (i.e., the person in the OR delivering anesthesia care, not the supervising anesthesiologists) can be substituted for the OR field to calculate turnovers. Depending on the workflow among ORs, this substitution can be preferable.

Facilities with OR information systems that do not have data review at the time of data entry often have datasets that contain errors or omissions, including lack of knowledge of the actual ORs in which some cases were performed. This can occur if cases are moved during the day without correcting the corresponding information systems, or if the times of OR entry or exit are incorrectly entered. This manifests as the false appearance of two cases overlapping in the same OR at the same time. The typical fix is to change the recorded OR of each case that overlaps to a unique unknown OR. For example, suppose that one case is listed as being performed in OR 1 from 10:00 h to 11:00 h and another in OR 1 from 10:30 h to 12:00 h. Among all cases in the dataset, the latter case is the 139th for which the true OR

is unknown. The second case can be considered to have been completed in the fictitious room "Unknown139." Making such a change affects calculated turnover times, as some turnovers between cases will be altered, and thus may affect OR allocations. Nonetheless, studies demonstrated that the impact of this adjustment on the labor costs that result from poor OR allocations is of negligible importance, for three reasons [42,43]. First, OR allocations are based on each service's total hours of cases, a large number, plus total hours of turnover times, a much smaller number. Second, for cases in an OR that have a preceding case and a following case, two turnover times are lost. Yet, the turnover time between the remaining cases is increased between the two cases surrounding the reassigned case to the default maximum turnover time [42]. Third, the effect of allocating OR time only in fixed increments (e.g., 8 or 13 h) is of larger importance.

Assessing trends, seasonal variation, and data errors

Use of complete enumeration assumes that there are no systematic differences among weeks in the expected OR workload (i.e., there are no trends or seasonal variation) [30]. National survey data show that these assumptions will hold for most facilities [44]. Raw data were reanalyzed from the 1994 to 1996 National Survey of Ambulatory Surgery. As a positive control, to insure that seasonal variation could be detected if present, the average number of myringotomy tubes inserted each day in ambulatory surgery centers of the United States was examined. As expected, myringotomy tube insertions peaked each winter, corresponding to the peak incidence of middle ear infections. Specifically, the average number of tubes inserted each day varied systematically among months for all 26 of the overlapping 11-month periods in the 36 months of the survey. In contrast, the average number of ambulatory surgery cases performed with an anesthesia provider each day in the United States per 10 000 persons was found not to vary systematically month to month on an 11-month basis.

Good routine practice is to test for statistically significant trends [45] or seasonality, to confirm that analysis is reasonable for each surgical suite. For example, the so-called "runs test" can be applied to the total labor cost over each consecutive 4-week period [30,46]. Calculate the total labor cost for each 4-week period. Subtract the median from each value. Delete zero differences. Assign a "+" to positive differences and a "–" to negative differences. A "run" is defined as a series of one or more consecutive values that are the same. Finally, compare the number of runs of +s and –s to a critical value from appropriate statistical tables. For example, if over 10 weeks the values were + – 0 – – – + – ++ there would be 5 runs (2 +, 1 ++, 1 – – –, and 2 –). At P<0.05, the expected number of runs is between 2 and 10, so the null hypothesis that there is a trend would be rejected. This test, the Wald–Wolfowitz one-sample runs test, is available in most statistics packages.

It is almost never necessary to incorporate methods appropriate for data with trends and seasonality into the analysis. When the runs test detects trends or seasonality, characteristically this reflects a problem with the data or special conditions [45] that needs to be modeled separately. For example, if a hospital opens a new three-room endovascular (interventional) suite in the middle of the data collection period, this may result in a positive trend in OR workload. The opening of a new surgery center may result in an abrupt decline in workload at the main facility [45].

In addition to using the runs test, plot each service's OR workload for the days of the week when the service is allocated OR time. The graphs are helpful to detect unrecognized errors in the data. For example, plotting OR workload for a service against time can show if a service had no cases listed for a day of the week for some part of the data period being used. This usually occurs when the data sent for analysis include one or more surgeons who recently left the facility and operated on the empty days.

Finally, look for the presence of many zero values in the histogram of OR workload for each combination of the day of the week and the service allocated OR time. This usually happens when the service's scheduling is characteristic of an individual surgeon rather than a group of surgeons. These "holes" often represent time when an individual surgeon is away (e.g., on vacation). These can be hard to identify in a graph of OR workload versus time. Such services may need to have their allocations of OR time combined with another service to achieve reliable staffing predictions.

Services with low OR workloads

Provided cases are scheduled sequentially into ORs (below), then services with average OR workloads that are consistently <8 h have no overutilized hours. Allocating OR time based on adjusted utilization does

not differ from doing so based on OR efficiency. Many facilities appropriately apply a minimum adjusted utilization for OR allocations [47,48]. For example, based on the relative cost ratio of 1.75 described above, if services' workloads were always the same each weekday, then the optimal (minimum) value would be 68% [47,48].

For example, a service's OR workload averages 6 h every Tuesday. The facility bases its decisions on the efficiency of use of OR time. The service's adjusted utilization is 75%. Thus, the service is allocated a single OR for 8 h. Because there are no overutilized hours, allocation based on OR efficiency is identical to allocation based on OR utilization. There are 0 h of underutilized time caused by OR allocation and case scheduling.

Each service not receiving an OR allocation on a given day (owing to low historical workload) can be combined into an "OTHER" service (i.e., open, unblocked, first-scheduled, first-served time). At facilities without substantial cross-training of staff, there may be different "OTHER" services for different nursing teams. The calculations of the preceding sections are repeated for the "OTHER" service(s) on each workday.

Importantly, do not simply measure the average OR workload of a service, observe that it is too low for an allocation of an 8-h OR for the day, and then automatically pool it into "OTHER" service time. Apply the graphical methods of the preceding section to insure that the reason for a low OR workload reflects an actual low workload, not a service that operates every other week on the studied day of the week [9]. Likewise, insure that incomplete data or a trend in OR workload is not being observed.

Using qualitative information to improve forecasts

Qualitative information not available from information system data should be used when finalizing OR allocations.

For example, a surgeon operates at an outpatient surgery center on Fridays in her 8 h of allocated OR time. For years, she has consistently performed 7.0 to 7.5 h of cases at the surgery center in her OR time. The OR allocations are being updated for the next quarter. Based on historical data, she would, of course, be allocated 8 h of OR time on Fridays. However, she is 8 months pregnant and has requested 3 months of maternity leave. She should not be allocated OR time during the next quarter because it would be underutilized, thereby reducing OR efficiency. Even without personally allocated OR time, she would continue to have open access to OR time on any future workday, if she were to change her mind and work for a few days during her period of maternity leave. Note that if she were not provided open access to OR time, then there would be an adversarial relationship between the facility not wanting to plan a "block" for her versus her desire to keep some block time to provide herself and her patients with some flexibility [36]. This highlights the fact that providing open access to OR time on any future workday generally increases OR productivity.

While applying qualitative knowledge, though, focus on the psychological bias that results in most of the inefficiency of use of anesthesia time, the bias being lack of use of the mathematics. The qualitative information should be used to update the *forecasts* of workload, not used to create an *ad hoc* process of converting from workload to OR allocations. We humans are good at forecasting changes in workload, not in making the mathematical conversions from mean workloads into appropriate OR allocations (staffing) [36].

Forecast remaining underutilized operating room time

A concern at some facilities is that underutilized OR time is needed for nonclinical, but nonetheless important, activities. For example, equipment for the next day's cases may be set up by nurses whose ORs finish earlier than the end of their shift. The nursing supervisors at such facilities may express concern that changing OR allocations to increase OR efficiency will impair processes that function well by taking advantage of existing underutilized OR time.

Expected underutilized time can be estimated empirically after future OR allocations have been determined. Applying the allocations, each historical day's resulting total underutilized hours are calculated. The statistical distribution of each day's total hours of underutilized OR time can be described using histograms or percentiles.

Case scheduling

Allocating OR time to increase OR efficiency is of little value unless cases are also scheduled into the OR time appropriately.

A series of thought experiments and computer simulations were performed to evaluate case scheduling based on maximizing OR efficiency [16]. The performances of different case-scheduling heuristics were compared. The analyses showed that managers can achieve efficient OR scheduling while leaving case-scheduling decisions to the convenience of surgeons and patients, provided three simple scheduling rules are followed. In other words, there are small differences in the resulting OR efficiency among different scheduling heuristics, with three exceptions.

The first of three scheduling rules is that a service should not schedule a case into another service's OR time if the case can be completed within its own allocated OR time [16].

For example, two thoracic surgeons are partners in a group that has been allocated 10 h of OR time on Tuesdays. One of the surgeons has scheduled 6 h of cases into the OR time, leaving 4 h of allocated but unscheduled OR time. A cardiac surgeon has scheduled 2 h of cases into his personally allocated 8 h of OR time. Nine days before the day of surgery, the second thoracic surgeon wants to schedule a new 2-h case. The available start time would be after her partner, who has already scheduled cases. The case would not be scheduled into the cardiac surgeon's OR time, even if the second thoracic surgeon wants to start earlier. The reason is that the thoracic surgeons have available OR time for the case.

The reason for this result is that OR allocations are calculated based on expected OR workload on the day of surgery. Services fill their allocated OR time at different rates [49]. Almost all facilities with allocated OR time follow the preceding scheduling rule. Thus, the importance of this finding was not that it showed a new way to schedule cases but that it showed that most facilities make decisions based on OR efficiency [16]. By definition, the decision would not represent a change in facility practice, but an unusual request of the second thoracic surgeon, because otherwise the thoracic surgeons would not have been allocated 10 h of OR time on Tuesdays.

The second of the three scheduling rules is that a case should not be scheduled into overutilized OR time if it can start earlier in another of the service's ORs [17]. This applies to services allocated two or more ORs. Suppose that OR workload is 23 h. The expected hours of overutilized OR time would be slightly less if two ORs were allocated for 13 h (total 26 h) versus three ORs for 8 h (total 24 h). This result would be less reliable if case scheduling did not result in similar packing of the cases into the allocated OR time [16,50]. Simulations show that usually it does.

For example, a service has been allocated OR 3 and OR 5 from 07:00 h to 15:00 h. One surgeon in the service has scheduled cases in OR 3 to finish at around 14:00 h; OR 5 is empty. A second surgeon in the service wants an afternoon start. He asks to start an elective 3-h case at 14:30 h in OR 3. Even though OR workload would be the same, scheduling the case into OR 3 would be expected to result in overutilized OR time and thereby reduce OR efficiency. His request should be denied. The surgeon should take the first case of the day and start in OR 5, or schedule the case on a different workday.

The preceding scenario matches what is done at most surgical suites. Cases are generally not scheduled into overutilized OR time when a service has another allocated OR that is empty. Consequently, as the first rule above, this rule shows that scheduling cases based on maximizing OR efficiency differs little from what is commonly done in practice [16]. Changes resulting from decision making based on OR efficiency generally do not affect case scheduling. Rather, they affect OR allocations (as above, and in the third rule regarding how OR time is released).

The third of the three scheduling rules is that if a service has already filled its allocated OR time, then, to maximize OR efficiency, its new case should be scheduled into another services' OR time instead of into overutilized OR time [16,50].

For example, a service has filled its allocated OR time but has another elective case that it desires to schedule. If the OR time of another service were not released, the case would be performed in overutilized OR time. OR efficiency is greater by performing that case in the OR time allocated to another service that otherwise would be underutilized on the day of surgery.

For example, a surgeon appears to be subverting the case-scheduling system for the "OTHER" service, which provides first-scheduled, first-served OR time. The surgeon seems to be creating fictitious patients to "hold" OR time for his cases (e.g., at the desirable 07:00 h start time). At the OR Block Committee meeting, a manager suggests that there be the policy that, when a case is cancelled, first access to cancelled OR time goes to other surgeons with waiting cases, not the surgeon canceling the case. That recommendation is not sound. When a service has filled its allocated OR time and has another case to schedule, OR efficiency is enhanced by releasing the OR time of the service expected to have the most underutilized OR time. No cases should be waiting to be scheduled.

To evaluate which service should have its OR time released, simulations were performed scheduling new hypothetical cases into actual OR schedules. Services fill their allocated OR time at different rates. Thus, theoretically, the service that should have its OR time released for a new case should be the service that is predicted, at the time the new case is booked, to be the service that will have the most underutilized OR time on the scheduled day of surgery. In practice, performance is only slightly worse (versus having perfect retrospective knowledge) by scheduling the case into the OR time of the service with the largest difference between allocated and scheduled OR time at the time when the new case is scheduled [49]. The latter is practically straightforward to implement.

In contrast, releasing the OR time of the service with the second most, instead of the service with the most, allocated but unscheduled OR time has a large negative effect on OR efficiency [49]. The reason is that usually a particular case can only be scheduled into one or two services' OR time without resulting in overutilized OR time. The differences among those few services in their amount of expected open OR time are often large. This occurs because day-to-day variability in the OR workload of services on a day of the week generally exceeds variability due to the timing of how quickly different services filled their allocated OR time.

The timing of when allocated OR time should be released has been studied [51]. Potentially, the scheduling office could wait to release the allocated OR time until closer to the day of surgery, when data may be available on subsequently scheduled cases, in order to improve the quality of the decision. Simulation results were equivocal as to the benefit of such a decision. Under two conditions, postponing the decision of which service had its OR time released for the new case until early the day before surgery had a negligible effect on resulting OR efficiency versus releasing the allocated OR time when the new case was scheduled [51]. This finding applies to an ambulatory surgery center with brief cases. At such facilities, typically there is only one good choice for the service to have its OR time released [49]. Thus, there is no good reason to wait in making the decision. This finding often also applies to large surgical suites in which cases are scheduled as if there were many smaller suites. For example, at a 30-OR surgical suite, one nursing and anesthesia team may staff the six ORs used for general and vascular surgery. From the perspective of releasing OR time for a new general or vascular surgery case, only six ORs are available, not all 30 ORs.

For example, a hospital contains a team cross-trained in neurosurgery and otolaryngology. One week hence, next Thursday, neurosurgery has been allocated one 10-h OR. Otolaryngology has been allocated one 10-h OR also. The otolaryngologists have scheduled 11 h of cases into their OR. A third otolaryngologist wants to schedule another 2-h case. The neurosurgeons have scheduled a case for 3 h from 07:00 h to 10:00 h. The otolaryngologist with the new case can book the case because the surgeons have open access to OR time on whatever workday they choose. Provided the otolaryngologist is available at 10:30 h, then the neurosurgeons' OR time would be released. There is no advantage to waiting to schedule the case. Yet, if the neurosurgeon with the 07:00 h to 10:00 h case was to schedule another case, the scheduling office should contact the otolaryngologist, and perhaps she would not mind starting her case later in the day.

Despite this consideration of how best to release allocated OR time, it is important to appreciate that results are *highly* sensitive to the OR time being allocated appropriately based on OR efficiency. Issues of when to release allocated OR time vastly pale in practical importance against OR allocation and staffing. Although OR management problems are observed on the day of surgery, often the root cause and only practical way to fix the problem is to plan OR allocations and staffing properly several weeks or months before the day of surgery [52]. The balance between the role of case scheduling versus OR allocations in causing inefficient use of OR time can be assessed for each facility by reviewing multiple examples, as in this chapter, and comparing each to the facility's current practices [53].

For example, OR information systems data are used to calculate OR allocations, which are then reviewed by the "block" committee. An ophthalmologist complains that his allocated OR time on Tuesdays has been "released" for 2 of the past 3 weeks. Each time, the otolaryngology service has filled its allocated 8 h of OR time and so has booked cases into his OR time. The ophthalmologist is upset that the schedulers are treating him unfairly by repeatedly releasing his allocated OR time. Although he schedules many cases a couple of days before the day of surgery, his OR workload is consistently at least 7 h each Tuesday. The ophthalmologist's concerns are well founded; this should not be happening. However, the problem is not that the schedulers are releasing his OR time. Rather, they are

making the proper decision to maximize OR efficiency. The problem is that the otolaryngology service should be allocated more than 8 h of OR time. This is either a failure of statistical forecasting of the otolaryngology service's workload, which is uncommon, or a failure in appropriating allocating OR time based on the forecasted workload, which is more common [36]. At facilities with frequent concerns about release of allocated OR time, be sure to focus on who is responsible for statistical calculations of the OR allocations and their use.

Although this chapter has focused on decision making before the day of surgery, the same principles apply to decisions made on the day of surgery [1,53,54]. The principles described can also be used to decide how cases are moved on the day of surgery [53,55], how staff are assigned on the day of surgery [56], and how cases are sequenced in each OR [57,58,59].

Impact of reducing times on productivity

Impact of reducing surgical and turnover times

The impact of interventions on labor costs can be forecast using each facility's own data, along with corresponding confidence intervals [9,14]. For example, turnover times can be reduced between each case [9,14]. Surgical times can be reduced to national average values for each procedure [15]. First case of the day starts can all be on time [9,48]. For all interventions, first the labor cost is calculated, assuming that OR time is allocated and cases are scheduled based on OR efficiency. Second, the intervention is performed, thereby reducing OR workload by service. Third, using the revised workload values, OR time is reallocated based on OR efficiency and the new estimates for labor costs projected. Fourth, the differences are calculated. By analyzing the differences in 4-week periods, to prevent effects of variation by day of the week, confidence intervals can be calculated for the differences [14,15,30].

For example, consider a hospital that allocates 8 h of OR time to each of many small services, each with an adjusted utilization of less than 85% [15]. Cases are being scheduled based on OR efficiency (i.e., sequentially into ORs [16]). Reducing OR times cannot result in reduced overutilized hours, because there are none. Labor costs will not be reduced (i.e., they are fixed to achievable reductions in OR times).

For example, a different hospital has few surgical services, most with more than one OR, and many ORs with workloads exceeding 8 h [15]. Then, reducing OR times can result in reductions in workload sufficient to reduce allocated OR time (e.g., an OR allocated for 10 h would now be allocated for 8 h). At this hospital, unlike the one in the preceding example, there would be financially important reductions in labor costs from reducing OR times.

Equivalent analyses can be performed at teaching facilities to calculate [15] the impact of longer OR times (due to factors such as teaching time and development of skills in trainees) [60,61] on labor costs.

These examples show that, generally, cost reduction from reducing OR or turnover times can only be achieved provided OR allocations are reduced [9]. The initial impact of reductions in OR or turnover times may be increased underutilized OR time and/or reduced overutilized OR time. This initial step is evident to clinicians. The secondary step is revisions of OR allocations based on the new values of decreased OR workload. The latter step provides for the large reductions in labor cost.

Usually, reductions in labor costs from reducing turnover times tend to be small. At four academic tertiary hospitals studied, reductions in average turnover times of 3–9 min would result in 0.8–1.8% reductions in labor cost [14]. Reductions in average turnover times of 10–19 min would result in 2.5–4.0% reductions in labor costs [14]. These analyses can be fruitful in educating stakeholders that achievable reductions in the times to complete tasks often have less effect on OR efficiency than does good management decision making.

Impact of not changing service-specific staffing

Some facilities do not make decisions systematically based on increasing OR efficiency and are unlikely to change their practices [36]. Then, the methodology above can be used to calculate the higher labor costs that the facility sustains from OR time not being allocated and cases not being scheduled based on OR efficiency [11,30,34].

For example, anesthesia group expenses exceed revenue at a facility. The calculation is performed using labor costs of anesthesia providers. The estimate of the resulting additional labor costs is used by the anesthesia group and hospital when negotiating appropriate administrative support agreement from the hospital [47].

Calculations of administrative support agreements can also apply to negotiations with medical schools, ambulatory surgical facilities, or a multispecialty group. At two academic medical centers, estimated annual excess labor costs were $1.6 million and $1.0 million, respectively [34].

Impact of not reducing the number of allocated ORs

Some organizations aim to adjust their OR allocations to be as close as possible to those that are expected to maximize OR efficiency while not reducing the number of allocated ORs. This approach does not result in maximal OR efficiency. Instead, this approach reflects organizational support for opening as many ORs as are available for first case of the day starts (e.g., to achieve on-time starts for surgeons) [62,63]. The mathematics can be weighted to allocate more ORs by repeating the analyses using a higher relative cost of overutilized to underutilized hours (e.g., 3:1). An increase in the relative cost gives an increase in how many ORs are allocated [9,19]. The smallest value is chosen for which the allocated number of staffed ORs matches the desired, usually current, number of ORs. This analysis is run separately for each day of the week [19].

Increasing the number of allocated ORs results in a slightly smaller percentage increase in OR labor cost than in staffing [19]. The reason is that opening more ORs than are needed to maximize OR efficiency does not change OR workload. Thus, the increase in allocated OR hours increases underutilized OR time and reduces overutilized OR time. The cost per hour of overutilized OR time exceeds that of underutilized OR time. Consequently, the percentage reduction in OR efficiency is less than the percentage increase in allocated OR hours. The same argument applies to labor costs.

Forecasting the time remaining in ongoing cases

The preceding sections have focused almost entirely on decision making before the day of surgery, because good decision making *cannot* be done on the day of surgery unless the OR allocations chosen months ahead are appropriate. As considered in the section Operating room efficiency on the day of surgery, above, when there is consistent overutilized time on the day of surgery, first and foremost this is a failure months before in statistical forecasting of workload and managerial decision making. However, to use those OR allocations in practice on the day of surgery, another set of data are needed: the forecasted time remaining in cases that are ongoing. In most hospital ORs, the cases running at the end of the day are those that took longer than scheduled [1]. Therefore, good decision making cannot be done in the late afternoon without estimating the time remaining in late-running cases. The solution to this problem is not intuitive.

Forecasting the time remaining in cases is one of the most important determinants of decision making on the day of surgery, as it affects decisions such as calling for the next patient, moving cases, and staff relief. Even where there is no bias (i.e., systematic difference) between scheduled times provided by surgeons and the actual durations from the OR information system (e.g., the average difference equals 0 min), there is substantial variance among historical case lengths for the same scheduled procedure or procedures that comprise a case.

Consider a laparoscopic small bowel resection scheduled for 2 h that has been in the OR for 0.5 h. The median expected time remaining is around 1.5 h. In contrast, suppose that the patient has been in the OR for 1.8 h. The median expected time remaining is not 0.2 h, but longer. The reason is that many of these resections took less than 1.8 h, so the median duration of the cases that took longer than 1.8 h is more than 2.0 h. The shorter-duration cases have been excluded. For some of these longer cases, the laparoscopic approach may have been abandoned in favor of an open resection owing to the presence of adhesions, or a complication ensued that required additional time.

For any given combination of surgeon and procedure, there is considerable variation between the time when skin closure begins and when the patient leaves the OR (e.g., from 15 min to 90 min) [64]. This "extra time" comprises the time for irrigation, inspection, and closure, for the patient to recover sufficiently from anesthesia to allow removal of the endotracheal tube, for monitors to be removed and intravenous lines secured, and for the patient to be transferred to the stretcher and transported out of the OR.

The time remaining in a case can be forecasted [64,65] using Bayesian methods by combining the scheduled OR time, historical case duration data, and elapsed times in the OR determined from real-time anesthesia information management system data. Practically, this requires computerization for two reasons. First, many cases running late at the end of the day include rare combinations of procedures with little

or no historical data [66–68]. These cases have a markedly disproportionate impact on the overall variability in decisions involving case durations on the day of surgery [68]. Second, accurate predictions require data about how long cases have been underway and in which OR they are being performed. That can be inferred automatically based on the identifier of the anesthesia information system workstation transmitting pulse oximetry, electrocardiogram heart rate, and end tidal CO_2 partial pressures [69]. The method of automatic forecasting of the remaining time works well even in the absence of any historical data, and automatically incorporates predictive variability in case durations due to changes from the scheduled procedure [64].

Summary

Operating room allocation is a two-stage process [10]. During the initial tactical stage of allocating OR time, considering OR hours to be fixed is reasonable. For operational decision making on a shorter-term basis, such a conceptual model produces results markedly inconsistent with how surgical suites are and should be run. Instead, consider the workload to be fixed on a short-term basis. Provide staff flexibly to match the existing workload, not vice versa. Do so by making operational decisions based on maximizing OR efficiency, as this is an important step to maximizing OR productivity.

References

1. F. Dexter, R. H. Epstein, R. D. Traub, *et al*. Making management decisions on the day of surgery based on operating room efficiency and patient waiting times. *Anesthesiology* 2004; **101**: 1444–53.

2. F. Dexter, L. O'Neill. Weekend operating room on-call staffing requirements. *AORN J* 2001; **74**: 666–71.

3. F. Dexter, R. H. Epstein. Holiday and weekend operating room on-call staffing requirements. *Anesth Analg* 2006; **103**: 1494–8.

4. Y. Xiao, P. Hu, H. Hao, *et al*. Algorithm for processing vital sign monitoring data to remotely identify operating room occupancy in real-time. *Anesth Analg* 2005; **101**: 823–9.

5. F. Dexter, A. Macario, F. Qian, *et al*. Forecasting surgical groups' total hours of elective cases for allocation of block time. Application of time series analysis to operating room management. *Anesthesiology* 1999; **91**: 1501–8.

6. R.T. Donham, W. J. Mazzei, R. L. Jones. Procedural times glossary. *Am J Anesthesiol* 1999; **23**(5 Suppl): 4–12.

7. D. P. Strum, L. G. Vargas, J. H. May. Surgical subspecialty block utilization and capacity planning. A minimal cost analysis model. *Anesthesiology* 1999; **90**: 1176–85.

8. D. P. Strum, L. G. Vargas, J. H. May, *et al.* Surgical suite utilization and capacity planning: a minimal cost analysis model. *J Med Syst* 1997; **21**: 309–22.

9. C. McIntosh, F. Dexter, R. H. Epstein. Impact of service-specific staffing, case scheduling, turnovers, and first-case starts on anesthesia group and operating room productivity: tutorial using data from an Australian hospital. *Anesth Analg* 2006; **103**: 1499–516.

10. F. Dexter, J. Ledolter, R. E. Wachtel. Tactical decision making for selective expansion of operating room resources incorporating financial criteria and uncertainty in sub-specialties' future workloads. *Anesth Analg* 2005; **100**: 1425–32.

11. R. H. Epstein, F. Dexter. Statistical power analysis to estimate how many months of data are required to identify operating room staffing solutions to reduce labor costs and increase productivity. *Anesth Analg* 2002; **94**: 640–3.

12. R. J. Sperry. Of economic analysis. *Anesthesiology* 1997; **86**: 1197–205.

13. R. E. Wachtel, F. Dexter, D. A. Lubarsky. Financial implications of a hospital's specialization in rare physiologically complex surgical procedures. *Anesthesiology* 2005; **103**: 161–7.

14. F. Dexter, A. E. Abouleish, R. H. Epstein, *et al.* Use of operating room information system data to predict the impact of reducing turnover times on staffing costs. *Anesth Analg* 2003; **97**: 1119–26.

15. A. E. Abouleish, F. Dexter, C. W. Whitten, *et al.* Quantifying net staffing costs due to longer-than-average surgical case durations. *Anesthesiology* 2004; **100**: 403–12.

16. F. Dexter, R. D. Traub. How to schedule elective surgical cases into specific operating rooms to maximize the efficiency of use of operating room time. *Anesth Analg* 2002; **94**: 933–42.

17. I. Ozkarahan. Allocation of surgical procedures to operating rooms. *J Med Syst* 1995; **19**: 333–52.

18. F. Dexter, A. Macario, R. H. Epstein, *et al.* Validity and usefulness of a method to monitor surgical services' average bias in scheduled case durations. *Can J Anesth* 2005; **52**: 935–9.

19. F. Dexter, A. Macario. Changing allocations of operating room time from a system based on historical utilization to one where the aim is to schedule as many surgical cases as possible. *Anesth Analg* 2002; **94**: 1272–9.

20. F. Dexter, J. T. Blake, D. H. Penning, *et al.* Calculating a potential increase in hospital margin for elective surgery by changing operating room time allocations or increasing nursing staffing to permit completion of more cases: a case study. *Anesth Analg* 2002; **94**: 138–42.

21. F. Dexter, H. Ledolter. Managing risk and expected financial return from selective expansion of operating room capacity. Mean-variance analysis of a hospital's portfolio of surgeons. *Anesth Analg* 2003; **97**: 190–5.

22. L. O'Neill, F. Dexter, R. E. Wachtel. Should anesthesia groups advocate funding of clinics and scheduling systems to increase operating room workload? *Anesthesiology* 2009; **111**: 1016–24.

23. A. Macario, F. Dexter, R. D. Traub. Hospital profitability per hour of operating room time can vary among surgeons. *Anesth Analg* 2001; **93**: 669–75.

24. L. O'Neill, F. Dexter. Tactical increases in operating room block time based on financial data and market growth estimates from data envelopment analysis. *Anesth Analg* 2007; **104**: 355–68.

25. J. T. Blake, F. Dexter, J. Donald. Operating room managers' use of integer programming for assigning allocated block time to surgical groups: a case study. *Anesth Analg* 2002; **94**: 143–8.

26. P. T. Vanberkel, R. J. Boucherie, E. W. Hans, J. L. Hurink, W. A. van Lent, W. H. van Harten. Accounting for inpatient wards when developing master surgical schedules. *Anesth Analg* 2011; **112**: 1472–9.

27. M. L. McManus, M. C. Long, A. Cooper, *et al.* Variability in surgical caseload and access to intensive care services. *Anesthesiology* 2003; **98**: 1491–6.

28. S. Gallivan, M. Utley, T. Treasure, *et al.* Booked inpatient admission and hospital capacity: mathematical modelling study. *BMJ* 2002; **324**: 280–2.

29. R. E. Wachtel, F. Dexter. Tactical increases in operating room block time for capacity planning should not be based on utilization. *Anesth Analg* 2008; **106**: 215–26.

30. F. Dexter, R. H. Epstein, H. M. Marsh. Statistical analysis of weekday operating room anesthesia group staffing at nine independently managed surgical suites. *Anesth Analg* 2001; **92**: 1493–8.

31. R. J. Casimir. Strategies for a blind newsboy. *Omega Int J Mgmt Sci* 1999; **27**: 129–34.

32. F. Dexter, A. Macario, R. D. Traub, *et al.* An operating room scheduling strategy to maximize the use of operating room block time. Computer simulation of patient scheduling and survey of patients' preferences for surgical waiting time. *Anesth Analg* 1999; **89**: 7–20.

33. F. Dexter, R. D. Traub, A. Macario, *et al.* Operating room utilization alone is not an accurate metric for the allocation of operating room block time to individual surgeons with low caseloads. *Anesthesiology* 2003; **98**: 1243–9.

34. A. E. Abouleish, F. Dexter, R. H. Epstein, *et al.* Labor costs incurred by anesthesiology groups because of operating rooms not being allocated and cases not being scheduled to maximize operating room efficiency. *Anesth Analg* 2003; **96**: 1109–13.

35. S. Freytag, F. Dexter, R. H. Epstein, *et al.* Allocating and scheduling operating room time based on maximizing operating room efficiency at a German university hospital. *Der Chirurg* 2005; **76**: 71–9.

36. R. E. Wachtel, F. Dexter. Review of behavioral operations experimental studies of newsvendor problems for operating room management. *Anesth Analg* 2010; **110**: 1698–710.

37. J. J. Pandit, F. Dexter. Lack of sensitivity of staffing for 8 hour sessions to standard deviation in daily actual hours of operating room time used for surgeons with long queues. *Anesth Analg* 2009; **108**: 1910–15.

38. F. Dexter, L. S. Weih, R. K. Gustafson, *et al.* Observational study of operating room times for knee and hip replacement surgery at nine US community hospitals. *Health Care Manag Sci* 2006; **9**: 325–39.

39. F. Dexter, D. Masursky, R. E. Wachtel, N. A. Nussmeier. Application of an online reference for reviewing basic statistical principles of operating room management. *J Stat Educ* 2010; **18**.

40. R. E. Wachtel, F. Dexter. Curriculum providing cognitive knowledge and problem-solving skills for anesthesia systems-based practice. *J Grad Med Educ* 2010; **2**: 624–32.

41. A. Junger, M. Benson, L. Quinzio, *et al.* An anesthesia information management system as a tool for controlling resource management of operating rooms. *Meth Inform Med* 2002; **41**: 81–5.

42. R. H. Epstein, F. Dexter. Uncertainty in knowing the operating rooms in which cases were performed has little effect on operating room allocations or efficiency. *Anesth Analg* 2002; **95**: 1726–30.

43. A. E. Abouleish, S. L. Hensley, M. H. Zornow, *et al.* Inclusion of turnover time does not influence identification of surgical services that over- and underutilize allocated block time. *Anesth Analg* 2003; **96**: 813–18.

44. F. Dexter, R. D. Traub. Lack of systematic month-to-month variation over one year periods in ambulatory surgery caseload application to anesthesia staffing. *Anesth Analg* 2000; **91**: 1426–30.

45. D. Masursky, F. Dexter, C. E. O'Leary, C. Applegeet, N. A. Nussmeier. Long-term forecasting of anesthesia workload in operating rooms from changes in a hospital's local population can be inaccurate. *Anesth Analg* 2008; **106**: 1223–31.

46. N. R. Farnum, L. W. Stanton. *Quantitative Forecasting Methods.* Boston: PWS–Kent Publishing Company, 1989; **57**.

47. F. Dexter, R. H. Epstein. Calculating institutional support that benefits both the anesthesia group and hospital. *Anesth Analg* 2008; **106**: 544–53.

48. F. Dexter, R. H. Epstein. Typical savings from each minute reduction in tardy first case of the day starts. *Anesth Analg* 2009; **108**: 1262–7.

49. F. Dexter, R. D. Traub, A. Macario. How to release allocated operating room time to increase efficiency. Predicting which surgical service will have the most under-utilized operating room time. *Anesth Analg* 2003; **96**: 507–12.

50. F. Dexter, A. Macario, R. D. Traub. Which algorithm for scheduling add-on elective cases maximizes operating room utilization? Use of bin packing algorithms and fuzzy constraints in operating room management. *Anesthesiology* 1999; **91**: 1491–500.

51. F. Dexter, A. Macario. When to release allocated operating room time to increase operating room efficiency. *Anesth Analg* 2004; **98**: 758–62.

52. F. Dexter, A. Macario, D. A. Lubarsky, *et al.* Statistical method to evaluate management strategies to decrease variability in operating room utilization. Application of linear statistical modeling and Monte-Carlo simulation to operating room management. *Anesthesiology* 1999; **91**: 262–74.

53. F. Dexter, R. E. Wachtel, R. H. Epstein. Event-based knowledge elicitation of operating room management decision-making using scenarios adapted from information systems data. *BMC Med Inform Decis Mak* 2011; **11**: 2

54. F. Dexter, A. Willemsen-Dunlap, J. D. Lee. Operating room managerial decision-making on the day of surgery with and without computer recommendations and status displays. *Anesth Analg* 2007; **105**: 419–29.

55. F. Dexter. A strategy to decide whether to move the last case of the day in an operating room to another empty operating room to decrease overtime labor costs. *Anesth Analg* 2000; **91**: 925–8.

56. F. Dexter, A. Macario, L. O'Neill. A strategy for deciding operating room assignments for second-shift anesthetists. *Anesth Analg* 1999; **89**: 920–4.

57. F. Dexter, R. D. Traub. Statistical method for predicting when patients should be ready on the day of surgery. *Anesthesiology* 2000; **93**: 1107–14.

58. F. Dexter, R. D. Traub. Sequencing cases in operating rooms: predicting whether one surgical case will last longer than another. *Anesth Analg* 2000; **90**: 975–9.

59. E. Marcon, F. Dexter. Observational study of surgeons' sequencing of cases and its impact on post-anesthesia care unit and holding area staffing requirements at hospitals. *Anesth Analg* 2007; **105**: 119–26.

60. T. J. Babineau, J. Becker, G. Gibbons, *et al*. The "cost" of operating training for surgical residents. *Arch Surg* 2004; **139**: 366–70.

61. S. Eappen, H. Flanagan, N. Bhattacharyya. Introduction of anesthesia resident trainees to the operating room does not lead to changes in anesthesia-controlled times for efficiency measures. *Anesthesiology* 2004; **101**: 1210–14.

62. R. E. Wachtel, F. Dexter. Influence of the operating room schedule on tardiness from scheduled start times. *Anesth Analg* 2009; **108**: 1889–901.

63. R. E. Wachtel, F. Dexter. Reducing tardiness from scheduled start times by making adjustments to the operating room schedule. *Anesth Analg* 2009; **108**: 1902–9.

64. F. Dexter, R. H. Epstein, J. D. Lee, J. Ledolter. Automatic updating of times remaining in surgical cases using Bayesian analysis of historical case duration data and instant messaging updates from anesthesia providers. *Anesth Analg* 2009; **108**: 929–40.

65. F. Dexter, J. Ledolter. Bayesian prediction bounds and comparisons of operating room times even for procedures with few or no historical data. *Anesthesiology* 2005; **103**: 1259–67.

66. F. Dexter, A. Macario. What is the relative frequency of uncommon ambulatory surgery procedures in the United States with an anesthesia provider? *Anesth Analg* 2000; **90**: 1343–7.

67. F. Dexter, R. D. Traub, L. A. Fleisher, P. Rock. What sample sizes are required for pooling surgical case durations among facilities to decrease the incidence of procedures with little historical data? *Anesthesiology* 2002; **96**: 1230–6.

68. F. Dexter, E. U. Dexter, J. Ledolter. Influence of procedure classification on process variability and parameter uncertainty of surgical case durations. *Anesth Analg* 2010; **110**: 1155–63.

69. R. H. Epstein, F. Dexter, E. Piotrowski. Automated correction of room location errors in anesthesia information management systems. *Anesth Analg* 2008; **107**: 965–71.

Chapter

7

Operations management and financial performance

Jeffrey Anderson MD
Seth Christian MD
Richard D. Urman MD, MBA

Contribution margin   68
Relationship between financial and
operational performance   68
Measures of financial performance   70
Capital structure   72

Measures of operational
performance   73
Process view   74
Process capacity and
bottlenecks   74

In its essence, operations management is the process by which one seeks to match supply and demand. This standard economic principle exists in all industries, whether it is the fast food restaurant, the big box retailer, or the emergency room of a community hospital. Matching supply and demand is problematic, however, as although the supply is relatively constant, demand can fluctuate greatly. For example, the ambulatory surgery center may be fully staffed for ten operating suites every Tuesday. On any given Tuesday, the number of cancellations may spike far above the mean, leaving empty operating suites attended by wage-earning employees. Conversely, the surgeon in one room may encounter difficulty during his or her first case of the day, causing the case to run significantly over its allotted time. The schedule of operations for the operating suite is then thrown off.

Operating rooms (ORs) are, in general, profitable. In the model of the free-standing ambulatory surgery center, the OR is a profit center. In many instances, however, the OR is just one part of a larger whole. So although the revenue stream is vital, running the OR efficiently with the lowest costs possible becomes increasingly important. The OR manager must, therefore, have a profound understanding of cost structures.

"Profit margin" is defined as the difference between revenues and costs. The profit margin can be increased by increasing revenues or, alternatively, decreasing costs. "Costs" can first be categorized as fixed, variable, or semi-variable. "Fixed costs" are costs the OR will incur regardless of volume of surgeries performed. Examples of such costs might include the salary of administrative staff. This cost will be in place whether the OR sees an increase in volume, no change in volume, or even a decrease in volume. "Variable costs" fluctuate based on the volume of cases performed. For example, as more surgeries are performed, more supplies are used, and supply costs increase. If there are no surgeries performed on a given day, no additional supplies will be used. Some costs are "semi-variable" or have elements of fixed and variable structures. An example of semi-variable cost is a full-time employee who is paid on an hourly basis. The first 40 h of their wages are more or less fixed. Any overtime pay, however, is a variable cost, which is dependent on OR volume.

All of the costs listed thus far are direct costs that are directly associated with the running of the OR. Costs can be attributed back to a source such as a thyroidectomy or other procedure. All hospitals and ORs also must factor in "indirect costs," or "overheads." Overhead costs are allocated costs that are spread among all departments or parts of a business. They often originate from support departments such as laundry, dietary services, and housekeeping. They cannot

Operating Room Leadership and Management, ed. Kaye A.D., Fox C.J. and Urman R.D. Published by Cambridge University Press. © Cambridge University Press 2012.

be directly attributed to the OR but must be factored into the OR budget.

The OR manager may not be able to influence overhead costs but does have a hand in establishing direct costs in the categories of supplies cost, practice management costs, and personnel costs. "Controllable costs" are costs that can be influenced by a manager's decisions. Staffing and supplies are often costs controllable by OR managers.

Supplies cost involves the materials needed by the OR to perform surgeries. This is a major component of the OR budget. Pressure exists to hold costs down as much as possible. Thus, this goal must be kept in mind all the way from purchasing the supplies to the analysis of the supplies' use. The OR must have vital supplies on hand at all times, but must avoid unused inventory, which raises costs without adding value.

Personnel costs include the nurses, surgical technicians, and aides in the OR and postanesthesia care unit. Anesthesia providers may also be included if they are employed by the hospital or surgery center. Personnel costs can make up to 60% of an OR budget. Thus, any variance in these costs can have a great impact on the profitability of the OR. Several strategies for reducing personnel costs have been utilized in the OR.

Contribution margin

In managerial accounting, a key concept to understand is the idea of the "contribution margin." This is a method of looking at the relationship between revenues and costs so that the manager can use them to make decisions regarding planning. The key attribute of this approach is the strict delineation between fixed and variable costs. The contribution margin is defined as the difference between revenues and variable costs.

Contribution margin = revenue – variable cost

The resulting amount, or contribution margin, is then applied to cover the fixed costs. If the contribution margin is greater than the fixed costs, the firm makes a profit. Conversely, if the contribution margin is less than the fixed costs, the firm suffers a loss. This is more easily understood if viewed graphically.

In Figure 7.1, the fixed cost is held fixed at $10 000. Total cost starts at $10 000 then has a positive slope up, based on variable costs. Variable cost is the difference between total cost and fixed cost. The point at which total cost and revenue are equal is the breakeven point, or the point at which the contribution margin covers the fixed cost exactly.

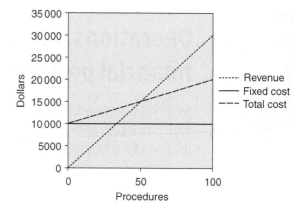

Figure 7.1 Contribution margin.

Breakeven point:
Total costs = revenues
or
Contribution margin = fixed cost

Any additional contribution margin will be applied to profit. The difference between the revenue and total cost line equals the profit (to the right) or loss (to the left). For this OR, the breakeven point (again, the point at which costs are covered by revenue) is 50 procedures. If this were the data for 1 week's time, the manager would know that as long as the OR were able to book and perform 50 procedures per week, the unit would be profitable. At any point below 50 procedures, however, the contribution margin would be unable to cover the OR's fixed expenses.

Relationship between financial and operational performance

Although OR managers are not typically responsible for overall financial and operational performance, they must be aware of at least a qualitative relationship between the financial and operational performance of the OR. In order to understand the relationship between operational performance and financial performance, OR managers must have a basic understanding of both financial and managerial accounting. Financial accounting is known as external accounting, because the principles of financial accounting aim to create standardized reports with the purpose of comparing organizations within an industry. Managerial cost accounting is known as internal accounting, because it is primarily used as a tool for managers to measure trends in financial performance internally.

Community Health Care System Balance Sheet

Assets (in thousands)		1998		1997
Current assets				
Cash	$	3364	$	5990
Cash equivalents	$	6032	$	4316
Account receivable	$	21655	$	22622
Uncollectable allowances	$	766	$	1046
Charity allowances	$	921	$	1257
Courtesy allowances	$	98	$	136
Doubtful allowances	$	144	$	201
Contractual allowances	$	4666	$	1086
Inventory and supplies	$	1745	$	2147
Prepaid expenses	$	1309	$	1544
Non-Current assets				
Property, plant, and equipment	$	62730	$	62452
Land and improvement	$	4545	$	3967
Building and equipment	$	116997	$	109648
Construction in progress	$	336	$	1087
Allowance for depreciation	$	59148	$	52250
Restricted assets	$	12344	$	12121
Other assets				
Miscellaneous assets	$	1392	$	830
Total assets	$	110571	$	112022

Liabilities and Equities (in thousands)		1998		1997
Current liabilities				
Account payable	$	7406	$	7895
Accrued liabilities				
Payroll expenses		2393		3684
Employee benefits		2253		2936
Other liabilities		2583		2823
Insurance costs		1768		1941
Current portion of long-term debt		1453		670
Non-current liabilities				
Long-term debt		37577		37833
Equity				
Retained earnings		55138		54240
Total liabilities and equity		$110571		$112022

Figure 7.2 An example of a balance sheet.

Financial accounting statements are composed of four basic documents: (1) the balance sheet; (2) the income statement; (3) the cash flow statement; and (4) the notes to the financial statement.

The balance sheet contains a categorized list of assets and liabilities at the end of an accounting period. It is a picture of the organization's financial position at one point in time, and is often considered the best single indicator of the financial condition of the organization (see Figure 7.2).

The income statement contains a list of all revenues and expenses (Figure 7.3). Revenue is generated from both patient care operations and nonpatient-care operations (parking, cafeteria, research grants, rental space, or equipment sales). Expenses include salaries, benefits, supplies, depreciation, and professional fees.

The cash flow statement contains a list of cash-producing and cash-consuming transactions for the accounting period (Figure 7.4). The cash flow statement shows the financial status in terms of cash flow,

Community Health Care System Income Statement

Revenues and Expenses (in thousands)	1998		1997	
Revenues				
Patient-care revenues	$	134 101	$	140 684
Other revenues				
Educational programs	$	887	$	886
Research and grants	$	973	$	2 417
Rentals space or equipment	$	2 421	$	971
Sales of medical and pharmacy items to non-patients	$	2 592	$	2 587
Cafeteria sales	$	802	$	801
Auxiliary fund raising and gift shop sales	$	1 143	$	1 141
Parking	$	1 058	$	1 056
Investment income on malpractice trust funds	$	973	$	971
Total revenues	$	144 950	$	151 514
Expenses				
Salaries and wages	$	667 165	$	67 893
Employee benefits	$	13 961	$	16 217
Professional fees	$	8 803	$	12 048
Supplies	$	33 269	$	33 316
Interest	$	4 004	$	3 857
Bad debt expenses	$	5 406	$	6 583
Depreciation and amortization	$	6 898	$	8 022
Restructuring costs	$	5 272	$	628
Taxes	$	252	$	913
Total expenses	$	145 033	$	149 477
Nonoperating gains (losses)				
Revenues from activities unrelated to patient care	$	812	$	833
Gains (losses) from investment of unrestricted funds	$	703	$	621
Gains (losses) from sale of property	$	(534)	$	(360)
Nonoperating gains (losses)	$	981	$	1 094
Excess of revenues and nonoperating gains over expenses	$	898	$	3 131

Figure 7.3 An example of an income statement.

rather than according to revenues and expenses in the income statement or accounting entries in the balance sheet.

The notes may include valuable information about the operational status of the organization. Much of the benefit derived from financial statements results from tracking trends in values from one period to the next.

Because health-care organizations function in different environments and may deliver different mixes of services to patient populations, operational indicators make diverse organizations more comparable. Many operational indicators are adjusted for case mix and prevailing local wages. Case mix adjustment is a mathematical correction made to account for differences in severity of illness between patient populations. Wage index adjustment is a mathematical correction made to account for differences in employee wages between geographic areas.

Measures of financial performance

In addition to the general observation of whether or not an OR is producing enough revenue to meet expenses, financial metrics or indicators can further describe the financial health of the entity. Such measurements describe an institution's ability to meet its responsibilities. For instance, a business can meet its short-term demands by taking on additional debt. This will allow the business to pay its bills at the end of a given month. This, however, is unsustainable in the long term. The business must be able to develop enough equity to meet these obligations. An inability to build such equity will hinder the business from making purchases,

Community Health Care System Cash Flow Statement

Cash Flow (in thousands)	1998
Cash Flow from operating activities and gains losses	
Revenues and gains greater than (less than) expenses and losses	$ 898
Adjustments to reconcile revenues and gains in excess of expenses and loses with net cash provided by operating activities and gains and losses	
Provision for bad debts	$ 5 406
Depreciation and amortization	$ 6 898
Change in assets and liabilities	
Patients accounts receivable with provision for bad debt	$ 4 439.00
Inventory and supplies	$ 402.00
Prepaid expenses	$ 235.00
Restricted expenses	$ (223.00)
Other assets	$ (562.00)
Account payable	$ (489.00)
Accrued payroll and employee benefits	$ (1 974.00)
Accrued interest	$ (173.00)
Other liabilities	$ (240.00)
Net cash provided by operating activities	$ 14 617.00
Cash flows from investing activities	
Purchase of property, plant, and equipment	$ (14 074.00)
Net cash used by investing activities	$ (1 453.00)
Cash flows from financing activities	
Repayments of long-term debt	$ (1 453.00)
Net cash provided by (used by) financing activities	$ (1 453.00)
Net increase (decrease) in cash and cash equivalents	$ (910.00)
Cash and cash equivaents at beginning of year	$ 10 306.00
Cash and cash equivaents at end of year	$ 9 396.00

Figure 7.4 An example of a cash flow statement.

developing new technology, or continuing to provide its current standard of service.

Specific financial ratios are also accepted indicators of financial performance (Figure 7.5). "Liquidity ratios" measure the ability to meet short-term obligations. "Capital structure ratios" measure ability to meet long-term obligations. "Profitability ratios" measure ability to generate retained earnings and thus to increase assets. "Activity ratios" measure the efficiency with which assets are used to generate revenues.

Indicators of financial performance expressed as ratios make the information easier to interpret and facilitate benchmarking between similar institutions.

Operating room managers understand that factors such as reduced OR costs, increased OR operational efficiency, and increased patient volume will improve financial performance.

Liquidity is the measure of an institution's ability to pay its debts or liabilities with its current assets. One can consider this to be "cash on hand." The amount by which assets exceed liabilities is known as "working capital."

Working capital = assets − liabilities

As an organization's liquidity increases, it has a greater ability to meet its liabilities. If an organization is managed poorly or is struck by unexpected financial hardship, a crisis can ensue when its bills cannot be paid. Such a crisis may be short lived or may be an indication of deeper financial problems. Liquidity is often studied in terms of ratios. The current ratio is the measure of current assets to current liabilities.

Current liquidity ratio = current assets / current liabilities

It is important to remember that current liquidity does not relate to assets that can be moved quickly to pay off liabilities. Although an organization's total assets may far outweigh its liabilities, the assets may be tied up in equipment, property, or long-term investments. Relative liquidity takes this into account. An extreme measure of relative liquidity is the "acid test." This measures assets that are actually cash or cash equivalents relative to liabilities.

Acid test = (cash + cash equivalents) / current liabilities

Community Health Care System Financial Performance Ratios

Ratio	Low	Middle	High
Liquidity			
Current	1.5	2	2.5
Acid test	0.2	0.25	0.3
Days in patient accounts receivable	40	55	70
Days of cash on hand	20	26	32
Capital structure			
Long-term debt-to-equity	0.6	0.7	0.8
Times interest earned	2.4	2.7	3.0
Cash flow-to-debt	0.1	0.2	0.3
Debt service coverage	3.1	3.5	4.0
Profitability			
Total margin	3%	4%	5%
Operating margin	2%	3%	4%
Return on equity	5%	7.5%	10%
Activity			
Asset turnover	0.8	0.9	1.0
Fixed asset turnover	1.5	2.0	2.5
Current asset turnover	3.0	3.5	4.0

Figure 7.5 Financial performance ratios.

Rarely is this ratio equal to one. Rather, a very high acid test ratio is approximately 0.3.

Another interesting liquidity ratio useful for making decisions and deciphering financial health of an organization involves the number of "days of cash on hand."

Days of cash on hand

= (cash + cash equivalents) / daily operating expenses (without depreciation)

Simply put, this measures the number of days the organization could meet its expenses using solely the cash it has on hand. This indicates an organization's ability to survive a sudden downturn in cash flows. For the manager, or even investor unfamiliar with operations management, this is a concept that can be missed. This is particularly true in the setting of the freestanding ambulatory surgery center. The capital to make a purchase may be available upfront (the building is financed, the equipment is purchased); however, the cash on hand is insufficient to maintain the operation should volume decrease due to market forces. A rudimentary example may be the ability to purchase the car, but being unable to buy the gas to make the vehicle run.

Capital structure

Even in health care, where the mission is often to serve and care for the patient, an OR must generate income.

Without doing so, the organization cannot buy equipment or hire additional personnel. As stated earlier, profit margin is the difference between total revenues and total costs. Profitability ratios indicate ability to generate income.

Total margin ratio = (income / total revenues) × 100%

The total margin ratio simply measures the amount of revenue that contributes to income. This can come from patient-care or nonpatient-care sources.

Operating margin ratio = (operating revenues – operating expenses) / total revenues

Operating margin excludes nonpatient care-related activities and focuses solely on the operational revenues from patient care. This is subsequently usually less than the total margin ratio. Within the OR the main mode of increasing operating margin is by decreasing expenses.

Return on equity = (income / equity) × 100%

Finally, return on equity is often considered the primary test of profitability. This measure relates income to equity or net assets of the organization. Equity is determined as the difference between assets and liabilities. The resulting number indicates the rate at which an OR or other organization produces profit relative to its net assets. A higher percentage indicates greater return on equity and thus greater profitability.

Table 7.1 Operational performance indicators and suggested example values

Occupancy	50%
Length of stay, case mix adjusted	4.5 days
Revenue per discharge, case mix, and wage index adjusted	$5000
Revenue per visit, wage index adjusted	$225
Cost per discharge, case mix, and wage index adjusted	$5000
Cost per visit, wage index adjusted	$225
Inpatient staff hours per discharge, case mix, and wage index adjusted	135
Outpatient staff hours per visit	6
Salary per full-time equivalent employee, wage index adjusted	$33 000
Capital costs per discharge, case mix, and wage index adjusted	$5400
Outpatient revenue	33%

Measures of operational performance

Although measures of financial performance are vital to determine the health of an organization's finances, they do not characterize the efficiency by which the organization provides services with the resources at hand. In an ideal model, an organization would utilize resources perfectly. In other words, the OR would consume exactly what is required for its services; no more, no less. Every additional suture required or labor hour needed above this point will decrease efficiency. A manager can work to increase operating income by increasing revenues or decreasing expenses. By and large, this overwhelming method for increasing income is by decreasing expenses. These fundamentals are analyzed much like the financial statements through the use of performance ratios (Table 7.1). These ratios are complicated by the fact that case mix is not universal across institutions. A case mix index is therefore applied that weighs a facility's cases and patient illness against an average. A similar index is utilized to adjust for wage differences between regions.

One indicator of interest is the revenue a facility generates per discharge. This can be used for inpatient hospitals as well as ambulatory centers. The net inpatient or outpatient revenues depending on the facility are divided by the number of discharges, adjusted for case mix and wage discrepancy.

Net patient revenues / (no. discharges × case mix index × wage index)

A similar indicator can be used to measure the costs incurred per discharge by substituting net costs for revenue. This is again adjusted for case mix and wage.

Net patient costs / (no. discharges × case mix index × wage index)

When operating within a large facility, it may be impossible to measure the OR's contribution to costs. Generally speaking, this contribution will be high and may make up the majority of the costs for a typical admission.

As labor costs often make up a large percentage of a facility's total expenditures, it is also important to analyze the efficiency by which labor is utilized. In an inpatient facility this is done by taking the number of full-time employees (FTEs) and multiplying them by 2080 (the number of hours worked in a year). This product is then divided, once again, by the number of discharges adjusted for case mix and wage.

(FTEs × 2080) / (no. discharges × case mix index × wage index)

The resulting value measures labor productivity. If the number of employees remains constant, a lower value indicates higher labor productivity. That is, labor is being utilized at a greater rate. As the number of discharges (patients) increases, labor productivity will be greater. Although this is generally a positive trend, it does not mean that costs may be lower. A facility may have higher labor productivity as fewer staff are required to see a set number patients, but if these employees are higher cost, overall labor costs may still be fairly high.

The average unit cost of labor can be measured by measuring the salary per FTE.

Total salary / (no. FTEs × wage index)

This indicator can be skewed higher or lower depending on the institution. A facility that utilizes fewer, higher-cost employees will have a higher average salary. This does not necessarily indicate greater total labor costs. Likewise, any institution that contracts for services such as dietary or housekeeping will have a greater average salary, as contracted employees are not factored.

Finally, a facility that provides both inpatient and outpatient services can analyze the contribution of outpatient services to overall revenues by calculating the percentage of revenue received from outpatients.

(Net outpatient revenues / total revenues) × 100%

If a facility is able to maintain a constant level of inpatient revenue stream, an increase in the percentage coming from outpatient services is generally a positive trend. This is secondary to fewer costs associated with such services. If, however, the increase in outpatient revenues is at the expense of inpatient revenues, the result is far less positive.

Process view

Any industry can be seen as more than the products it produces. It is important to examine the processes by which supply is generated. The process is the accumulation of multiple steps or activities. When one analyzes an OR, it is often done from the perspective of the patient. That is, the patient is the unit of measurement. As the patient works his or her way through the process of outpatient surgery, they will experience many activities, including: registration, pre-admit testing, preoperative nursing care, preoperative assessment, transfer to preoperative holding area, procedure in OR, recovery room, outpatient surgery, and finally home. The time the patient spends in each of these activities is called the activity time. If there are gaps in between the activities, the patient is then waiting. This allows one to describe supply–demand mismatches. Waiting times are a consequence of finite supply. In a hospital with unlimited ORs, surgeons, nurses, and anesthesiologists, the patient's waiting time would be zero. Unfortunately, this is rarely the case.

Process performance can be analyzed using three measurements: "inventory," "flow time," and "flow rate." Inventory is the total number of units within the process at any one time. Flow time is the amount of time required for one unit to flow through the entire process. Flow rate is the rate at which units are passed through the process in flow units per unit time

(units/hour or day). In the OR, the number of patients awaiting surgery, receiving surgery, and recovering from surgery is the inventory. The flow time is the average time for a patient to make it through from registration to discharge. The flow rate is usually the number of patients who receive surgery per day. The maximum flow rate is also known as the capacity for the process – that is, the greatest rate at which patients receive surgery and are discharged home. If you are able to increase capacity, supply will be able to meet demand under a greater number of circumstances. These three measurements are related to one another through Little's Law:

Average inventory = average flow rate × average flow time

Process capacity and bottlenecks

Process capacity, or maximum flow rate, is the maximum amount a process can produce during a certain period of time. This is the amount the process can produce even if the process generally produces less than the capacity. One of the foremost goals of operations management is to maximize capacity. One does so by first analyzing the process itself to seek out limits to capacity. These limits may be physical, such as having ten ORs, or related to labor, such as lacking an extra nurse for the recovery room. The point at which the process stalls, slows, or is limited by the flow time through an activity is the known as the "bottleneck." The bottleneck's capacity is, in turn, the process's capacity. This is the rate-limiting step.

Let's look at a simplified example of process analysis applied to the OR. The process is made up of many steps or activities, starting with the patient arriving at registration. First the patient must register to be admitted. This step is staffed by three employees and takes an average of 15 min per patient. Second, the patient is admitted to outpatient surgery, where nursing staff check vitals, start IVs, draw any ordered tests, administer medications, etc. Six nurses, who can see two patients at a time, staff the unit. It takes the nurse 30 min to complete this step. Third, once the patient is called for, he or she is moved to the preoperative holding area, where a nurse checks all consents, anesthesia providers meet and evaluate the patient, and the surgeon checks on the patient. Up to ten patients can be in the preoperative holding area at any one time, and they stay for approximately 30 min. Fourth, the patient

Table 7.2 Process analysis in the OR

Activity	Inventory	Flow time (h)	Capacity (patients/h)
Registration	3	0.25	3/0.25 = 12
Outpatient surgery	12	0.5	12/0.5 = 24
Preop holding	10	0.5	10/0.5 = 20
OR	20	2.0	20/2 = 10
PACU	8	1.0	8/1 = 8
Outpatient surgery	10	0.5	10/0.5 = 20

is brought to the OR for surgery. This facility staffs 20 locations with an average procedure time of 2 h. Fifth, the patient is moved to the postanasthesia care unit (PACU) for recovery, where he or she is monitored by nursing staff. The PACU is staffed with four nurses, who can each take two patients. Average time to discharge a patient after arrival is 60 min. Sixth, once the patient is discharged from the PACU, he or she returns to outpatient surgery for monitoring and discharge. Owing to the staggered nature of postoperative arrival back in outpatient surgery, the unit is staffed with five nurses, who can again take two patients at a time. The average stay is 30 min. So, in this example there are six distinct steps that must happen in order.

Table 7.2 lists all the locations/steps in the order that the activities are performed. The inventory is the maximum number of patients that can be in the activity at any one time, while the flow time is the average time the activity takes. Using this information we are able to calculate the capacity for each step. Although the inventory of the registration is lowest among the activities, the flow time is also the shortest. Conversely, flow time is longest in the OR itself, but the high level of inventory allows for higher capacity. The activity with the lowest capacity turns out to be recovery in the PACU, at eight patients per hour. It is the bottleneck, or rate-limiting step. Additional ORs can be opened or registration staff hired, but the maximum capacity will not improve above eight patients per hour.

By analyzing the process, we can seek to determine the bottleneck. In our example, if the manager worked to relieve the bottleneck in the PACU by increasing staffing or decreasing flow time, he or she could work to improve the process capacity.

We can also look at the utilization of a process. That is, how much production is made relative to the maximum production possible.

Process utilization = flow rate / process capacity

We can then analyze why a process may not be 100% utilized. This may be demand limited if flow rate is decreased owing to a lack of demand for the unit produced: for instance, the ORs being underutilized because the number of surgeries booked is low. Going back to our hypothetical OR, if the flow rate is less than eight patients per hour, the PACU is no longer limiting flow through the process. The decreased utilization is due to demand rather than supply. If we then look at each step within the process we see that the activity with the highest utilization will be the bottleneck of the process.

If we were to find that the process flow rate was six patients per hour even though our bottleneck capacity was eight patients per hour, our process utilization would stand at 75% (Table 7.3). The PACU still stands as our bottleneck, as it has the highest activity utilization of the process, but at this time it is not limiting the OR's production.

If, on the other hand, the process were running at capacity of eight patients per hour with patients waiting to be transferred to the PACU, the process utilization would be at 100%. The OR Manager now has the opportunity to effect change. An additional PACU nurse is hired and efforts to improve efficiency within the PACU decrease the flow time from 60 to 45 min.

Now more patients are able to complete the process, capacity has increased to 12 patients per hour (Table 7.4). The PACU is no longer the bottleneck. The ORs and registration are now limiting capacity.

One of the main goals of the OR manager is to identify sources of inefficiency that reduce capacity and then to resolve these issues. The manager must seek to identify the bottleneck and work to relieve

Table 7.3 Process capacity of eight patients per hour

Activity	Inventory	Flow time (h)	Capacity (patients/h)	Utilization (%)
Registration	3	0.25	3/0.25= 12	6/12 = 50
Outpatient surgery	12	0.5	12/0.5 = 24	6/24 = 25
Preop holding	10	0.5	10/0.5 = 20	6/20 = 30
Operating room	20	2.0	20/2 = 10	6/10 = 60
PACU	8	1.0	8/1 = 8	6/8 = 75
Outpatient surgery	10	0.5	10/0.5 = 20	6/20 = 30
		Process flow rate = 6 patients/hour	Process capacity = 8 patients/hour	6/8 = 75

Table 7.4 Process capacity of 12 patients per hour

Activity	Inventory	Flow time (h)	Capacity (patients/h)	Utilization (%)
Registration	3	0.25	3/0.25 = 12	12/12 = 100
Outpatient surgery	12	0.5	12/0.5 = 24	12/24 = 50
Preop holding	10	0.5	10/0.5 = 20	12/20 = 60
OR	20	2.0	20/2 = 10	12/12 = 100
PACU	10	0.75	10/0.75 = 13.33	12/13.3 = 90
Outpatient surgery	10	0.5	10/0.5 = 20	12/20 = 60
		Process flow rate = 12 patients/hour	Process capacity = 12 patients/hour	12/12 = 100

it – otherwise the OR will be forever limited by that step. Increasing staffing or equipment to every other activity in the process will do nothing but decrease efficiency while increasing cost. However, if one is able to take a process analysis view of the OR, such decisions can be made without missing the true source of the problem. Such a misstep can have the potential to be costly, such as allocating resources towards additional housekeeping staff in hopes of improving turnover times, when the nursing shortage in the PACU has patients recovering in the OR.

Suggested reading

P. C. Brewer, R. H. Garrison, E. W. Noreen. *Managerial Accounting*, 13th edn. New York: McGraw-Hill/Irwin, 2010.

G. Cachon, C. Terwiesch. *Matching Supply with Demand: An Introduction to Operations Management*, 2nd edn. Boston: McGraw-Hill, 2006.

R. A. Gabel, ed. *Operating Room Management*. Chicago: Butterworth-Heinemann, 1999.

A. P. Harris, W. G. Zitzmann. *Operating Room Management: Structure, Strategies, & Economics*. St. Louis: Mosby Year Book, 1998.

Chapter

8

Reengineering operating room function

Nigel N. Robertson MB, ChB, FANZCA

Introduction   77
Efficiency, productivity, and design   77
The OR design process   80
"Waste" management in the OR   87

Building life span and
renovation   93
From plans to procedures   93
Summary   94

Introduction

Operating rooms (ORs) are rightly regarded as important drivers of the productive potential of any health-care organization. They are often the greatest source of revenue within a hospital system but also have a high cost base that presents an element of risk to the organization if not managed effectively.

Globally, health-care systems are under ever more pressure to deliver greater efficiency, productivity, and – above all – quality of care within constrained budgets. Operating rooms are increasingly seen as "outliers" by funders and regulators measuring performance improvement through transformational process redesign methodologies such as Lean Six Sigma (LSS).

Modern industrial and commercial complexes are designed and built to seamlessly integrate into the process and functional objectives of the organization. Many examples of such workplaces are available as video clips on the web; readers are particularly directed to one such clip featuring the Volkswagen Phaeton plant in Germany (www.youtube.com – search "VW phaeton factory").

Much of the current hospital stock was built in the 1950s to 1980s. Clinicians were not involved in high-level design until the layout of the building had been determined. By then, it was too late to optimize the OR design and co-locations; many an architect's plan placed the intensive care unit (ICU) at a remote location from the OR, much to the chagrin of the putative operators!

The objective of this chapter is to briefly discuss the meaning of efficiency in the context of ORs, outline the concept of LSS, variability, and waste in OR processes and describe ways in which architects and clinicians can work to design facilities that will be fit for purpose. The building process is described and also how to stay in touch with the process to achieve best outcomes. Communication platforms in the OR are also described. Refurbishment of existing buildings is a particular skill, and there is some discussion on this aspect within the chapter. It should be made clear from the outset that there is no single best way to design the OR suite; solutions are contextual – it depends how the organization and clinicians plan to use the unit. Space precludes the creation of an OR design manual; this chapter, however, gives clinicians and managers a toolkit with which to benchmark their facility.

Efficiency, productivity, and design

What does the term "efficiency" mean in the OR? Stakeholders in a health-care system define efficiency in the OR with a range of responses (Figure 8.1) that are discussed in detail in other parts of this book. The objective of delivering efficiency at its simplest level is to produce a realistic schedule that fits the resource available; the schedule for the day has a reasonable probability of filling the OR session without finishing early, finishing late, or cancelling any patients, as described by Pandit et al. [1]. It sounds so simple.

Operating Room Leadership and Management, ed. Kaye A.D., Fox C.J. and Urman R.D. Published by Cambridge University Press. © Cambridge University Press 2012.

Table 8.1. A scoring system for OR efficiency (A. Macario. Are your operating rooms efficient? A scoring system with eight performance indicators. *Anesthesiology* 2006; **105**: 237–40.)

Metric	Points		
	0	1	2
Excess staffing costs	>10%	5–10%	<5%
Start-time tardiness (mean tardiness of start times for elective cases per OR per day)	>60 min	45–60 min	<45 min
Case cancellation rate	>10%	5–10%	<5%
PACU admission delays (% of workdays with at least one delay in PACU admission)	>20%	10–20%	<10%
Contribution margin (mean) per OR hour	<$1000/h	$1000–2000/h	>$2000/h
Turnover times (mean setup and cleanup turnover times for all cases)	>40 min	25–40 min	<25 min
Prediction bias (bias in case duration estimates per 8 h of OR time)	>15 min	5–15 min	<5 min
Prolonged turnovers (% of turnovers that are more than 60 min)	>25%	10–25%	<10%

OR, operating room; PACU, postanesthesia care unit.

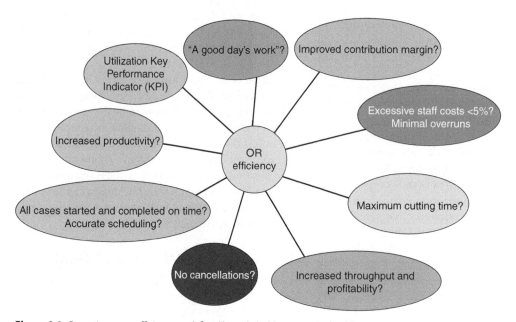

Figure 8.1 Operating room efficiency, as defined by stakeholder groups in the OR.

A number of measures of OR activity have been proposed over the past two to three decades, but most of them have significant limitations and can either be manipulated or include major correction factors to enable a merger of quantitative and qualitative datasets. These are discussed in more detail elsewhere in this book.

Recently, Macario produced a scoring system for OR efficiency (Table 8.1) that utilized existing data and assigned points to eight metrics that he deemed

to be important end points of OR efficiency [2]. These included excessive staffing costs, start time tardiness, turnovers, contribution margins, postanesthesia care unit (PACU) admission delays, and cancellations. Efficient units scored more points, and in his editorial Macario succinctly described real-life metrics that all OR clinicians recognize.

Pandit and his colleagues have also developed an elegant model that uses simple data, available in all OR suites, to create a measure of "productive potential" for an OR team [3].

It is important to understand measures of efficiency when designing ORs. Some of the preceding discussion will perhaps have delivered some clues as to the reasons for this; "turnover times" and "PACU admission delays" have an impact on OR efficiency, however it is defined. We therefore need to explore how the design of OR facilities affects these production metrics.

Over the past decade, many health-care organizations have sought to streamline their operations by adopting methods developed for industry and commerce, such as LSS processing and queueing theory. These have become very attractive to managers, chief executives, and boards as a way to bring some order to the apparently chaotic nature of health care.

There is, however, little evidence of systemic success in the literature thus far (although many anecdotal examples are quoted). Skeptics point to the unique variability within health care compared with car production lines, for example, as a potent reason to resist adoption of LSS in health care. However, as Dr. Litvak at the Institute of Healthcare Improvement and others have pointed out, there are two types of variability: natural and artificial [4]. The former relates to the randomness of patient arrival into the system, the complex and variable nature of their illness, and the length of the treatment episode. This variability may add cost but cannot be eliminated.

Artificial variability, however, is usually the result of a systems limitation or bottleneck, such as a poorly drafted elective surgical schedule or a building capacity and design problem. This form of variability can and should be eliminated.

Waste

Elements of LSS and variability methodology in health care constitute a common theme of waste in the system. The following discussion will focus on waste in the OR and how this relates to the design of the OR facilities.

The NHS Institute for Innovation and Improvement in the UK defined seven forms of waste as applied to the health-care context [5]:

- overproduction – undertaking activity in batches or "just-in-case;"
- inventory – refers to materials and also to patients; usually a symptom of poor supply chain or admission/discharge process;

- waiting – can apply to patients, staff, material, or equipment;
- transportation – excess or inefficient movement of patients or material;
- defects – any defect that impacts on a process, including patient cancellation;
- staff movement – relates to organization and layout of facility and also to information solutions;
- unnecessary processing – using complex facilities or equipment to undertake simple tasks.

When these elements are applied to the OR, we start to see the importance of developing an integrated view of design and process.

Waste in the OR suite – design is a contributor

This concept of waste allows some themes to emerge for both clinicians and managers concerned with OR efficiency. These may now be applied to the OR setting (Figure 8.2):

- overproduction – example: batched patient arrivals for OR sessions;
- inventory – example: poor storage layout/ inadequate capacity, leading to uneven supply chain;
- waiting – example: poor scheduling, prolonged turnover, tardiness, PACU capacity;
- transportation – example: poor layout of OR suite, co-location of related units such as ICU, PACU, sterile supplies; elevators remotely located;
- defects – example: cancellations, missing patient information, equipment failure, surgical site infection;
- staff movement – example: store rooms remote from OR, lack of surgeon workspace during turnover, use of information technology (IT) solutions;
- unnecessary processing – examples: repeated patient checks in the OR, nonvalue-added preoperative testing, ambulatory cases in tertiary center OR suites.

The first two elements of the design journey are now described: an outline of efficiency and productivity in the OR; and the concept of systematic waste that is influenced by the design of the OR suites. Taking these forward, we can then start to formulate a design process that will produce a facility that is fit for purpose (Figure 8.3).

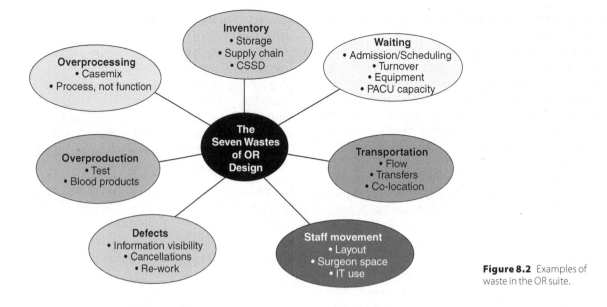

Figure 8.2 Examples of waste in the OR suite.

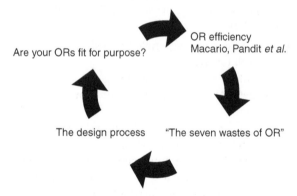

Figure 8.3 The design cycle for OR construction.

The OR design process

Who is involved?

Anyone who has built a house will recognize that there are many parties involved: owner, bank, local authority, builder, architect, and others.

Hospitals are enormously complex facilities and require input from a bewildering range of stakeholders (Figure 8.4). Clinicians may have limited experience dealing with many of the representative professions and trades involved, but it is important to be part of the design team from the earliest opportunity to insure that clinical concerns are met as the process evolves. A tender process will result in selection

of a "design and build" team and a project management team that will usually be responsible for delivery of the facility.

Clinicians should be seconded to the latter team from the outset. Crucial decisions that impact on the whole life of the building are often made within the first few weeks and months of the project. Initial footprint and layout plans are often tied to tender documents and budgets. Plan redraws become problematic once the organization and project team has locked them in to target timelines and payment schedules.

Ideally, staff clinicians should be involved and seconded to the project team. The organization must recognize the value of this addition to the team and provide cover for the clinical commitments of their staff.

Clinicians attached to the project team bring authenticity to the design. They can enlist their colleague "champions" to develop a very clear vision of the design features required to support the function of the facility. In our project, I was the design coordinator for the OR suites, and this involved "360" meetings with many stakeholder groups such as:

- clinical user groups;
- project executives and board members;
- government/funder representatives;
- consumer representatives;
- construction and project management team members;
- architects;

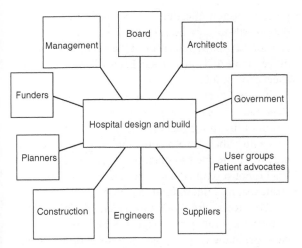

Figure 8.4 The important stakeholders involved in a hospital design and build project.

- engineers/IT consultants/electrical engineers;
- building and workforce migration specialists.

Many weeks and months of discussion and negotiation are the norm, and it is crucial to gather information, keep an open mind, be nonjudgmental, and, above all, focus on the solution.

Relatively few clinicians have the task of designing an OR facility during their career, and therefore it may seem a daunting prospect.

Site visits

A useful benchmarking exercise is to visit other recently constructed facilities. The architects engaged on the project will be specialized in the design of hospital facilities and will have previous projects available for scrutiny. These visits are vital for the success of the project for the following reasons.

- A modern hospital facility is substantially different from the current aging hospital stock. A visit demonstrates what is now possible in design and function.
- Architects tend to template the current project from recently completed works. Visiting other hospitals designed and built by the same group will help to develop the vision of the facility and also foster understanding of how they develop a project design.
- Assessment of the environmental aspects of the facility – size and shape of the rooms, corridor widths, storage, color scheme, acoustic

management, etc. – is mandatory. These are all contributors to the "feel" of the building.

- Fixtures such as pendants and booms or minimally invasive surgery (MIS) ORs can be critically appraised from a clinical perspective, with feedback from clinical staff rather than sales pitch from the company representative.
- A useful if informal cost/utility analysis can be completed on site with the staff and managers.
- Staff working in the facility can be asked to give feedback, both on their design process and an informal "post-hoc" audit of the unit. This is especially valuable for benchmarking.
- Meetings with management representatives can be scheduled to gain further feedback on strengths and weaknesses of the design.

Site visits during a project may result in significant variance to the proposed design that may require careful negotiation with architects and funders.

Process mapping

The success of the project depends on this step. It is crucial to construct a clear picture of the expected caseload, case mix, model of care, and clinical pathways for the planned facility.

If the project is a redevelopment (new hospital building within an existing complex), most processes and pathways will have evolved to fit the old facility. User groups should be given the tools to redesign the capacities and flows to match best practice, and for many this is a potentially stressful exercise requiring good leadership. Professional facilitation and change management will be required. Cultures also become established and may need some transformational change to maximize the benefits of the new facility. This should be tackled early and facilitated.

There are several process issues that have a significant bearing on design.

- Basic demographic statistics
  - Patient numbers
  - Surgical specialities
  - Future population growth/health requirements
- Proposed model(s) of care
  - Hospital inpatient, ambulatory
  - Planned surgery/unplanned/trauma
    - Dedicated unplanned surgery OR required?

- Variable utilization targets, efficiency, urgency
- Clinical pathways
  - Preadmission process
  - Planned/unplanned surgery pathways
  - Postoperative care/discharge

What will emerge is a comprehensive plan describing how the facility is to be used. That plan will then determine the overall size of the unit, the numbers and dimensions of the ORs, the size and configuration of the admission and postoperative facilities, and the requirements for staff amenities. In reality, of course, this cannot be 100% accurate given the forecasted nature of future health requirements, but the exercise of compiling a process map is invaluable when discussions commence with architects and planners and this allows staff to revalidate their own practices and benchmark off other similar organizations.

The key is to build as much flexibility into the design as possible. Most buildings have a working life of 40–50 years. Planners are not able to predict all future developments over this time span, and therefore the building will almost certainly be modified. The best designs are simple, flexible, and also fit for purpose.

Getting started

The project director will map out a process leading to sign-off for the developed design plans that will be converted into building drawings (Figure 8.5). The first step will be high-level floor plans outlining the location of wards and other units within the building. The architects will then meet with the user groups to agree a "schedule of accommodation." This is a set of documents detailing the size, shape, services, fixtures, and fittings of every room in the OR suite, down to the last power and data outlet. It is this information that the architect will use to draft the initial plans, and it goes without saying that a great deal of thought and work is required to get this correct.

The schedule will also detail the width of corridors and size of storage facilities. There are two points to remember here. The first is that storage space is often a victim of "value management," or what is more commonly known as staying on budget; adequate, well-placed storage is essential. The second point is that circulation space (corridors, reception space, etc,) should constitute approximately 35% of the total floor area of the unit (Ian Moon, architect, and McConnel, Smith and Johnson architects, Sydney, Australia,

personal communication). The schedule of accommodation will usually be presented in data-sheet form, specific to a particular room type such as an OR, an office, or a PACU bed-space. Each will have a unique sheet code number.

The architect will want a great deal of detail at this stage; success is facilitated by a clear process map and vision of the functional aspects of the proposed unit. Remember that, as with house building, architects can only design to the brief that they receive. If a detailed brief is not submitted and agreed, a stock solution will ensue that may not be fit for purpose.

Architects use computer-aided design (CAD) software to draft plans (Figure 8.6). These software packages allow very complex designs to be clearly displayed and can be redrafted relatively quickly to reflect changes. Object CAD software can now develop 3D computer models of facilities, and more recently building information modeling (BIM) has been developed as an approach to integrate design, function, budgets, and progress updates to give the project team real-time data on which to base necessary changes more efficiently. Clinicians on the project team should become familiar with these valuable tools.

A set of preliminary design plans will follow, based on the schedule of accommodation. This will be the basis of ongoing discussion and negotiation until sign-off is achieved. Involve all interested stakeholders in this stage, including surgeon representatives (often the most intermittent attendees), infection control, and the radiology service.

Issues to be decided will include:

- size and shape of the ORs and their position in the OR suite;
- environmental considerations – windows, natural light, acoustic solutions;
- position of fixtures, fittings, and services such as power, gases, and communications within rooms;
- advanced features such as magnetic resonance imaging (MRI) and MIS equipment and interventional radiology; special floors and set-downs may be required;
- support rooms for the OR (scrub bay, setup room, anesthesia induction room, cleanup room);
- location, as well as size, shape, and visibility, of the reception area and control hub for the OR coordinators and managers;
- storage areas – floor area, shape, sterile/nonsterile, co-location to ORs, shelving – fixed/mobile,

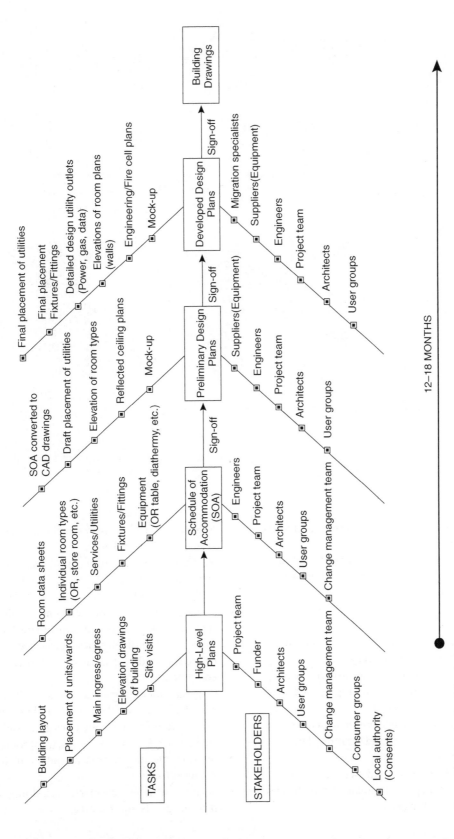

Figure 8.5 High-level building design process map.

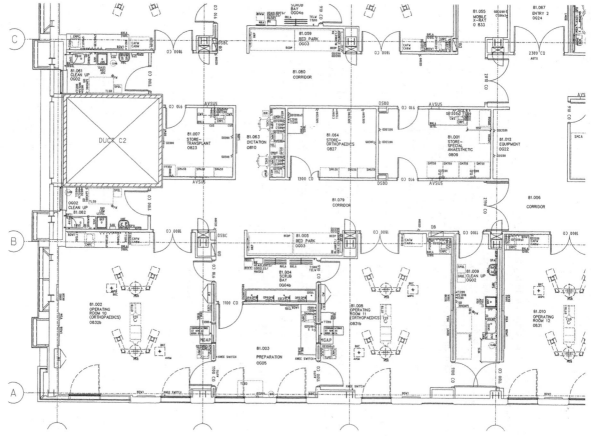

Figure 8.6 This is a developed design CAD drawing of part of the 8th level of Auckland City Hospital, New Zealand, showing the OR suite. The ORs are situated around the perimeter of the building to maximize natural light use. Reproduced with the permission of McConnel, Smith and Johnson P/L, Architects, Sydney, Australia.

required services such as IT, and power outlets for charging equipment;

- admission and postanesthesia units – location, floor area, number of patient spaces, staff base positions, fixtures and fittings;
- procedure areas for anesthesia blocks, minor procedures;
- pharmacy supply – satellite pharmacy, mobile solution, controlled drug management;
- ingress and egress routes – how the access ways are designed for patients, staff, supplies, and equipment; emergency egress;
- fire and smoke damage prevention measures;
- fire and smoke cell design and location of fire alarm control panels;
- electrical safety measures and methods – line isolation monitor (LIM), residual current devices, equipotential earthing studs;

- infection control measures, including ventilation systems and room design;
- electrical supply safety, including generator-supplied circuits, uninterruptable power supply (UPS) circuits, location and number of outlets;
- sterile supplies and processing unit – within unit or remote? (many will be remote from the OR suite); transport of sterile supplies – dedicated elevators?;
- corridors – width, clear, or allow storage of equipment?;
- single corridor design or sterile core with outer corridor for nonsterile traffic – this has major implications for many other design considerations;
- staff amenities – changerooms, meal room, offices, internet café, meeting rooms, dictation area, washrooms;
- ancillary services – cleaners, trash storage and pick-up, goods inwards area;

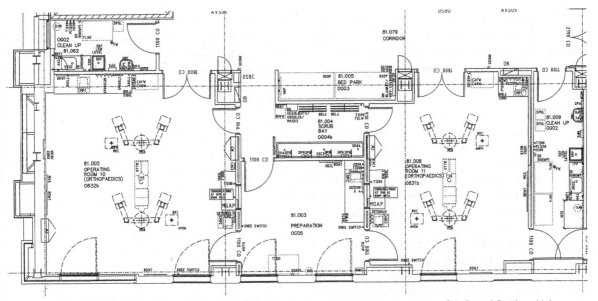

Figure 8.7 Preliminary design CAD drawing of an individual OR "pod." Reproduced with the permission of McConnel, Smith and Johnson P/L, Architects, Sydney, Australia.

- links to co-located units such as ICU, high-dependency unit (HDU), etc.;
- hospital/OR interface and substerile areas; scrubs-only areas.

Clearly, to consider all of the above (and this is not exhaustive) the users will need well-conceived plans of how the unit is to be used. Again, flexibility is the key, coupled with simplicity of design.

Throughout the process, matching of design proposals to the agreed flows and functional mapping will pay dividends. Many iterations of the plans will be circulated before sign-off; keep track of the current version to avoid confusion.

A useful exercise is a mock-up of the OR design. This can be done either in a rented industrial space or at the architect's office and will allow users and other stakeholders to view full-scale facilities and the configurations of rooms; this may avoid costly redraws of final building plans.

Operating room dimensions

There is an inexorable trend toward larger ORs as the operating team "footprint" becomes ever larger and more complex. A wide array of designs, sizes, and shapes have been described, including the so-called "barn operating rooms," where several OR areas are clustered in one physical space, separated only by retractable curtains and each with a discrete ventilation unit (Figure 8.7).

Not all ORs need to be 860 sq. ft. (80 m²), an area commonly quoted in some discussion documents. The ideal size of the room depends on the type of surgery that is proposed (and therefore the surgical footprint), the presence of ancillary facilities such as anesthesia induction rooms, and the flow within the OR itself. The configuration of the immediate OR area will also determine the numbers and positions of doors, regarded as dead space by architects when planning the configuration of a room.

At Auckland City Hospital, the largest OR is 700 sq. ft. (65 m²), and orthotopic liver transplants are comfortably undertaken in a 650 sq. ft. (60 m²) square-sided room. These rooms accommodate the surgical footprint, all of the ancillary equipment (such as C-arms and microscopes), and still have circulation space around the perimeter.

To retain flexibility, a general rule is to keep the OR fixtures such as cupboards and benches to a minimum, unless the OR is going to be used for one type of surgery only (examples would be ophthalmology surgery or endoscopic ambulatory surgery). Relatively "empty" rooms are beneficial for cleaning and infection control purposes.

Special consideration will have to be given for MIS rooms, including those housing robots. These may include such additions as specially strengthened areas on a wall on which to mount plasma screens, an adjacent area for a robotic control console, and added systems cabling behind the walls and in the ceiling space. Such MIS rooms have a software control hub that may need to be located in an adjacent space, and proprietary cabling may be required.

Utilities

Special mention should be made about the provision of power, gases, and communications in the OR.

Utility services become more complex as rooms become larger and more sophisticated. A model of utility supply must be agreed that will service the functions of the room as early as the schedule of accommodation stage. This includes the number and distribution of electrical outlets and their power source. Most, if not all, circuits will be routed through the hospital generator backup supply; a subgroup will also be routed via a battery bank that will provide UPS in the event of generator failure. This supply has a finite capacity, and users will be advised by the engineers how to match the battery bank capacity to the requirements of the unit.

Many ORs now have their power, gas, and data cabling delivered via a boom or pendant, in order to deliver the services to the center of the room and have some ability to locate the services to suit the patient orientation within the OR.

Each boom or pendant needs to be positioned appropriately in the room. There is no "correct" position, and the users need to model the room function and decide on:

- symmetrical versus asymmetrical position within the room;
- position relative to the operating table;
- articulated or fixed-arm boom/pendant, stalactite pendant;
- a solution for the anesthesia machine – freestanding on the floor, docked and lifted on the pendant, or fully pendant-mounted;
- numbers and types of power points, gas outlets, vacuum and gas scavenging connection points, and data connection sockets.

Space precludes more detailed discussion on this issue here. Most booms and pendants will have a life span of up to 20 years. Some forward thinking and engineering will reduce the chance of a costly upgrade by requesting extra data cabling and draw lines within the housing so that new cabling can be added later without major refit work. Any proprietary cabling for monitoring systems needs to be specified and supplied by the relevant company. Booms or pendants may also be used in ICU, cardiac catheter rooms, and the emergency department; the tender process will require a solution that has the flexibility to suit all locations, and other user groups will be involved in the tender process.

Operating room ventilation systems

It is only 30 years ago that some ORs had no dedicated ventilation system, and more "mature" readers may remember rooms that had opening windows to cool the rooms in summer! Many variations of design have been used since then, ranging from horizontal flow units through laminar, ultra-high-flow systems, to the down-flow hepa-filtered units of today. Engineers and designers have produced well-researched computational flow dynamic (CFD) or airflow models that appear to deliver the best ventilation and decontamination of the surgical field.

Space precludes detailed discussion on this subject. The main principles are given below.

- The OR is a plenum, relative to the corridors and ancillary rooms – that is the pressure inside is higher than outside.
- Every room should have an individual air handling unit that has independent temperature and humidity control.
- The current best model is a ceiling-mounted down-flow system with a hepa-filtered array above the patient and team with high- and low-level exhausts positioned on the ceiling and opposite walls in the room for even venting.
- The area of the filter array should match the surgical footprint if possible.
- Down-flow rates from the filters above the patient are more important than room air changes per hour (the traditional measure of effectiveness).
- High-flow rooms with large arrays should be used for surgery such as joint arthroplasty, but traditional "laminar flow" with a curtain around the surgical footprint is not necessary. Indeed, evidence is emerging in the literature of possible inferior outcomes in arthroplasty patients with excess surgical site infection rates from laminar flow rooms.
- The smooth downdraught of air will be disrupted by objects such as lights, booms, and surgical personnel and therefore will not completely wash the surgical site in a laminar fashion.

- Ventilation systems do not, of themselves, prevent infection. They produce an incremental effect in conjunction with other well-documented measures outside the scope of this chapter.

Sterile supplies and instrument processing

Formerly, OR suites had an instrument-processing and -sterilizing unit attached and were designed around a sterile processing core. Many modern facilities, in contrast, have remote surgical sterilizing departments (SSDs), and there are some examples of clusters of regional hospitals being supplied from a single remote, factory-like SSD by truck.

The design of the OR suite determines how the surgical instruments are managed. For example, if a single corridor design is designed to allow natural light into the ORs, this mandates the use of sealed case-carts to achieve separation of clean and used instruments.

A dedicated means of transportation of instruments to and from the SSD is recommended, and a backup route should be formally identified. Users also need to agree on the proportion and type of instruments that can be stored in the OR suite once processed versus those that need to be ordered from the SSD sterile instrument store as required. Flash sterilizers have been extensively used in the past but are not now regarded as best practice and should not be included in the design brief. A software solution linking the procedure booking with the surgeon preference list and the picklist in the SSD is essential, along with a smart storage solution.

The sterile supply chain and process requires a strong systems approach. Clinical staff should sign off the instrument and equipment orders, but it is immensely wasteful of time and energy to have them find missing instruments or correct errors in the picklist.

Admission unit

Ideally an admission unit should be central and close to the organizational hub of the OR. It should be easily accessed by patients and their families and be of sufficient size to cope with peak traffic. This usually occurs between about 06:00 and 08:00 h depending on the OR start pattern (same start or staggered start), which will determine the required capacity of the unit.

The admission unit can be co-located with the PACU and inpatient preoperative area to facilitate staffing flexibility and cross-functional use of space. Consult rooms or cubicles should be included for interviews, surgery-site marking, and last-minute examinations in private. Storage facility for patient records and property is essential. Access to patient records, labs, and a picture archiving and communication system (PACS) is essential for clinicians, especially if the patients have been pre-assessed outside the facility.

Postanesthesia care unit

The floor area and location of the PACU is vitally important. Patient and staff flows through the unit require formal mapping, and the interface to the rest of the building must be determined. Access to ICU and ingress for services including radiology and cardiology for postoperative investigation purposes need to be addressed. It should include a clinical station that is centrally located, capacious, and has good visibility across the unit.

Fixtures such as booms or pendants to deliver utilities into the bed space may be considered.

The PACU may be the best site for a sub-pharmacy, and it should also have its own storage area.

In large units, the recommended ratio for PACU spaces to ORs is 1.5:1, and the bed-space area should be approximately 85 sq. ft. (8–9 m²), including circulation space. In ambulatory units this ratio can be less, as patients usually progress more rapidly to a step-down unit or may bypass PACU completely. The capacity to provide patient privacy, at least visual, is important. Users may request a subgroup of HDU-type spaces with enhanced monitoring capability for extended PACU stays.

"Waste" management in the OR

Let us now return to the concept of waste in the OR process and how design may be used to mitigate this.

To recap, the seven wastes cited above are:

- waiting;
- transportation;
- defects;
- staff movement;
- inventory;
- overproduction;
- unnecessary processing.

The reader will note the change of order of the individual elements; this reflects their impact on OR suite efficiency.

Waiting

Waiting is probably the biggest source of waste in the OR. In its broadest sense, it can be embedded within all aspects of OR activity, from the admission process to PACU capacity or equipment delivery, and generally can be translated into delay or tardiness in the OR pathway.

Many groups have published papers on start times, turnover, and OR scheduling, over the past decade in particular, and the underlying objective of most has been to improve efficiency, complete more cases in a given time, reduce waiting and delays, and improve profitability by increasing contribution margins.

Areas that have been explored include:

- development of robust pre-assessment models to reduce admission times and avoid cancellations on the day of surgery;
- accurate scheduling of surgery, using historical data, to reduce tardiness and session overruns;
- solutions to shorten the turnover time between cases and improve first-case start times;
- modeling of flows through the PACU to determine capacity and minimize bed block;
- evolution of roles and responsibilities of staff to achieve greater flexibility and productivity in the workforce;
- storage, maintenance, and processing solutions for equipment and consumables.

Building design can reduce waiting and delays. The list below shows where design features in the OR suite support and facilitate improvements in flow and productivity:

- an admission unit within the suite to process pre-admitted patients on the day of surgery;
- working in parallel (see below) at the start of the day and also between cases to minimize nonoperative time;
- a PACU that is correctly located and sized to deal with the OR workload and has a discharge pathway or step-down unit to smooth flow out of the OR suite;
- well-positioned and designed storage areas.

Working in parallel – one size fits all?

Many older hospitals (particularly in the UK and Australasia) were designed and built with anesthesia

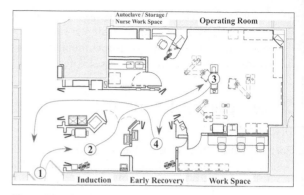

Figure 8.8 The operating room of the future; a self-contained pod of perioperative spaces, including a workspace for staff. Sandberg *et al. Anesthesiology* 2005; **103**: 406–13.

induction rooms. Induction rooms went out of vogue in many places but recent work has been exploring their place in modern practice. Induction rooms are one potential solution in the quest to reduce turnover and nonoperative times, but there are others. Marjamaa *et al.* compared five scenarios in a computer simulation [6]: the traditional model of sequential induction and surgery in the OR; use of induction rooms; use of a centralized induction area; use of an anesthesia induction team; and finally the more traditional approach to parallel processing, having four OR teams for three surgeons. They found that all of the parallel solutions outperformed the traditional model and that increased costs of personnel were balanced by increased revenue. They commented that cases of less than 2 h' duration benefit most from parallel tasking and that the best model for quality of care was the model of one anesthesia team following the patient though the whole process.

Sandberg *et al.* constructed the "operating room of the future" at Massachusetts General Hospital, with the express intent of running activities in parallel and reducing nonoperative time [7] (Figure 8.8). Patients were transferred from main admission to an induction area within the OR pod, where anesthesia was induced prior to transfer to the OR. Postsurgery, early recovery occured in a dedicated space within the pod, prior to transfer to the main PACU by perioperative nurses. This model, in conjunction with advances in technology such as mobile operating table tops and a reengineered work process, led to enhanced performance, saving around 38 min per case. Increased staff costs were largely offset by increased revenue.

Two other design models are worthy of comment. The first is the inclusion of a regional block area. This can be utilized well before the scheduled start of the operating list to insert and establish both central neuraxial and major peripheral nerve blocks and can either be staffed by the attending anesthesia team or by a separately rostered "block" team. This area is best co-located near the PACU to maximize staffing flexibility and requires adequate space and lighting to perform procedures, as well as equipment such as ultrasound imaging devices and ready access to resuscitation equipment.

The second design is a more radical solution to working in parallel and consists of an instrument preparation room attached to the OR, where the sterile instruments can be decanted and set up by the scrub personnel, either while the previous patient is emerging from anesthesia and the room is being cleaned and set up, or while a prolonged anesthesia induction and setup is undertaken in the OR. The preparation room ventilation is supplied from the same OR air handler and pressures are set such that the prep room is a plenum relative to the OR, thereby eliminating atmospheric contamination from the OR. The advantage of this model is that the patient is induced in the OR by the anesthesia team and is not moved during anesthesia. Once the patient is fully prepared and positioned, the decanted instrument trolleys are wheeled from the ultra-clean prep room into the OR and final patient checks, skin prep, draping, and surgery proceed. This is the design used at Auckland City Hospital (see Figures 8.7 and 8.9).

Using a combination of these models, Smith *et al.* set out to reduce nonoperative time and increase throughput for joint arthroplasty cases by utilizing an induction room for block insertion, a sterile setup area for instrument decanting, and a reengineering of roles within the OR team. This group achieved a 50% reduction in nonoperative time and higher throughputs that generated a positive margin greater than the incremental cost, making it a cost-effective solution [8].

It appears, then, that a parallel tasking solution is desirable – but which one? This is clearly a crucial question for any design team, as the chosen solution will require a supporting architectural design and real estate with appropriate engineering and utility services to be successful. It should be emphasized that all of the above solutions rely not only on redesign of the facility but also reengineering of processes and reassignment of staff roles. The project group should

therefore select a solution that best fits the proposed model of care.

Induction rooms seem to be most effective for relatively short cases, with shortened nonoperative times allowing extra cases to be completed in the allocated session time. For longer and more complex cases, instrument preparation rooms may be more effective, in conjunction with a regional anesthesia block insertion area. The solution is contextual and in theory may produce a mixed design model, with some ORs equipped with induction rooms and others with instrument preparation rooms in the same suite.

Transportation

Unnecessary transportation of patients, equipment, or consumables is extremely wasteful. When applied to OR design, this means ensuring that internal co-locations fit the flow of patients through the OR suite. For example, the admission unit should not be remotely located from the ORs and the PACU should be centrally located within the suite. An important but somewhat counterintuitive concept is that vertical adjacencies may be more convenient than horizontal ones in large facilities. Staff changerooms or patient admission units may be better positioned on an adjacent floor rather than at great distance on the same floor.

Operating room user groups must also decide how patients are going to be transported to and from the ORs. Routes from the emergency room and radiology need to be mapped and optimized. Bilateral meetings with the emergency room, ward, and radiology user groups are mandatory for success.

Patient transfer solutions should also be considered here. Mobile operating patient trolleys and OR table tops are available to minimize the number of patient transfers during the OR stay. These will shorten case times and potentially reduce staff injuries from manual handling of patients.

Transportation of instruments and equipment is a major logistical exercise. Many OR suites do not have the storage capacity to hold all of the instrument inventory; most are held in a clean "warehouse" facility in SSD and transported to the OR either as part of a consignment for a given session or within a case cart for an individual case.

As outlined above, the SSD is often remote from the OR suite in modern facilities, and this necessitates a robust transport solution, such as dedicated elevators or corridors into the OR suite. A secondary or step-down sterile store within the OR suite acts

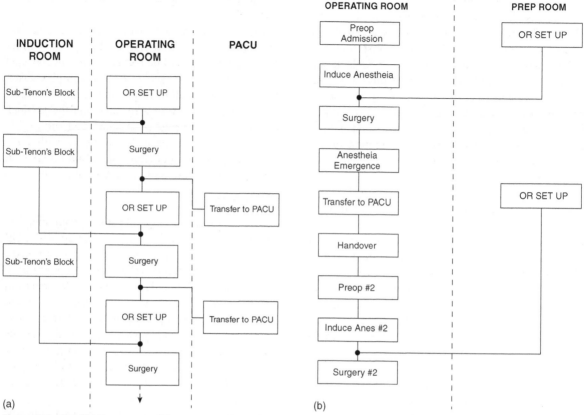

Figure 8.9 (a) and (b) These are two different process maps of OR procedures with parallel task solutions. Induction rooms are used for short rapid-turnover cases whereas instrument-preparation rooms are used for longer, more complex cases.

as the receiving area for the sterile instrument pack, and final adjustments can be made prior to transfer to the OR.

Laboratory specimens either should be processed in the OR suite (blood gas analysis or thromboelastography) or transported efficiently to the lab, for example by compressed air tube network. The route and mode of transport for emergency supplies such as blood products should also be mapped.

Staff movement

In larger OR suites, staff may spend considerable time transferring patients, sourcing supplies, and travelling to and from staff amenities, changerooms, etc. During the early planning stages, take some time to map out staff flows during the working day. The architect's plans (Figure 8.10) will end up with a myriad of coloured lines as different staff members in the user group map their day, but it will yield very valuable information, detailing how the staff will need to move within

the unit, and may lead to rearrangement of subunits to minimize unnecessary movement. The solution will be optimized only in conjunction with a review of staff roles and process reengineering.

Surgeons have gaps in their operating day during the nonoperative phase of the OR list. Office space close by the OR (see Figure 8.8) will allow them to complete some office work and also help to keep them in close proximity and available for the next case. This need only be an alcove with a desk and IT hub but will be appreciated and cost-effective. The communication platform in the OR suite will be covered later in the chapter.

Most other innovations to reduce waste in this area are outside the scope of this chapter and will be dealt with elsewhere in the book.

Reducing defects

Reducing defects is a key feature of LSS processing and in the OR relates to issues such as patient cancellation,

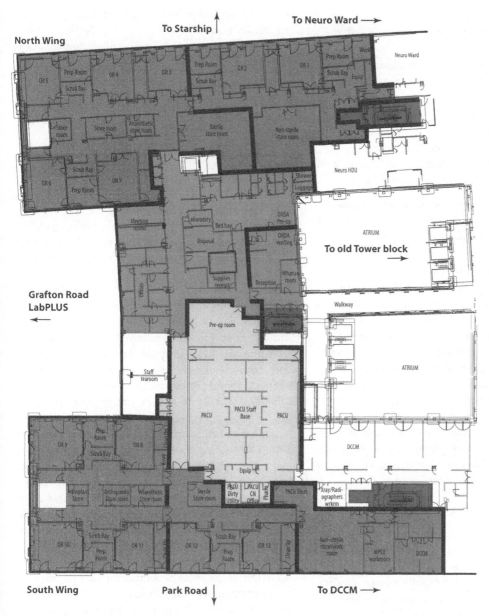

Figure 8.10 This shaded plan is used to map out transport flows and staff movement. The main ingress/egress routes are center right. There is a single-corridor design. The admission and PACU areas are central and the ORs and staff areas are on the perimeter of the building. Reproduced with the permission of McConnel, Smith and Johnson P/L, Architects, Sydney, Australia.

wrong-site surgery, equipment defects, incorrect information, and scheduling errors. Access to patient information to reduce cancellation and re-work has been discussed above.

Most of the measures to reduce defects involve reengineering, and redesigning processes and building design features are mostly related to flow and capacity. Are the admission unit and the PACU large enough cope with peak traffic? How is the ICU

capacity calculated to prevent bed block and OR cancellation?

Inventory and storage

This aspect of design and planning will be mostly about the interface between the ORs, materials management, goods inwards, and SSD; representatives of these services should be involved in planning.

The goals are:

- to establish storage floor area and location in the OR suite;
- to map out transport of instruments and consumables to and from the storage areas;
- to delineate sterile and nonsterile storage areas;
- to negotiate a robust supply chain and minimize inventory held in-house;
- to perform a "5S – sort, set, shine, standardize, sustain" exercise to optimize layout, shelving solution, and sustainability of design in the storage areas.

This section also includes pharmacy imprest and supply chain mapping. A satellite pharmacy will save time and effort for the OR and anesthesiology staff.

Overprocessing/overproduction

These two wastes are probably of least relevance to OR design. They refer mainly to process issues but can be of relevance in terms of matching process to design. An example of waste here would be an admission unit that was too small to deal with batched admissions at 06:00 h for the start of the day. The solution is that either the unit has to be designed to fit the process or the process has to be altered to support, for example, staggered OR starts.

Overprocessing refers to developing an overcomplicated process when dealing with a simple problem and has little relevance to building design, other than mapping out flows through the unit and as a general principle when signing off plans.

Communication platforms in the OR

With the advent of health information technology (HIT), the handling of data and information in health care has been revolutionized over the past decade. Patient records are rapidly becoming digitized (as are laboratory and radiology data) and stored in vast data warehouses. Clinical records departments are fast becoming IT portals instead of storage facilities.

Within the OR suite, IT platforms are used for:

- logging patient procedures and time stamps for throughput and financial management;
- promulgating the OR workload with scheduling software;
- ordering sterile supplies and instruments;
- creating electronic health records during procedures (both surgical and anesthesia), including dictation of procedure record;

- computerized provider order entry for medications;
- accessing patient information, including labs and radiology;
- image generation and management from MIS rooms, including real-time Internet transmission;
- generating reports of OR activity for staff/management/board;
- logging incidents for investigation/audit;
- researching patient pathology or drug information via the Internet and online library.

It will be apparent from the above list that the physical design of the network within the building and the OR suite is vitally important. It is the OR process that should dictate the IT requirements and design, rather than the converse.

Developments in HIT move with great rapidity, making future proofing the network problematic. However, if the building is designed with future modification in mind, the network will be relatively easily upgraded.

Currently, most hospitals are constructed with a core network of fiber-optic conduit interfacing with copper cabling to individual outlets. Wireless and mobile solutions are also becoming more prevalent, as are "cloud-computing" solutions, in which software platforms and data storage are supplied by a third party. Data warehousing and large servers will often be offsite and should be considered as a continuity issue for ORs.

Timely access to primary-care patient information for hospital staff remains a challenge. Here HIT applications will certainly enhance overall care and reduce re-work. During the design drawing phase, users will need to specify how the IT solutions will be used (the bullet-point list above includes potential uses), and therefore which network components are required.

Contemporary ORs may have as many as five or six hardware units within them (PCs, PACS, image management systems), all requiring intranet cabled or wireless connections. As wireless and cloud solutions develop, hardware and cable requirements should diminish.

Another mode of communication within the OR is the call system for house staff or orderlies and in the event of a critical incident. The physical design of the call buttons and their location in the OR need some thought, as does the method of communicating with and requesting assistance from outside the OR; this can be auditory, visual, or both.

Visibility of information within the OR will help to reduce both unnecessary staff movement and defects. If, for example, the registered nurse in the OR can see the instrument picklist from SSD online for the next case, he or she will not have to leave the OR to verify availability in person. If the anesthesiologist can see the labs and echocardiography report of the next patient online in the OR, a delay or cancellation may be avoided.

Building life span and renovation

Future proofing the design

Throughout this chapter, the emphasis has been on simplicity and flexibility. Most buildings completed today will have a useful life of 40–50 years and will almost certainly require alteration and refurbishment at some time. The preferred building format at present is to have a structural lattice of concrete or steel beams with concrete or steel beam floors at about 5-m intervals and suspended false ceilings to give room heights of about 3 m. The room design and layout within this lattice is usually achieved with a plasterboard or dry-wall solution. This gives the building great flexibility of design and allows alterations to be easily completed. The ceiling space contains much of the infrastructure installations such as air-handler units, plumbing, gas piping, and fixture supports and can be accessed easily for upgrades and repairs.

Future proofing the capacity of the building is also desirable. Population-based intervention rates almost inevitably lead to expansion of the facility but initial fit-out of all spaces may not be justified in the first few years. Modern building design allows that spaces such as future ORs can be built to a shell stage with services to the space but no fit-out of walls, ceiling, or fixtures, saving initial cost and matching expansion costs to increased revenue at a later stage. The space can be utilized as storage until required. Fit-out can often be achieved with little or no disruption to activity as the external cladding of the building can be removed to facilitate building and installation work.

Many buildings are also designed to support the construction of an additional floor, if required at a future date.

The relatively open design of modern buildings also means that refits of IT hubs and networks are comparatively straightforward.

Renovating an existing building

Renovating an existing building presents a fresh set of potential barriers to success, as the building frame is likely to feature:

- solid wall construction, requiring major demolition work;
- very limited ceiling space for infrastructure refit, such as air-handler units;
- low ceiling height – problematic for modern ceiling-mounted fixtures such as pendants/booms or operating lights;
- limited ducting for utility upgrades;
- poor flow design and co-locations of rooms;
- limited OR and PACU floor area;
- remote staff amenities.

Careful evaluation early in the project will determine whether the building can be made "fit for purpose." It may be more cost-effective to demolish and build new.

If the decision is to renovate, all of the considerations for a new build pertain, but good problem solving may be required to remediate the building limitations. Often, the full extent of required work is not apparent until the actual demolition and construction has commenced, and therefore the project team needs to build flexibility into the project schedule as well as contingency funding if required for extra works.

Renovation solutions rarely achieve all the design objectives possible in the new building, but with an expert design and build team a satisfactory outcome is possible. Many older buildings will have redundant areas, often vertically adjacent to the proposed renovation that can, when refitted with modern transport solutions, become useful ancillary space for the OR suite. Relocating the SSD off-floor will liberate valuable clinical space within the OR suite, for example. Construction of enlarged air-handler units and cabling for fixtures in the limited ceiling space presents a particular challenge, but again, careful design with the engineers will yield acceptable solutions.

From plans to procedures

Staying in touch

Clinical user groups commonly comment on exclusion from the building process once the design drawings had been signed off. There is usually an 18-month to 2-year construction and fit-out phase for a large installation, and user groups must remain in touch with the process. They will mostly be involved in planning any migration program but should also be taken on site visits on a regular basis.

Clinicians seconded to the building project need to remain involved as integrated members of the team. Engineering schedules will require review, and real-time problem solving is an almost everyday event, as those who have been involved in a domestic building project will attest.

Translation from drawing to framing is never 100%, and careful site visits will pick up inaccuracies, such as a missing doorframe or a floor construction anomaly. Horizon-scanning for new technology should continue throughout the project, as last-minute infrastructure may be required before walls or ceilings are finalized. Budget and timeline variances may require clinician input to problem solve and prioritize negotiable and non-negotiable positions that only clinical experience and contacts can finesse.

Tenders for fixtures such as booms and equipment such as case-carts and anesthesia machines also require attention, with clear, agreed tender processes and objectives.

Handover of the facility from the construction team requires many hours of work to complete facility and utility systems checks prior to migration. Clinical engineering and infection control units must formally sign off the facility as fit for use.

Migration

The organization will hire a specialist migration team to move staff and patients into the new building. This process will take up to a year before the moving date to plan, and clinical scenarios should be modeled to cover any eventuality, including systems failures. Trialing the new ORs prior to moving date is essential, as is a formal sign-off of all the systems and utilities in the OR suite. Successful migration requires meticulous planning and execution and almost merits a dedicated chapter.

Summary

In this chapter, we have explored the concept of design for OR efficiency. We have looked at the potential for good design to reduce or eliminate wasteful process in the OR and we have suggested steps for a successful design process.

The clear message here is that the design of the OR suite should:

- reflect and support the flows and processes, as determined by the organization;

- establish simplicity and flexibility as the two main guiding principles;
- provide a safe environment that fosters quality health outcomes.

The theme throughout has been that design, process, and function cannot and should not be considered as separate entities; they are integral parts of hospital building solutions that, today more than ever, are required to deliver productive, efficient, and effective health outcomes.

Acknowledgments

I thank Associate Professor Simon Mitchell and Drs. Charles Bradfield and Chris Chambers for their editorial and proofreading skills and Ms Diane Newby and Ms Karen Patching for their help in preparing the illustrations.

References

1. J. J. Pandit, S. Westbury, M. Pandit. The concept of surgical list "efficiency": a formula to describe the term. *Anaesthesia* 2007; **62**: 895–903.

2. A. Macario. Are your operating rooms efficient? A scoring system with eight performance indicators. *Anesthesiology* 2006; **105**: 237–40.

3. J. J. Pandit, D. Stubbs, M. Pandit. Measuring the quantitative performance of surgical operating lists: theoretical modelling of "productive potential" and "efficiency". *Anaesthesia* 2009; **64**: 473–86.

4. E. Litvak, M. Long. Cost and quality under managed care: Irreconcilable differences? *Am J Manag Care* 2000; **6**: 305–12.

5. NHS Institute for Innovation and Improvement. The seven wastes of Lean. NHS Institute for Innovation and Improvement, 2008. Available from: www.institute.nhs.uk/quality_and_service_improvement_tools/ (last accessed May 2, 2012).

6. R. Marjamaa, P. Torkki, E. Hirvensalo, O. Kirvela. What is the best workflow for an operating room? A simulation study of five scenarios. *Health Care Manag Sci* 2009; **12**: 142–6.

7. W. Sandberg, B. Daily, M. Egan, J. Stahl, J. Goldman, R. Wiklund, D. Rattner. Deliberate perioperative systems design improves operating room throughput. *Anesthesiology* 2005; **103**: 406–18.

8. M. Smith, W. Sandberg, J. Foss, K. Massoli, M. Kanda, W. Barsoum, A. Schubert. High-throughput operating room system for joint arthroplasties durably outperforms routine processes. *Anesthesiology* 2008; **109**: 25–35.

Chapter

9

Operating room design and construction
Technical considerations

Judy Dahle MS, MSG, RN
Pat Patterson

Introduction   95
Strategic program planning   95
New construction or renovation?   96
The planning and design team   96
Phases of a project   97
Considerations for operational processes   98
Design of individual ORs   102
Equipment planning   103

Infection prevention during
construction   104
Interim life safety measures   104
New technology/integrated ORs   105
Hybrid ORs   105
Design considerations for ambulatory surgical
centers   106
Summary   106

Introduction

For most operating room (OR) leaders, the planning and design of a new surgical suite happens only once or twice in their careers. More than likely, these responsibilities will be added to their normal duties. These complex, multiyear projects are demanding, and there is a great deal to learn and apply within a short time. The projects call for a variety of strengths, including strong organizational skills, the ability to collaborate with other disciplines, and the ability to manage complex projects with deadlines.

Surgery is always a team effort. That's particularly true for an OR design and construction project. The success of the entire project, from the initial meetings to the final approval and move in, depends on the collaboration among multiple disciplines. That includes not only the clinical disciplines of surgery, anesthesia, nursing, and related disciplines but also the design and construction professions. Working with a multidisciplinary team can be a major benefit because it provides a support system for decision making and an educational opportunity for the OR manager and the entire surgical team. Whether the OR director is a novice or experienced, a key to staying organized is to break the project into phases and to develop a checklist for each phase.

Several essential resources can provide guidance throughout the project. These include the *Guidelines for Design and Construction of Health Care Facilities* from the Facility Guidelines Institute [1], *Planning, Design, and Construction of Health Care Facilities* by the Joint Commission [2], and guidelines and standards of the Association for Professionals in Infection Control and Epidemiology [3], among others.

Strategic program planning

The building or remodeling of OR suites is a demanding and expensive undertaking. Whether the project is to renovate a current suite or build new ORs, it is important to think about the organization's long-term direction and how that will influence the design and efficiency of the surgical suite. The challenge for management and the design teams is to envision how surgery will be performed in the future. How will new and emerging technology affect the services provided? How will work processes be affected by technology? What will the patient population be like within the next five to ten years? Will the hospital's admissions have a higher percentage of geriatric patients requiring complex surgical care? Are there programs in the community promoting diet and weight loss, which may bring

Operating Room Leadership and Management, ed. Kaye A.D., Fox C.J. and Urman R.D. Published by Cambridge University Press. © Cambridge University Press 2012.

a new bariatric program to the hospital? It is crucial for the organization to define its goals and strategies clearly so that the design team may plan for OR processes that will support an efficient, safe, and cost-effective care delivery system for many years.

The first step in the planning process may be to conduct a needs analysis that will help drive decisions throughout the process. In a needs analysis, all of the surgical, anesthesia, and support services identify goals and discuss their anticipated needs for the future. Multiple meetings are needed to gather input from each surgical specialty and anesthesia providers. As part of the analysis, management must identify the reason for the construction: is it to expand space for increasing surgical volume, to redesign the facility for emerging technologies, to better compete with neighboring facilities, to anticipate new services, or to respond to changes in the health-care delivery model?

The OR leadership team plays a crucial role in strategic planning. They will be asked for data regarding types and volume of procedures. Operating room directors experienced in this process also recommend gathering detailed financial and market information, including trends, projections for volumes, and case types as well as profitability information [4].

Many more questions need to be addressed during the planning phase, such as:

- What are the market demographics?
- What will provide the competitive edge?
- What level of technology will be required?
- What are the pros and cons of the technology costs?
- How much functional space is needed for each OR suite?
- Will there be specialty rooms?
- How much storage will be required?
- Where will storage be located?
- What will the traffic flow be like and how efficient will it be? [4]

Detailed questions for each area, specialty, and technology will be addressed later in the design process, when the masterplanning and design concepts are in place. An effective planning process is essential for the success of the completed project. A successful project will have been designed to be flexible and adaptable for the future. Although trends cannot be predicted with certainty, detailed multidisciplinary planning can help to avoid major design mistakes.

New construction or renovation?

As part of the planning process, management may want to evaluate whether to build new OR suites or renovate existing space. A variety of conditions affect the feasibility of renovation, such as:

- the amount and type of space available for renovation;
- mechanical and electrical system limitations;
- ability to work within the existing building's boundaries;
- location of columns and structural walls;
- location of vertical penetrations, such as mechanical shafts, elevators, and fire stairs.

In some cases, organizations can renovate and convert existing space for less money than they can build new space. Often, renovation costs may exceed new construction costs because of unforeseen conditions, phasing, scheduling, or logistical complexities. There are several issues to consider.

- Converting existing space to new functions frequently requires working with room dimensions, structural grids, and building configurations that force compromises to meet the needs and goals of the project.
- Remodeling often triggers the need to upgrade existing structures to meet current building code requirements. This in turn increases construction costs.
- Renovation can cause disruption of ongoing normal operations and require the relocation of services. Coordination of temporary relocation of services and the sequencing of events on the overall time line may make remodeling more time-consuming than new construction.
- A renovation project may trigger correction of accessibility deficiencies in areas of the facility remote from the proposed renovation.
- A partial renovation can result in the need for dual systems, which may increase operating costs and staff confusion [2].

The planning and design team

The planning and design team should consist of a core group that will remain consistent throughout all phases of the project. The team needs a level of ownership and commitment to the project. The organization's representatives should be a multidisciplinary group from the relevant areas of the facility. The professional consultants on the team include those who will execute the planning, design, and construction. The size of the team varies with the complexity of the project. Additional members function in an advisory role and may attend only certain meetings that require their expertise.

Core members include:

- a representative from administration;
- physicians;
- nurses;
- infection preventionist;
- facilities planning/engineering;
- architects;
- engineers;
- finance.

Members who provide additional input at times throughout the project:

- contractor;
- equipment/technology planners;
- materials management;
- laboratory staff;
- support services;
- pharmacy staff;
- interior designers;
- landscape designers for new facilities.

An empowered leader from the organization needs to be selected and given the responsibility to keep the process moving forward, on time and within budget. The leader will establish the communication process. This person needs to have facilitation skills and to be a good manager of people, flexible, and responsive to sudden changes.

One person from the consultant role, usually an architect, will take the leadership role for coordinating the members representing consulting services. Frequently, this person is helpful in determining when to ask the advisory or additional members to participate in meetings.

A representative of the architectural firm usually takes the minutes of each meeting, which initially may be weekly, and distributes them to members of the planning and design team. In addition, the architect in collaboration with the organization's representatives develops and maintains an organizational tool such as a project evaluation and review technique (PERT) chart. A PERT chart diagrams the project activities and identifies critical tasks, milestones, projected timelines, and primary responsibility for each of the activities. This

tool is helpful for the entire team to identify delegated tasks, tasks not assigned, and tasks that may delay the project.

The organization develops a budget as part of the initial preplanning that is revised as the project moves forward and changes are made. The budget is developed in several segments: construction costs, equipment costs, professional fees, escalation fees, and contingency costs. As a guide, a project cost checklist is available for download from Joint Commission Resources at www.jcrinc.com/PDC09/Extras.

The nurse leader is the clinical expert on the team. All team members look to the nurse leader for recommendations and input about the appropriateness of the design with respect to regulatory requirements from accrediting bodies, state health departments, and others; space allotment; patient safety; and interdepartmental functions, to name a few of the areas of expertise. It is nursing's opportunity to design an environment that is safe for patients and staff, is efficient, meets the needs of the physicians, and meets the mission and vision of the organization.

The nurse leader has a prominent role as a member of the planning and design team. Initially, this may seem like a daunting task that adds to an already full workload. Although the project may seem overwhelming to a nurse leader who is not familiar with design and construction, it provides a great leadership opportunity. Involving everyone who will be directly affected by the construction and will be working in the new or remodeled area is essential. Collaborating with staff members in the process allows them to feel a sense of ownership in the building effort [5]. Communication about the project with nursing, physician, and support staff helps decrease the staff's stress about the project and brings helpful ideas to the design process. The staff can provide valuable ideas in relation to storage and supply access, types of case carts, OR furniture, and cabinets as well as the location of electrical outlets, data ports, and other design items that affect patient flow. Direct-care providers can provide the best input regarding design aspects that will improve safety and efficiency. Nurses who are participating in design and construction for the first time will find that the design team members are willing to share their expertise.

Phases of a project

Design and construction projects typically follow six phases.

Planning

The planning phase includes the wish list considerations, masterplanning, setting the vision, and the needs analysis. This is the time to gather input from each specialty and to hold meetings with the staff to find out what they envision for the new OR and what the positive and negatives of the current OR may be.

Site visits to other facilities are helpful because they provide OR leaders with an opportunity to see completed ORs and talk to the personnel to learn what works well in their facility and what they would have done differently. It is helpful to take a multidisciplinary group on the site visit.

Schematic

The schematic phase involves drawing a rough outline of the project, including a preliminary room layout, structure, and scope of the project. At this time, the architect begins to prepare diagrams that display the major functions, the structural components, and the approximate size needed for the various functions. The planning and design team members provide important input at this time. There are frequent meetings during this phase with brainstorming and many probing discussions with the architectural firm. A detailed list of ideas is collected, and the architect will develop more in-depth drawings from each of these sessions.

Design development

In design development, details are added to the design drawings, including electrical outlets, data ports, furniture location, fixtures, and details regarding casework, hardware, and decor. This phase takes several meetings, with frequent revision to the plans. The design team should ask many questions and review the plans closely. Every detail of the finished facility needs to be included at this time. The final design is reviewed by the planning team. Then the key decision makers from the organization approve and sign the final plans before they are converted to construction documents. Once this phase is completed, making revisions incurs additional costs.

Construction documents

During the construction documents phase, all aspects of the design are converted into building plans that a contractor can use to estimate costs, identify issues, and plan construction activities. These documents will be used throughout the construction phase and are used to obtain building permits for the project. At this point, the organization discusses contract conditions with the contractor and the architect. Roles and responsibilities of all participants are defined. During this phase, the design team does not meet as often, and there may be less communication between the architect and other team members. At this time, the architectural firm is detailing the drawings in preparation for the bidding process with the builders.

Construction

During the construction phase, the OR suite is actually built. Before the construction begins, the design team should meet with the contractors to discuss final preparation. These discussions need to include site security, contractor education, storage of materials, barrier placement, infection prevention, and the communication process to be used during the project. Frequent visits to the site, when appropriate, by planning and design team members is advisable. It is important to ask questions at this time. Sometimes what the team saw on the drawings does not look the same during construction. Ask for clarification and explanation of the construction process. Weekly construction meetings provide an opportunity for effective communication and education throughout the project.

Commissioning

Before taking ownership of a building, project, or renovation, the organization must make sure: all specifications are met; all requirements are in order for licensure; and all systems, components, equipment, are operational [2]. Plumbing; electrical systems; heating, ventilating, and air conditioning (HVAC) systems; fire alarms; and safety systems will be tested at this time.

Considerations for operational processes

General considerations for OR suites

The size and location of the surgical suite will be determined by the level of care provided. The number of ORs and postanesthesia care unit (PACU) beds and the size of the support areas are governed by the expected workload. Current and future workloads by specialty should have been determined during the preplanning and planning phases (Table 9.1).

Table 9.1 OR design: General principles

Make each OR at least 600 square feet, larger for cardiovascular, orthopedic, and other complex procedures. (The *Guidelines for Design and Construction of Healthcare Facilities* recommend a minimum of 400 square feet of clear floor space for general ORs, with a minimum of 600 square feet for ORs performing surgical procedures that require additional personnel and/or large equipment, such as some cardiovascular, orthopedic, and neurosurgical procedures.)

Make the ORs identical to avoid staff having to adjust to new positions and item locations.

Install adequate wiring, ventilation, and structural reinforcement to accommodate equipment.

Design ORs for multiple uses because case loads and surgical techniques may change.

Include communication tools such as wall monitors and e-mail stations in OR design.

Make storage space adequate and rapidly accessible; avoid distant storerooms, or expect more onsite hoarding of supplies.

Design logistics for smooth supply transport and protection of sterile items.

Design patient transport routes and waiting locations to provide comfort, privacy, and the growing trend toward the presence of family members.

Source: Reprinted with permission from *OR Manager*. 2011;27(5):13. Copyright 2011 Access Intelligence. All rights reserved.

The major physical activities of the surgical suite are divided into unrestricted, semi-restricted, and restricted areas.

- The unrestricted area includes a central control point established to monitor the entrance of patients, personnel, and materials. Street clothes are permitted in this area. The preoperative holding area is classified as unrestricted, which allows family members the option of remaining with patients before surgery.
- The semi-restricted area includes the peripheral support areas of the surgical suite. The area has storage for clean and sterile supplies, work areas for storage and processing of instruments, scrub sink areas, and corridors leading to the restricted areas. This area is limited to personnel and patients and requires surgical attire.
- The restricted area includes ORs, procedure rooms, and the clean core (the clean supply and instrument area). Surgical attire is required, and masks are required where there are open sterile supplies and scrub persons [1].

Evidence-based design

Evidence-based design (EBD) is a recent concept fostered by the Center for Health Design (www.health-design.org) [6]. In EBD, design and construction are based as much as possible on research evidence, with the goal of producing the best possible outcomes for patients, families, and staff while improving the process of care. The evidence suggests that standardization is one aspect of design that improves patient safety by reducing the risk of errors. For example, when facilities such as ORs are oriented the same way, the staff knows where equipment and supplies are kept. The surgical team knows how the patient will be oriented in the room, reducing the risk of wrong-side surgery. Less time is spent looking for supplies and equipment, which reduces rework, minimizes fatigue, and allows caregivers to focus on direct patient care. Standardization also improves efficiency and productivity and lowers costs [6].

Patient flow considerations

The smooth flow of patients from the admitting area to the preoperative holding area, to the individual OR suite, and into the PACU depends partially on an efficient facility design. The planning for patient flow should consider the experience not only of patients but also of family members who accompany the patient on the day of surgery. Patients need to be prepared and wait for surgery in a private environment, where the family may stay with them until they are taken into the OR. There also needs to be a quiet area where medical staff can discuss medical issues with the patient and a quiet, comfortable area where families can wait during the procedure. New facilities are often designed with family waiting areas that have features such as natural light, comfortable furniture, data ports and wireless Internet access, and play areas for children.

The decision for private rooms or bays in the preoperative area is influenced by the size of the area, the ability to provide patient care efficiently, and the impact of the choice on staffing levels. A common design for patient cubicles is three walls with a curtain across the foot of the bay. This allows patient privacy but provides efficiency and visibility for the nursing staff.

The immediate preoperative area (holding area) needs space to accommodate both patients on stretchers and ambulatory patients who are seated. This area needs to be under the direct visual control of the nursing staff. Provision needs to be made for patients with transmissible infections, developed in collaboration with the infection prevention department. Consideration also needs to be given to the patient mix and the surgical program. Space may be needed for additional equipment, depending on the surgical program planned.

The planning phase for the preoperative space is an opportunity to evaluate spaces that may be used as cross-functional areas during the day. For example, a portion of the PACU may be used as part of the preoperative holding area during the first part of the day. This arrangement can contribute to efficient staffing, particularly if the staff is cross-trained for both preoperative and postanesthesia care, and may decrease the amount of space required for the preoperative holding area.

The planning phase is also the appropriate time to design the communication and documentation systems for the new area, which can have a positive impact on efficiency, safety, and patient and staff satisfaction. The use of information technology can make for a quieter work area, fewer interruptions, and an opportunity for more efficient patient flow. These are examples of how information technology may provide for an improved environment:

- airport-style tracking systems enable the staff to see the status of individual OR suites, help the staff to anticipate the patient flow, communicate with other departments such as the critical care unit, and keep families informed of patients' progress;
- wireless communication systems using small phones or badges may be installed to facilitate communication among the nursing staff;
- audiovisual systems allow surgeons to communicate with the radiology and pathology departments more efficiently and clearly.

Design of postanesthesia care areas

There are specific space requirements for both Phase I and Phase II recovery areas. The Phase I level of care

applies to patients in immediate postanesthetic recovery in which a 1:1 or 1:2 nurse:patient ratio is maintained, depending on the patient's status, until the patient meets the "critical elements," as recommended by the American Society of PeriAnesthesia Nurses. During Phase II, care focuses on preparation of the patient and family for discharge to home or extended care [7].

The *Guidelines for Design and Construction of Health Care Facilities* [1] recommend a separate area for Phase 1 and Phase II postanesthesia care, such as a separate step-down area, but this is not always possible because of space. The first concern is to follow the appropriate level of care while maintaining patient privacy.

Maintaining privacy in the preoperative and postoperative areas is a challenge because of limited space. Many facilities have cubicles with three walls and a sliding glass door or a privacy curtain. Others provide separate enclosed patient rooms for preoperative care and discharge preparation, but this design does not provide the flexibility required for efficient patient flow and presents a staffing challenge.

There are general requirements such as medication stations, handwashing stations, a nurses' station, charting facility, and storage allocations [1]. Involving the PACU staff in planning this area is beneficial because they can provide valuable information about what functions well in the current facility and what does not. The design of the PACU also depends on the functional program. Examples of issues to be considered are whether the PACU will accommodate pediatric patients, intensive care patients, and family visitation and whether the area will care for inpatients as well as outpatients.

Materials flow

Surgery consumes a large volume of supplies and instrumentation. How these materials are supplied and distributed through the facility has a major bearing on the surgical suite's overall efficiency and on the cost of care.

The flow of materials needs to be planned so that the movement of clean and sterile supplies and instruments is separated from contaminated items and waste by space or traffic patterns [8]. The clean storage space needs to be in a moisture- and temperature-controlled area that is free from cross-traffic. The soiled area cannot have direct connection with the ORs. Involving the staff from materials management and sterile processing as well as the OR staff who are most directly involved in supply distribution is important to planning a successful materials flow.

There are several issues to consider for surgical supplies.

- How will supplies be received in the surgical suite? Is there a separate area outside the suite to break down shipping containers so that only the clean inner packaging enters the suite?
- What supply chain system will be used for delivery, control, and replenishment of supplies?
- How will supplies be transported to the surgical area and to the individual ORs?
- How much and what type of storage will be needed to accommodate this system, both in the suite and in the individual ORs? Where will sterile supplies be stored so that their sterility is not compromised?
- After surgery, how will soiled trash be removed from the suite and stored so that patients and clean areas are not exposed to contaminated materials?

There are also several issues to consider for surgical instrumentation.

- Where will instrumentation be processed? In some hospitals, sterile processing is performed within the semi-restricted area of the surgical department. In this case, the size and location of the clean and soiled workrooms will be determined in the functional program. In other hospitals, sterile processing is performed outside the suite. In this case, direct but separate paths should be planned between the surgical suite and sterile processing area for both clean and soiled instrumentation. For example, the surgical suite may be on a floor above the sterile processing area, with dedicated clean and soiled elevators connecting the two units.
- Will the surgical suite perform sterilization on an emergency basis? If so, sterilization facilities need to be provided in an area readily accessible to the ORs that complies with guidelines for immediate-use steam sterilization (formerly called flash sterilization). Immediate-use sterilization refers to the processing of items intended to be used immediately and not stored. This process requires the same critical reprocessing steps as any other sterilization cycle, including cleaning, decontamination, and transport of sterilized items [9].

Equipment storage

Equipment storage is always a challenge. Today's surgical procedures require a variety of large, portable equipment such as X-ray machines, stretchers, fracture tables, and warming devices. All of these must be stored in locations that are convenient to the ORs but must be kept out of corridors and away from traffic [1]. If the surgical suite will be large with specialized ORs, the storage spaces should be readily accessible to the specialized rooms. In new construction, recessed space is frequently planned outside each OR for the storage of a stretcher. Other areas may be designed for large items such as X-ray machines. In developing the functional program, the planning and design team should list all of the equipment the surgical suite is likely to include and how frequently it is used. That list should be available for reference as the design is developed.

Staff support areas

The design of staff support areas can have a major impact on staff satisfaction. These areas include places for changing from street clothes to surgical attire and a lounge for breaks and lunch. The changing areas are required to have lockers, showers, toilets, handwashing stations, and space to change clothing [1].

The lounge area is intended to minimize the need for staff to leave the surgical suite for breaks and meals and to provide convenient access for both the OR and the PACU staff. The decision about whether to have a combined or separate lounge for physician, nursing, or ancillary staff usually depends on the amount of available space and the philosophy of the organization. There are also regulations for these areas that vary by state and locality.

Although much of the surgical suite design focuses on functionality and efficiency, the design of staff support areas should also consider comfort and aesthetics. The staff's participation is essential in planning an area that will suit their needs. A combination of eating area, lounge, and kitchen is most desirable. If there is an opportunity, the lounge should have windows to allow for natural light and an outside view. Selection of furniture is important for comfort and function. Color selection should consider gender as well as generational, cultural, and geographical preferences.

Ancillary department coordination

The physical relationship between the surgical suite and supporting departments is an important consideration. The planning teams needs to consider the surgical program and identify all of the services that may be required for each specialty. Generally, the ORs should be located close to the emergency department, radiology department, cardiac catheterization laboratory, and clinical and pathology laboratories. The PACU should be located so that patients can be transported easily to the intensive care units. Representatives from pharmacy, interventional radiology, and any department that routinely provides services to the surgical department should be included in discussions about location and information technology that may assist in the coordination of care.

Design of individual ORs

Space requirements

A general operating room is required to be at least 400 sq. ft. with a minimum clear dimension of 20 feet between fixed cabinets and built-in shelves, according to the *Guidelines for Design and Construction of Health Care Facilities* [1]. Operating rooms for surgical procedures requiring additional personnel and/or large equipment such as cardiovascular, orthopedic, and neurological procedures, require 600 sq. ft. Many hospitals are designing all of the operating rooms to accommodate the latest technology and equipment, allowing for flexibility in scheduling procedures into any room. The larger rooms, in addition to accommodating the many pieces of equipment today's surgery requires, provide adequate room for the staff to move, allowing for better staff circulation and greater efficiency. Larger rooms also allow clearance for patient transport and the movement of portable equipment. In addition, they provide space for a sitting workstation, where clinicians can document care electronically and manage controls for digital imaging and other technology.

Ceiling-mounted booms

The use of ceiling-mounted booms in ORs enables equipment and related cords to be kept off the floor, decreasing clutter and allowing for safer movement around the room [10]. In new construction, the space above the ceiling can be designed to include conduit to accommodate utilities and the necessary cabling for equipment mounted on the booms. If the ORs are being remodeled, engineers must assess the ceiling structure to determine the weight-load capabilities before planning to install ceiling-mounted booms. It is a good idea to provide additional capacity to meet future needs.

Retractable utility columns for anesthesia providers provide an efficient, well-organized service area at each end of the room. The columns house medical gases, phone jacks, and data connections. The columns do not eliminate the need for a small anesthesia cart but provide another means to keep the floor free of cords.

Proper placement of ceiling-mounted equipment booms is crucial. Booms should be placed on the side of the room away from the OR door, where patients enter the room. The articulating arms need to move freely and not interfere with movement of the surgical lights. Physicians and staff who perform minimally invasive video-guided surgery can provide valuable insight on placement of booms and should be involved in site visits to view established facilities. Computer-aided design and simulation are also helpful in visualizing the placement of booms.

Configuration of the OR

During the design process, it is helpful to create a schematic drawing of the individual OR and trace all of the paths personnel may travel during a procedure. The room plan should be evaluated for how it will function during the setup phase of surgery as well as when the sterile back table has been moved into place during the procedure. Scenarios should also be created for other mobile equipment that comes into the room during surgical procedures. This same process should be used to plan the placement of storage cabinets, workstations, wall-mounted view boxes, whiteboards, and other stationary devices.

Door placement should be designed to maintain a sterile work zone in relation to the OR bed. There are two doors, one for transporting the patient and personnel and the other for access to the substerile area or central core. The main door should be located to facilitate the transport of the patient by stretcher or by patient bed. The most efficient door placement is to the left of the patient's head. It is also advisable to design all of the OR rooms so that the approach to each room is the same. Consistency in design improves safety and efficiency.

Placement of electrical and data outlets is crucial for the OR's functionality and efficiency. Even if there are ceiling-mounted booms, additional outlets are required throughout the room. The architect and electrical engineer can provide guidance to the design team about electrical loads per outlet and the types of outlets required. Outlets that will be used in the event of a power failure when the OR is on an auxiliary system are required to be clearly marked. The clinical staff on the design team can provide valuable information about the location of these emergency outlets. It is convenient if electrical outlets can be placed at a higher-than-normal elevation on the wall. Despite wireless technology, hardwiring is still necessary for backup data access. It is a good idea to plan for the future during the construction process by providing for additional electrical and data capacity. It is less expensive to run additional conduit at the time of construction than to add it a few years later, when it may require taking an OR out of service for upgrading.

Substerile space requirement

In many OR suites, a substerile room is located between each two OR rooms and enhances the rooms' function. Substerile rooms, used for immediate-use sterilization, are typically equipped with a steam sterilizer, a countertop, and built-in storage for supplies [1]. The substerile area may also be in the clean core if the clean core is directly accessible from the ORs. In this case, the substerile area needs to be accessible without traveling through any ORs.

Interior finishes

Interior elevation drawings will include information about design elements such as cabinets and other casework, wall service details, equipment mounting locations, sinks, plumbing fixtures, and other details [11]. The purpose for cabinets needs to be defined. What will be stored in the cabinets? Do the cabinets all need to be built in, or should some storage be mobile? Cabinet surfaces need to be chosen, keeping in mind the surface's durability and ability to withstand frequent cleaning.

Wall finishes must also last through rigorous cleaning yet be smooth and seamless. The color needs to be pleasing and relaxing. Floors must be durable, non-skid, capable of handling the movement of heavy equipment, and ergonomically comfortable for staff. Many flooring options are available, including terrazzo, tile, sheet vinyl, and newer products. The design team's interior design representative can provide samples of materials and discuss the pros and cons of each product.

Equipment planning

Outsourced equipment planners

Equipment planning is an essential and time-sensitive element of the planning, design, and construction process. Timing for equipment delivery should be planned so that equipment arrives at the correct time for installation and so that unnecessary storage is not required because equipment arrives too early. To determine the equipment space, design needs, and budget, an equipment list should be developed as part of the planning phase. The equipment list is necessary not only for the design process but also as a budget guide.

Researching equipment options, cost, and availability can be time-consuming. One option is to hire a company that specializes in planning and purchasing equipment for health-care facilities. The equipment planner then meets with the project representative to learn about the needs of the project and propose the role the planner can provide. The hospital decides what level of services to contract for with the equipment planners, weighing the cost of these services against the hospital's own resources for equipment planning.

There are several options when using an equipment planner. The planner can collaborate with the team to identify all of the equipment, from large equipment such as sterilizers, X-ray units, lasers, and OR lights to smaller items such as carts and stools. The planner researches product availability and costs and obtains product information and installation details for the contractors, and then assembles the information in a binder or reference file. In addition, the equipment planning firm can either purchase the equipment itself or coordinate with the hospital's purchasing department. The equipment planner can develop a timeline with the vendors and schedule deliveries according to the construction timeline.

Purchasing protocol

Whether or not an outside equipment planner is used, the hospital's materials manager needs to be an advisor to the design team, and a decision-making protocol needs to be established for the project. An effective method is needed for evaluating equipment and determining its value related to improvements planned in areas such as patient and staff safety, patient outcomes, best practice, and regulatory requirements. Decisions are needed early in the design process about whether to acquire new or refurbished equipment, purchase through existing group purchasing contracts, and who will be responsible for each element of equipment planning and acquisition.

A data sheet for each room is used to identify and record types and locations of all necessary room elements and systems. The data sheet may also indicate who will be responsible for purchasing and installation of each element, or this may be completed on a separate document. A sample data sheet may be downloaded from www.jcrinc.com/PDC09/Extras/. Data sheets also can function as checklists to confirm all details have been completed prior to the room being used.

Infection prevention during construction

Part of the planning for construction includes plans for managing potential risks to patients, staff, and the public during the project [12,13]. At the beginning of the planning phase for a construction project, the hospital needs to plan for infection control by conducting an infection control risk assessment (ICRA) [1]. The goal of the ICRA is to mitigate the risk of harm to the patients, staff, and others within or near the construction project. Depending upon the scope of the project, some potential risks are dust and fumes, mold, fungi, water contamination, hazardous material, noise, and vibrations.

The ICRA is a multidisciplinary, documented assessment process to identify and mitigate risks of infection that could occur during construction. This assessment is part of the integrated facility planning, design, construction, and commissioning activities. The ICRA team consists of members with expertise in infection prevention and control, direct patient care, facility design, construction, HVAC, and plumbing systems. The scope of the project dictates whether other members are needed [1].

The OR manager on the design team is responsible for participating in the ICRA and monitoring adherence with the infection control plan and regulations. A challenge is to make sure the staff understands these risks and that the contractors understand how to work safely in the hospital environment, especially when close to patient care areas [12,14].

Important resources are the Centers for Disease Control and Prevention's *Guideline for Environmental Infection Control in Health-Care Facilities* [15], the Facility Guidelines Institute *Guidelines for Design and Construction of Health Care Facilities* [1], the Joint Commission's book, *Planning, Design, and Construction of Health Care Facilities* [2], and the Association for Professionals in Infection Control and Epidemiology standards and guidelines [3].

Interim life safety measures

In addition to infection prevention, the team needs to assess and manage other risks that may arise during construction, such as protecting patients from fire, smoke, and toxic fumes. They must also consider risks that may arise after the structure is occupied. Health care must meet the needs of three populations: families/visitors, patients, and staff, particularly patients who are unable to leave their beds, the OR, or the hospital [16].

During the project, part of the planning team's responsibility is to plan for compliance with interim life safety measures (ILSM). The National Fire Protection Association 101 (NFPA 101) is part of the interim life safety measures [17]. The NFPA 101: Life Safety Code is used in every US state to address minimum building design, construction, operation, and maintenance requirements necessary to protect building occupants from fire, smoke, and toxic fumes. Life Safety Code® is a registered trademark of NFPA. The Life Safety Code can be used in conjunction with other building codes or alone in jurisdictions without a building code. The Centers for Medicare & Medicaid Services (CMS) and the Joint Commission refer to NFPA 101, as do federal, state, and local fire officials.

Among life safety issues that may need to be considered during construction are the need to redirect occupants because of blocked exits, to alter fire safety systems temporarily, and to construct fire barrier walls altering traffic patterns. Plans to mitigate these and other hazards need to be developed and communicated throughout the affected areas of the hospital. Plans for managing emergencies also must be established before construction begins.

Throughout project planning and construction, the OR manager needs to anticipate potential safety hazards that may surface. An unexpected utility shutdown, for example, is a serious safety concern. As part of the ILSM plan, the manager should be prepared to educate the construction team about the importance of planning for and communicating about any type of event that could potentially affect patients, families/visitors, and staff.

New technology/integrated ORs

Advancements in technology have allowed ORs to integrate systems that manage information, audiovisual signals, and radiographic imaging inside and outside of the OR suite. There is some indication that integrated technology can enhance the efficiency of certain aspects of surgical procedures. Small studies have found that compared with a conventional OR, intraoperative efficiency was improved in a dedicated minimally invasive surgery (MIS) OR with permanently fixed equipment [18,19]. Researchers have also found neck flexion and surgical spine rotation for surgeons and nurses were significantly reduced in a dedicated MIS room. Some of this technology not only enhances efficiency but also improves patient safety through improved and timelier communication among care providers.

Questions that arise during the planning and design of a new suite include how much technology is needed in every room, how much of this technology needs to be integrated, and whether the technology installed today will be compatible with the next phase of technology. To answer these questions, the OR planning team needs to perform extensive research, make site visits, interview other clinicians who have developed integrated ORs, learn from their experience, and develop a list of pros and cons.

General questions for planning for new technology include:

- Will the technology integrate with the hospital's systems?
- How will the technology affect existing processes?
- Will automation actually be more efficient or will it add unnecessary steps to an existing system?
- How many ORs need an imaging system?
- What types of procedures will be performed in these rooms?
- Is an anticipated new service or procedure volume driving the design plan?
- Should the rooms be flexible or specific for certain types of procedures?
- Are all the rooms equipped to handle the new technology?
- If a robotic surgical system is a potential addition, how many surgeons will use it, and will it be cost-effective?
- Will technology be ceiling mounted or floor mounted?
- Will the equipment be wired or wireless?

Hospitals that decide to build integrated OR(s) should involve stakeholders to identify the goals and desired outcomes of the project to achieve and determine the best return on investment. They also often decide to engage the advice of an unbiased consultant. Organizations that subscribe to services offered by the nonprofit ECRI Institute (www.ecri.org) can seek its advice for unbiased technical information.

Hybrid ORs

Hospitals with large volumes of cardiac and neurosurgical procedures are likely to consider developing a hybrid procedure room. These technologically advanced rooms, which combine surgical equipment and instrumentation with a fixed and dedicated imaging system, are intended for complex surgical and interventional procedures that require advanced imaging. Examples are hybrid coronary revascularization procedures, percutaneous cardiac valve replacement, and complex brain and spine cases [20].

Evidence on clinical benefits is limited, but some reports indicate that advantages may include shorter patient recovery time as a result of less physiological stress because multiple procedures can be performed in the same episode, streamlined care delivery, better cross-specialty communication, and potential for revenue growth as conventional ORs and interventional rooms are freed for other procedures [21,22].

Because hybrid rooms are not only technologically but operationally complex, planning requires the collaboration of multiple disciplines. This includes not only the surgical and interventional disciplines but also administrative and clinical staff, facilities personnel, biomedical engineers, information technology specialists, and equipment vendors. It is also important to include others who are critical to the room's functioning, particularly anesthesia providers, imaging support personnel, and perfusionists [20].

There are several general questions to address in planning.

- Will a hybrid OR be supported by existing interventional and surgical caseloads?
- How will a hybrid OR affect the utilization of other interventional suites and ORs?
- Can a hybrid OR be installed in existing space or will substantial renovation or new construction be needed?
- Is the hybrid OR best located in the interventional or surgical departments? Generally, interventional

suites do not have the required ventilation, scrub area, sterilization area, or access to surgical equipment and instrumentation. It may be less expensive and easiest to install the hybrid OR in the surgical suite, where those support services are already in place.

- What infrastructure will be needed? Consider in particular the size of the room, ceiling height, and weight-bearing capacity of the ceiling and floor.
- How will the room's space be organized? Consider the positioning of equipment and lights, air flow, and the pattern of movement for patients and personnel. It is helpful to construct a mock-up of the room to allow clinicians to test the configuration of space and equipment. Planning teams often also choose to visit existing facilities to learn what works well and does not work well for them [20,23].

Design considerations for ambulatory surgical centers

In an ambulatory surgical center (ASC), where patients arrive soon before surgery and are discharged soon after, the admission process and patient flow are prime considerations. The facility needs to be planned so the admission process is convenient for the patient and efficient for physicians and staff. Surgical scheduling and the preoperative assessment program need to be planned so that procedures can be scheduled easily, the preoperative assessment is safe as well as convenient, and a limited number of patients are waiting in the admitting area at any one time. Preoperative and postoperative areas also need to be planned to balance the need for privacy with smooth, safe, and efficient patient flow.

For an ASC project, it is advisable to have an architect who specializes in the design of outpatient facilities, specifically surgery centers. The design team needs to include members who understand the importance of efficient patient flow.

The detailed size and facility requirements for an ASC can be found in the *Guidelines for Design and Construction of Health Care Facilities* [1]. In general in ASCs, the OR size is smaller than in a hospital, and hallway dimensions vary by location. The NFPA Life Safety Code and infection prevention and control requirements apply to the design and construction of an ASC just as they do to a hospital.

The facility's entrance forms the patient's and family's first impression of the ASC's services. The facility needs to be designed so that patients: can easily enter the building, whether they are ambulatory or have assistive devices (such as crutches, a walker, or wheelchair); can easily find their way; and are protected from the elements. A separate exit and patient pick-up area are needed to prevent preoperative patients and postoperative patients from using the same passageways and/or elevators. The pick-up area needs to be convenient for drivers to access and protected from the elements.

Support services should be planned during the initial phase of the design process. The planning team should conduct a needs assessment for ancillary services such as laboratory (both clinical and pathology), radiology, medical records, central supply, sterile processing, and materials management should be developed as the functional program is designed. The amount and flow of materials are crucial because ASCs often have limited space.

Summary

The information provided in this chapter is intended to guide the OR manager and the surgical team through a design and construction project in the surgical arena, whether the project is small or large. Although the project may appear overwhelming initially, breaking it into phases can make it more manageable. Collaboration among multiple disciplines and input from the end users will greatly assist in a successful outcome.

The essential resources, *Guidelines for Design and Construction of Health Care Facilities* from the Facility Guidelines Institute [1], *Planning, Design, and Construction of Health Care Facilities* by the Joint Commission [2], and guidelines and standards of the Association for Professionals in Infection Control and Epidemiology [3], among others, can provide strong support during all phases of the project.

With these resources as well as a team of qualified professionals and the close involvement of end users, OR leaders can participate in designing and building a project that will meet the quality and safety expectations of patients and clinicians as well as help to fulfill the organization's vision and mission.

References

1. Facility Guidelines Institute. *Guidelines for Design and Construction of Health Care Facilities*. Chicago, IL: Facility Guidelines Institute, 2010.

2. Joint Commission. *Planning, Design, and Construction of Health Care Facilities*, 2nd edn. Oakbrook Terrace, IL: Joint Commission, 2009.

3. Association for Professionals in Infection Control and Epidemiology. Guidelines and Standards. Available from: www.apic.org (last accessed May 2, 2012).

4. D. J. Worley, S. Hohler. OR construction project: from planning to execution. *AORN J* 2008; **88**: 917–41.

5. C. Saver. Tips for surviving an OR building project. *OR Manager* 2008; **24**: 18, 21.

6. Center for Health Design. Available at: www.healthdesign.org (last accessed May 9, 2012).

7. American Society of PeriAnesthesia Nurses. *Perianesthesia Nursing Standards and Practice Recommendations 2010–2012.* Cherry Hill, NJ: ASPAN, 2010.

8. Association of periOperative Registered Nurses. *Perioperative Standards and Recommended Practices.* Denver, CO: AORN, 2011.

9. Association for the Advancement of Medical Instrumentation, Accreditation Association for Ambulatory Health Care, Association of Perioperative Registered Nurses, Association for Professionals in Infection Control and Epidemiology, ASC Quality Collaboration, International Association of Healthcare Central Service Materiel Management. *Immediate-use steam sterilization.* Arlington, VA: AAMI, 2011. Available from: www.aami.org (last accessed May 10, 2012).

10. G. Brogmus, W. Leone, L. Butler, *et al.* Best practices in OR suite layout and equipment choices to reduce slips, trips, and falls. *AORN J* 2007; **86**: 384–94.

11. American Society for Healthcare Engineering, Association for Professionals in Infection Control and Epidemiology, Society for Healthcare Epidemiology of America. Joint ASHE, APIC, and SHEA response to electronic faucet technology. June 23, 2011. Available from: www.apic.org (last accessed May 10, 2012).

12. J. M. Bartley. APIC state-of-the-art report: the role of infection control during construction in health care facilities. *Am J Infect Control* 2000; **28**: 156–69.

13. J. M. Bartley, R. N. Olmsted, J. Haas. Current views of health care design and construction: practical implications for safer, cleaner environments. *Am J Infect Control* 2010; **38**: S1-12.

14. J. Greene. Preventing infection during OR construction. *OR Manager* 2006; **22**: 14, 16, 19.

15. Centers for Disease Control and Prevention. *Guideline for Environmental Infection Control in Health-Care Facilities, 2003.* Atlanta, GA: CDC, 2003. Available from: www.cdc.gov/HAI/prevent/prevent_pubs.html (last accessed May 10, 2012).

16. R. L. Peck, S. Powers-Jones. *Staying up-to-date on life safety. Healthcare Building Ideas[serial online].* November 1, 2010. Available from: www.healthcarebuildingideas.com/print/article/staying-date (last accessed May 10, 2012).

17. National Fire Protection Association. *NFPA 101: Life Safety Code.* Quincy, MA: NFPA, 2009.

18. M. J. Van Det, W. J. Meijerink, C. Hoff, *et al.* Ergonomic assessment of neck posture in the minimally invasive surgical suite during laparoscopic cholecystectomy. *Surg Endosc.* 2008; **22**: 2421–7.

19. K. C. Hsiao, Z. Machaidze, J. G. Pattaras. Time management in the operating room: an analysis of the dedicated minimally invasive surgery suite. *JSLS* 2004; **8**: 300–3.

20. J. Van Pelt. Hybrid ORs: what's behind the demand? *OR Manager* 2011; **27**: 7–10.

21. J. Bonatti, E. Lehr, M. R. Vesely, *et al.* Hybrid coronary revascularization: which patients? When? How? *Curr Opin Cardiol* 2010; **25**: 568–74.

22. J. Mathias. Planning and staffing a hybrid OR. *OR Manager* 2011; **2**: 10–12.

23. J. A. Urbanowicz, G. Taylor. Hybrid OR: is it in your future? *Nurse Manage.* 2010; **41**: 22–7.

Chapter

10

Operating an ambulatory surgery center as a successful business

John J. Wellik CPA, MBA

The history of ambulatory surgery   108
Additional factors driving the growth of ASCs   109

Types of ASCs   110
Getting started   110
Monitoring performance   115

The history of ambulatory surgery

Early ambulatory surgery

In the early 1800s all surgery was "outpatient surgery"

Ambulatory surgery can be traced back to the roots of surgery itself. In the 1800s, surgeons would perform surgery in the home of the patient, and with the exception of alcohol and restraints, very little was done to dull the pain. Anesthesia as we know it did not exist for these surgical operations. Drugs such as nitrous oxide and ether had been used recreationally for some time, but physicians did not apply the analgesic and amnestic effects of these agents to the practice of medicine for many years.

Early anesthesia was associated with significant morbidity and mortality

In 1842, a dentist by the name of Horace Wells witnessed a public demonstration of nitrous oxide in Hartford, Connecticut, and later realized that he might be able to use nitrous oxide to extract teeth with very little pain. Wells eventually had one of his own teeth extracted under nitrous oxide anesthesia, but it took several years before nitrous oxide was fully accepted by the medical community [1]. Unfortunately, early anesthetics, including nitrous oxide, had significant morbidity and mortality [2].

Advances in medicine necessitated hospital-based surgery

For nearly a century, advances in surgery and anesthesia necessitated that procedures take place in a controlled environment that could only be offered by a large hospital. Even as early as 1927, some physicians, such as Ralph Waters, argued that their techniques were safe enough to be performed outside the hospital. Waters wrote in his memoirs that his techniques of measuring blood pressure and heart rate frequently made his procedures safe, and that his office-based practice avoided the obstacles of a hospital operating room (OR) as well as patient and surgeon inconveniences [2].

The evolution of modern ambulatory surgery

The concept of ambulatory surgery was revisited in the 1950s

It was not until the 1950s, as a result of a hospital bed shortage, that Canada began revisiting the idea of performing ambulatory surgery. Canadian physicians began performing hernia repairs in the outpatient setting as early as the 1950s. The idea of ambulatory surgery did not become popular in the United States until the 1960s, when John Dillon and David Cohen at the University of California Los Angeles (UCLA) created an outpatient surgery service. Although Canada began performing outpatient surgeries because of a hospital

Operating Room Leadership and Management, ed. Kaye A.D., Fox C.J. and Urman R.D. Published by Cambridge University Press. © Cambridge University Press 2012.

bed shortage, Dillon and Cohen were more interested in the economics of ambulatory surgery and the potential financial implications [2].

Anesthesiologists pioneer the first freestanding ambulatory surgery center

Two anesthesiologists in Phoenix, Arizona, John Ford and Wallace Reed, were also interested in ambulatory surgery because of the potential for improvements in cost containment, reimbursement, efficiency, and convenience. In 1971, John Ford and Wallace Reed created the Phoenix Surgicenter, which is credited with being the first freestanding ambulatory surgery center (ASC) in the United States [2]. The primary goal was to achieve maximum efficiency and patient throughput. To decrease overhead and costs to the patients, they eliminated all unnecessary services that existed in standard hospitals (i.e., cafeteria, transport personnel, excessive laboratory testing).

Several changes were necessary for ambulatory surgery to become practical

Although physicians were realizing the potential benefits of ambulatory surgery, the practice of medicine was not capable of implementing the concept. Specifically, most surgeries were still very invasive, and anesthetic techniques had complication rates far too high for routine same-day discharge. For this reason, relatively few ASCs were built until the mid-1980s, when several things happened: (1) accreditation programs and standards were established; (2) the US government accepted ASCs and established Medicare reimbursement rates; (3) advances in the field of anesthesiology dramatically reduced the anesthesia-related morbidity and mortality; and (4) development of new surgical instruments such as lasers, enhanced endoscopic techniques, and fiberoptics reduced the trauma and recovery time associated with many surgical procedures [3].

In 1980 the United States had approximately 275 ASCs, and approximately 15% of all surgeries were done in outpatient facilities [3]. By 1990, the number of ASCs had grown to 1450 and the flurry of ambulatory surgery organizations continued to expand. The Society for Ambulatory Anesthesia (SAMBA) was created, and new drugs were being created to further facilitate ambulatory surgery. Ketorolac, the first parenteral nonsteroidal anti-inflammatory drug (NSAID) approved for severe postoperative pain, was reported

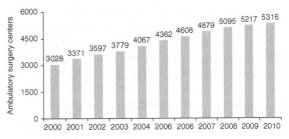

Figure 10.1 Number of outpatient surgery centers, 2000–2010. Source: Medicare Payment Advisory Commission, *A Data Book: Healthcare spending and the Medicare Program, June 2007 and June 2011.*

to provide the analgesic potency of morphine without associated respiratory depression [4]. By the year 2000, there were approximately 3000 Medicare-certified ASCs and the number continued to grow throughout the decade, increasing over 75% to 5316 by the close of 2010 (Figure 10.1).

Although the new regulatory environment and medical advances helped establish an environment for ASCs to reap the benefits envisioned nearly 40 years ago, these were not the only factors for the explosion of ASCs across the country.

Additional factors driving the growth of ASCs

Procedures in ASCs cost less

As mentioned earlier, ASCs were designed to maximize efficiency, eliminate unnecessary services, and decrease costs. ASCs are now widely acknowledged to be a cost-effective alternative to the higher-cost inpatient setting. Hospitals have to pay higher overhead, administrative, and facility development costs, which make their per-procedure costs higher than those of ASCs. For this reason, managed care companies, self-insured employers, and government payers prefer to have patients go to lower-cost ASCs [5].

Patients value the convenience of ASCs

Ambulatory surgery centers are designed to be more convenient for the patient. The architectural layouts are usually designed to maximize throughput. Administrative paperwork is minimized to facilitate faster admission. Family members are allowed to be with the patients during the recovery period, and patients are allowed to leave ASCs relatively quickly after surgery. The US Department of Health and Human Services Office (DHHS) of the Inspector General surveyed Medicare beneficiaries who had one of four procedures in an ASC and found that 98% of the people were satisfied with their experience [6].

Surgeons value the efficiency of ASCs

Efficiency is particularly important to surgeons. It takes much less time to prepare an OR in a specialized ASC for the next patient than in a standard hospital. Improved efficiency allows the surgeon to treat more patients in the same amount of time than he or she would be able to do in a hospital; some surgeons maintain that they can do three times the number of procedures in an ASC as they could in a hospital setting [3]. According to the Federated Ambulatory Surgery Association (FASA) Outcomes Monitoring Project, 75% of ASCs started more than 95% of their cases on time [6]. Many doctors prefer working in an ASC because they can set the standards for staffing, safety precautions, postoperative care, etc, rather than having these things decided for them by a hospital administrator. Physicians also prefer the greater flexibility in scheduling and more consistent and reliable nurse staffing [5].

Types of ASCs

Practice based

Practice-based ambulatory surgery centers are commonly owned and operated by a specific physician group practice. Practice-based ASCs are equipped and staffed for a single medical specialty and are usually located in or adjacent to offices of a physician group practice. Practice-based or single-specialty centers often require lower capital and operating costs than freestanding ASCs.

Freestanding

Freestanding ASCs are typically owned by a group of local investors, physicians, and/or an investment company. Such ASCs generally serve a broader group of physicians, which compromises the flexibility of scheduling and increases overhead, but adds diversity of revenue levels and patient mix.

Hospital joint venture

Surgery centers operated through a hospital joint venture include a hospital or health system in their ownership hierarchy. These ASCs may have been built by the participating hospital as a separate facility dedicated to ambulatory services or, as is becoming increasingly more common, resulted from a merger between previously freestanding and/or practice-based ASCs with large health-care providers.

Getting started

Legal structure and ownership

Ambulatory surgery centers are typically organized as some type of limited liability entity, which affords the individual investors a limitation on personal liability associated with the financial obligations of the center. Limited liability companies (LLCs) are the most common type of legal entity used for an ASC, although limited partnerships may offer some advantages over LLCs in certain states.

As noted previously, there are different types of ASCs and, accordingly, the ownership of the entity will depend upon the type of facility. Practice-based centers may be owned by the group practice or by individual physicians within that practice. Freestanding centers may have ownership split among a number of group practices and/or individual physicians as well as third-party management or development companies. Centers joint ventured with a hospital will include an interest owned by an entity affiliated with the hospital or health-system partner.

Anti-kickback and "Stark Law" considerations

The ownership and operation of ASCs is subject to comprehensive federal and state regulations. Although the specific provisions of the Social Security Act prohibiting physician referrals to facilities in which they or family members own a financial interest, commonly referred to as Stark Law, generally do not apply to ambulatory surgery services, the overall "anti-kickback" provisions of federal criminal law do apply and must be considered when structuring ownership allocation and investment protocol in a surgery center. These regulations prohibit payment or receipt of any consideration in exchange for referring patients for services that are reimbursed under a federal health-care program, notably Medicare and Medicaid. The Health and Human Services Office of the Inspector General (OIG) has published regulations outlining certain safe harbors under the anti-kickback statute, including safe harbors applicable to surgery centers. This safe harbor generally protects ownership or investments in surgery centers and payments that are a return on that investment for physicians who refer patients to the center or perform procedures on patients who are referred to the center, if certain conditions are met. These conditions include the following criteria:

1. at least one-third of each physician investor's medical practice annual income must come from performing outpatient procedures that are approved by Medicare for reimbursement in an ambulatory surgery center;
2. at least one-third of the Medicare-eligible outpatient procedures performed annually by each physician investor must be performed at the surgery center in which the investment is made.

The safe harbor guidelines also allow nonphysician investors who are not employed by, nor in a position to provide any goods or services or refer patients to, the center or the physician investors. Surgery centers that include ownership by a management company, which is typically compensated with a percentage of the center's revenue, or by a hospital, which is likely to be in a position to refer patients to the center or its physician investors, would not satisfy all of the requirements of the safe harbor provisions. However, it should be noted that the safe harbor provisions do not expand the scope of activities that the anti-kickback statute prohibits and the OIG has acknowledged that legitimate surgery center arrangements exist that do not meet all of the safe harbor criteria. Thus, although failure to meet all the safe harbor criteria does not mean that any given surgery center structure is in violation of the law, such structures could be subject to greater scrutiny by regulators.

Governing board

The organizational documents of the legal entity should outline the specifics of the facility's governance, i.e., number of board members, election protocol, subcommittees, etc. Identifying initial board members with a mix of business, clinical, and interpersonal skills is critical to the successful start-up of the center. Any compensation arrangements for the board members should be mindful of the safe harbor guidelines discussed above. Given that the physician investors, who are the most likely candidates for board positions, may also be the largest utilizers of the facility, any compensation for board service should be clearly tied to time

spent on governance issues and be subject to reasonable periodic maximums in order to avoid the appearance of payment for volumes of patient referrals to the center.

Regulatory approval and licensing

Certificate of need requirement

Health-care regulations in certain states require that, prior to the construction of new health-care facilities or the introduction of new services, a designated agency must determine that a need exists for those facilities or services. This process is often referred to as a certificate of need (CON) application, which can be time-consuming and expensive. Not all states have CON laws, and for those that do the requirements and process varies, with some providing thresholds for capital expenditures or scope of service that may exempt smaller and/or single specialty surgery centers from the CON review process.

Medicare provider application

In order to participate in Medicare, an ASC must satisfy regulations known as conditions for coverage. For a new facility, this is typically accomplished through a direct survey coordinated through the Center for Medicare Services (CMS) after submission of a Medicare provider application. Diligent completion of the application and coordination with CMS on scheduling the survey to coincide with the anticipated facility opening date are critical to avoiding delays in obtaining the Medicare provider number. Although receipt of that provider number directly impacts payment for services performed for Medicare and Medicaid patients, private managed care payers typically will not finalize reimbursement contracts until the facility obtains its Medicare certification.

Business plan

Specialties, types of procedures

Determining the surgical specialties to be accommodated will drive many of the specific assumptions involved in preparing a comprehensive business plan. The number and size of operating and procedure rooms will drive the overall space requirements for the facility. Specific procedures to be performed will dictate the equipment and instrument requirements and budget as well as the staffing plan.

Managed care contracting strategy

A number of surgery centers in recent years have adopted "out-of-network" strategies, whereby the facility chooses not to enter into contracts with some or all private managed care payers. In extreme examples, the facility does not apply for Medicare certification. These facilities rely on individual patient payments, or more typically, receipt of out-of-network reimbursement from the patients' insurance carriers. Traditional preferred provider network plans (PPOs) historically have paid a lower percentage of charges to providers of services to their members who do not contract with the carrier. However, with no contracted fee schedule, centers executing these out-of-network strategies have often been able to realize higher reimbursement per case at the lower out-of-network percentage of gross charges reimbursement than if they had contracted with the carrier. As the number of facilities pursuing such a strategy has grown, so too have the efforts by the managed care companies to limit their exposure to these facilities. These efforts include: (1) alerting state regulators to practices in which a patient's financial responsibility, which is typically higher due to the higher co-pay percentage and/or deductible for services provided by an out-of-network provider, is waived; (2) providing reimbursement directly to the patient instead of the provider, resulting in the facility needing to collect from the patient well after the date of surgery; and (3) refusing to provide any reimbursement for services provided by specific facilities.

Regardless of an in- or out-of-network approach, estimating reimbursement levels, or net revenue, is one of the most critical steps in developing a pro forma income statement to be included in a business plan. Assumptions regarding the anticipated payer mix within the specific geographic and demographic mix of patients must be made. Understanding the existing payer mix for the practices of the surgeons who will be utilizing the facility is one potential starting point. This is also one area in which working with a management company and/or a hospital partner can be a key differentiator. Not only will those resources be able to assist with a better understanding of the probable payer mix, they may also be able to assist with negotiating higher reimbursement rates through specific provisions of the contracts with the individual payers.

Managed care contracts for ASCs typically will provide for a percentage of Medicare reimbursement as a starting point in setting contracted reimbursement rates for a facility. Achieving as high a multiple or percentage of Medicare rates as possible for those types of procedures that the facility anticipates performing the most should be a key goal in negotiating contracts. Additionally, "carving out" specific procedures that are likely to be a focus of the facility and/or are significant with the practices of key physician utilizers should be another goal in contract negotiation. Specifying set reimbursement rates or higher percentages of Medicare for those procedures can have a dramatic impact on the profitability of the facility. Similarly, establishing mark-up percentages on implantable items should be a consideration.

Location

Proximity to the practice offices of identified physician partners is likely to be one of the key drivers in selecting a search area for a new surgery center. Vacant land or a site available for redevelopment is the most viable alternative, as retrofitting an existing building and transforming it into an efficient surgery center is typically not practical. Proximity to the hospital where the physician partners perform surgery currently and where they will probably continue to perform their inpatient cases is also a consideration. There are advantages and disadvantages to surgery centers located on or adjacent to a hospital campus. Although it may offer convenient access for the surgeons, particularly if they also have their practice office on the campus, it also may bring many of the detractions from patient and staff viewpoints, notably traffic congestion, parking difficulty and expense, and suboptimum discharge logistics.

Site plan

As noted in the introduction to this chapter, efficient patient flow was one of the primary drivers in Dr. Ford and Dr. Reed's design of the first freestanding surgery center in the United States. That goal carries forward to today. The ideal floorplan provides for logical and efficient physical movement of a patient from check-in to discharge with convenient access for staff to cover both preoperative preparation and postoperative recovery. All sterile areas should be confined to contiguous space in the middle of the patient flow. The exterior site plan should allow for staff parking and entrance near the lounge or locker rooms with ample patient parking near the reception and discharge areas, which should be in close proximity to each other but visibly separated for patient privacy and comfort.

Financial pro forma

The specific components of the financial pro forma will be discussed in the next section of this chapter. The pro forma provides the basis for determining the amount of external financing required and is also a key requirement in working with lenders to secure the financing.

Key components of the financial pro forma

Case volumes

Estimating case volumes and the ramp-up in those volumes during the center's start-up phase is the critical first step in putting together a financial pro forma. Identifying the individual surgeons who are committed to utilizing the center from its inception can be a starting point in arriving at the volume estimates. The routines or practice flows of those surgeons and further, how they, and their scheduling staff, are willing to alter it with the opening of the center must be analyzed. Depending upon where each surgeon is planning on moving cases from, there will probably be pressure to maintain volumes at the facilities they are currently utilizing. These pressures may be unspoken and/or subtle but they should not be underestimated. Preferences in scheduling of OR time as well as the availability of key staff could be altered. Similarly, the influence of the surgeon's scheduler should not be underestimated. Ideally, the surgeon will drive the decision on the volume and types of cases to be scheduled at the new center, but the surgery center staff should work to develop relationships with the key contacts at each surgeon's office.

The number of operating and procedure rooms contained in the facility will ultimately have an impact on the capacity of the case and procedure volumes to be budgeted for the facility. Initially, however, the capacity of the facility is not likely to be a determining factor in estimating case volumes. Rather, the case volume estimates arrived at by analyzing the probable changes in practice patterns for the early surgeon utilizers should drive the decisions on when to "open" how many ORs. Staffing and equipping only those operating and procedures rooms necessary to handle the initial case volumes will be key to controlling the start-up expenses of the center.

The managed care contracting strategy discussed earlier will also have an impact on initial case volume estimates (as well as the more obvious reimbursement amounts per case to be discussed in the next section). Going with a complete out-of-network strategy discussed earlier, in which Medicare certification in not pursued, allows a center to plan for, and ultimately schedule, cases without consideration of whether the managed care contracts will be in place to facilitate payment. An "in-network" strategy will necessitate projecting the timing of finalizing contracts with the individual insurance companies in determining the ramp-up in cases for insured patients.

Revenue per case

The amount of revenue collected per case will be driven by the specific cases performed and the source of payment for each of those cases. The amount of revenue actually collected is often referred to as "net revenue," whereas the amount billed is referred to as "gross revenue" or "gross charges." The gross revenue for a facility will be driven by the "charge master," which will need to be established within the patient accounting system utilized by the facility for tracking patient billings and collections. Most ASCs set their gross charges on a "bundled" basis per procedure, in which there is one all-inclusive charge for a given procedure, rather than the unbundled, detailed line item charge process typically utilized in an inpatient setting. This approach is driven by the reimbursement schedule utilized by Medicare for ASCs, which in turn is often the basis for managed care contracts, as discussed previously in the Managed care contracting strategy section of this chapter.

The most precise approach to estimating gross and net revenue would be to develop a matrix of anticipated procedures by physician and by reimbursement source. Depending upon the number of anticipated physicians who will utilize the facility and their surgical specialties, this approach may not be practical. A reasonable alternative for a multispecialty ASC would be to arrive at average gross charges by specialty (orthopedic versus gastrointestinal, etc.) and then estimate average reimbursement percentages by payer type (e.g., contracted, out-of-network, workers' compensation, self-pay, Medicare). If implants are anticipated to be a significant component of cases performed at the center (orthopedic, spine, pain stimulators, etc.), the net reimbursement for those items needs to be included in the revenue calculations in order to develop reasonable estimates of anticipated cash-flow requirements and sources.

Fixed versus variable costs

Fixed costs

The fixed costs of a facility are those that do not fluctuate based on activity volumes. The most significant of this type of cost is the cost of the facility itself – either rent or a mortgage payment if the facility is owned by the partnership and leveraged. Equipment costs are typically fixed costs as well, most frequently financed through secured leases or bank loans. The third type of fixed cost is associated with the core staffing of the facility – the administrative or management overhead positions as well as the minimum clinical staffing levels required regardless of the number of cases the facility performs. Determining this staffing level and the timing of hiring each position will be one of the keys to controlling start-up losses and cash-flow demands.

Variable costs

Variable costs are those that fluctuate (or should fluctuate) based on case volumes. Clinical staffing above the core staffing levels is typically the most significant variable cost, and the cost that needs to be managed most closely in order to control the profitability of the facility as volumes fluctuate. This can be managed in a number of ways, and each has its advantages and disadvantages. Using contract or agency nurses provides the most flexibility in managing hours, as these arrangements allow for staffing as close to an "as needed" basis as possible. However, the per-hour cost of agency nurses will probably be the highest of any of the alternatives. Additionally, availability of specific individual nurses is not assured with this approach, leading to "learning curve" inefficiencies, frustration of the surgeons in working with new staff, and worst of all, potential clinical quality issues.

Identifying a sufficient number of dedicated staff willing to "flex" their hours based on case volumes provides the most consistency in the workforce dynamics at the facility. In order to retain these individuals, it may be necessary to guarantee a certain number of hours each pay period and/or confirm that they will continue to qualify for full-time status for benefit purposes. Maintaining benefits, particularly health-care coverage, is frequently a determining factor for an employee staying in a position. However, the costs to the center for this coverage are significant and can become unreasonable on a cost-per-hour basis if the level of productive hours is consistently below a full-time load.

An alternative to using agency staff to supplement the facility's full-time staff is to develop a group of individuals who are willing to work on an as-needed basis, often referred to as PRNs. These individuals are employees of the facility being paid hourly rather than through an agency, typically resulting in lower hourly rates. Similar to full-time staff, however, the PRN employees may need a commitment of a minimum number of hours per pay period or per month in order to commit to remaining available for work when needed.

After personnel costs, drugs and medical supplies is the other significant cost item that will be driven by case volumes. Standardizing as many items as possible by working with the utilizing surgeons will help with controlling the required investment in supply inventory and also build purchasing leverage with larger quantities. Consistent and complete utilization of preference cards, whereby the surgeons specify supplies to be used for a given type of case, will further assist with controlling supply levels and limiting wasted supplies. Various types of "packs" are available that contain the supplies typically utilized for different types of cases. Although these offer convenience and may simplify the ordering and inventory monitoring processes, they can also increase the amount of wasted supplies and overall supply costs.

Depending upon the types of procedures performed, implantable supplies or devices can be significant drivers of supply costs. Individually expensive items should be stocked on an as-needed basis for specific cases, or on a consignment basis, allowing for payment to the distributor or manufacturer only when the items are used for a case. As previously noted, insurance contracts should allow for reimbursement of many implantable items at a multiple or percentage of costs in addition to the contracted payment rate for many procedures. Maintaining logs detailing receipt and use of these items will insure accurate reimbursement as well as prevent theft or loss due to expiration.

Financing

Facility

Finish-out costs for a surgery center are significant, typically two or three times the cost of constructing the "shell" of a new facility. Real-estate developers or landlords will often roll the cost of the finish out into the lease rate for a facility, although the "cap rate" used may not be attractive, given that the owner will factor in payment risks as well as a return above their cost of capital.

Another consideration that will impact the monthly and annual cost of rolling finish-out costs into a facility lease rate is the term over which the costs are being amortized. The lease term required in order to achieve a manageable rent level may be for a longer period than the surgery center investors are willing to commit. An approach to arriving at an equitable lease rate for a newly developed surgery center would be to develop an initial rate that is a blend of a shorter amortization period, perhaps 10 or 15 years, for much of the finish out with the core facility construction costs amortized over 20 or 25 years. Lease renewal options should factor in this blended approach, with an appropriate reduction in rate after the finish-out costs have been amortized.

Equipment

Rolling the finish-out costs into a broader financing agreement that also covers the initial equipment is another approach. However, including more than tangible, movable equipment in a financing agreement will increase the interest rate as well as the likelihood of the requirement of personal guarantees from the individual physician investors in the surgery center. Guarantees, while an obvious financial encumbrance for the initial physician investors, can also become a practical and administrative burden for the surgery center business or legal entity as physician owners leave or change ownership interests. The requirement of a debt or lease guarantee will also be an impediment to bringing in new physician investors. Approaches to mitigating these concerns include ensuring that any guarantees are pro rata based on ownership and also "burn off" provisions that provide for elimination of the guarantee over time assuming satisfactory payment experience or other criteria.

Working capital

In addition to funding the finish out and tangible surgical and business office equipment, funds will also need to be available to cover preopening operating expenses, notably payroll and supplies as well as rent and other fixed costs. Accurately projecting the opening date and tying hire dates and supply receipts to this date will mitigate the preopening expenses and related cash flow requirement.

Monitoring performance

Once the ASC is operational, monitoring its performance will help insure that it remains viable. As the number of ASCs has proliferated, more are failing during their early years of operation. Inadequate discipline in monitoring key metrics and taking appropriate action based upon what those metrics are saying was probably a significant contributor to many of these failures.

Operating metrics

Operating room utilization and scheduling efficiency

Available OR time is the overriding resource constraint for an ASC. Accordingly, managing utilization of the center's ORs will be a determining factor in its success. Developing and adhering to scheduling protocols is a first step. The computerized patient accounting system used by the facility should have an application to facilitate scheduling of OR time, but regardless of whether the computer system is used or more rudimentary paper schedules are the approach, the protocol for scheduling cases should be clearly documented and thoroughly communicated, both to the center's staff as well as to the schedulers at the physician offices for the center's key surgeons.

The components or considerations of the scheduling protocol should include the following.

- What are the acceptable communication channels for requesting OR time? Having a dedicated scheduling phone line that will not be tied up with other center calls will help insure availability of the line when a surgeon's office wants to schedule a case and that the request gets to the correct person at the center. Although multiple employees could have the ability to add a case to the schedule, it should be clear who at the center "owns" the schedule. If schedule requests are accepted via facsimile, again there should be a dedicated fax line to receive these requests and clear procedures on who is responsible for monitoring these incoming fax transmissions and confirming receipt with the surgeon's office. If email or other electronic means (e.g., the center's website) are allowed for scheduling, considerations for ensuring Health Insurance Portability and Accountability Act (HIPAA) compliance are required as well as the follow-up and confirmation procedures noted for scheduling via fax.
- How will block scheduling be handled? Surgeons who intend to be heavy users of the center will probably want to "block out" or reserve

certain consistent, recurring periods of time on the center's schedule to insure they have available OR time for their patients. Although this practice can be a huge plus for the center from an OR utilization viewpoint, it can quickly turn into a utilization, and political, nightmare. On the plus side, reserving blocks of OR time indicates an intended practice pattern whereby the surgeon communicates his or her intent to bring a significant number of cases to the center. Presumably, the surgeon's scheduler knows of the blocked time and will schedule all eligible patients accordingly. The situation turns problematic when multiple surgeons want to block the same prime, early morning time slots as well as when they fail to consistently book cases within their reserved time frames. Mitigating these challenges is another of the many areas in which encouraging the physicians to help manage each other will often yield the best results. The physician governing board should set and help enforce the procedures for prioritizing block schedule requests and releasing uncommitted blocks timely to insure that the benefits of blocked time exceed its disadvantages.

- How much time will be scheduled for each case? One of the primary advantages to a surgeon in using an ASC versus a hospital environment is the predictability of ORs being available when scheduled. Maximizing this advantage requires accuracy in scheduling. Thorough and precise communication with each surgeon and their staff regarding expectations on required OR time for each type of case will contribute to establishing baselines in scheduling. Tracking of actual times against that scheduled will allow for refinement of the scheduling based on experience. Monitoring and recording whether cases start on time, with standard reasons if not, is a key metric to track and report to the center staff and the physician governing board. Elimination of physician controllable delays (e.g., surgeon not arriving as scheduled) is another area in which "self-policing" among the physicians is most effective.

- How much time will be allowed for between cases? Turnaround time between cases is another key metric to be tracked and shared with the center staff. Keeping that time as short and consistent as possible requires clearly documented procedures and duty assignments.

Staffing management

As previously discussed, staff costs are the largest variable cost within the facility. Accordingly, managing hours is the most critical area in controlling expenses of the center. The best metric for monitoring how effectively the center is managing its staffing is worked hours per case, which should be tracked and charted on a daily basis. In order for the metric to be actionable, the clinical staff hours should be segregated from the business office and management staff. Maintaining consistent worked hours per case as volumes fluctuate is an indicator that staff hours are being managed effectively. This is only possible if the scheduling protocols mentioned earlier are followed and the turnover time between cases is effectively managed.

The ratio of contract or agency hours to total clinical hours is another staffing metric to track on a daily basis. As discussed earlier, use of agency nurses allows for the most flexibility in staffing but typically at the highest incremental cost per hour and also at the risk of reducing physician satisfaction as well as clinical quality. Accordingly, seeing recurring spikes in contract usage other than on days with unusually high case volumes could indicate issues with managing staff absences, whereas seeing consistent use of contract hours would indicate the potential need for adding "permanent" staff.

Supply management

After staff costs, medical supply costs will be the second highest variable cost. Working with the physician leadership to establish the center's master supply list and minimizing variances from that list due to individual physician preferences is often one of the more challenging tasks in controlling costs. However, reaching a consensus among the physician leaders on basic supplies with reasonable per unit costs can have a significant impact on the profitability of each case while also minimizing the cash required to stock multiple versions of the same item.

Using preference cards for each case can be an effective tool to assist with purchasing supplies and also for monitoring exceptions from the master supply list requested by individual physicians. At the most basic level, a preference card would include all the supplies that a specific physician requires (or requests) for a specific type of procedure. Templates of these cards can be maintained either manually or on an automated basis through the computer system used by the facility. The need for any modifications to the template for a specific patient can be confirmed when scheduling the case with the physician's office.

Although supplies other than implants are typically included in the bundled facility charge for a given procedure, recording actual supply use after completion of a case and pricing out those supplies will facilitate benchmarking of supply costs between physicians performing the same procedures. This allows the physicians to work together on identifying supply-cost-saving opportunities to enhance the center's profitability.

Financial metrics

The center's monthly financial reports should facilitate monitoring of key financial metrics in comparison to the budget and historical performance. The sample income statement in Figure 10.2 outlines some of the more critical metrics and provides some typical observations based on the month's results.

In addition to monitoring and taking appropriate action based on the center's income statement metrics, the balance sheet also deserves some attention. Cash is likely to be the most important line item on the facility's balance sheet to the physician investors; however, managing it requires focus on several other line items, notably: accounts receivable, inventory, accounts payable, and cash distributions.

Accounts receivable

Utilizing tools within the center's patient accounting computer system will be key to managing the center's accounts receivable. With respect to monitoring the center's summary balance sheet, ensuring that accounts receivable per the balance sheet equals the total reported by the detail of patient balances maintained within the patient accounting system at each month end is a key control. Discrepancies could reflect receipts that are deposited but not posted to the appropriate patient balance in the patient accounting system or, more concerning, receipts that have been posted to a patient's account but were not subsequently deposited to the center's bank account.

The accounts receivable aging report provided by the patient accounting system will categorize patient balances into "buckets" by the number of days that have elapsed (e.g., less than 30, 30 to 60, 60 to 90, etc.) since the date of service. The system should also facilitate categorization of the balances between amounts due directly from the patient (deductible, co-pay,

etc.) and the amounts due from the insurance carrier. Proper presurgery screening procedures should facilitate collection of a majority of the amounts due directly from the patient on or before the date of surgery. Procedures for timely and consistent follow-up for any remaining patient balances should be clearly documented and adhered to in order to minimize any write-offs incurred by the facility. These procedures should also outline when, or if, a patient account should be turned over to a collection agency and written off as a bad debt. Decisions also need to be made as to whether the facility will offer payment terms to the patient for their responsibility. This has become a more common request with the higher deductible and co-pay levels that employers and insurers are transferring to individuals. Third-party financing companies have developed programs specifically for health-care providers and may provide an attractive alternative to requiring center employees to deal with this aspect of the patient relationship.

For insurers with whom the center is "in network," the majority of amounts due should be collected within 30 days of the date of service. Significant delays beyond that time frame would indicate issues with the accuracy of filing claims and/or following the process required by the insurer. Monitoring the day's sales outstanding (DSO) in accounts receivable is a good metric to track on a monthly basis to insure collections are being received on a timely basis. The metric is calculated by determining the average daily net revenue and then dividing the month end accounts receivable by that amount. Using the most recent 2 months of revenue will level out daily fluctuations and also provide for the normal collection lag. For example, if net revenue for January and February totaled $450 000 and February's accounts receivable balance was $270 000, the DSO would be 35 (i.e., $450 000 divided by 59 days equals average daily revenue of $7627, which when divided into the $270 000 accounts receivable balance yields the DSO metric of 35 days.)

Inventory

There are different approaches to accounting for inventory within a center's financial statements. Technical accounting rules would require that all supplies be recorded to inventory on the balance sheet when purchased and then recorded as expense when used for a surgical case. While most patient accounting systems do provide for tracking depletion

Center Name
Income Statement Variance Analysis
Month ended MM/DD/YYYY

	Actual	Budget	Prior Year	Variance Budget	%	Variance Prior Year	%
Cases	346	295	249	51	17.3%	97	39.0%
REVENUE							
Gross patient revenue	$510,551	$438,075	$266,609	$72,476	16.5%	$243,942	91.5%
Contractual adjustments	237,502	232,180	146,690	5,322	2.3%	90,812	61.9%
Net revenue	**273,049**	**205,895**	**119,919**	**67,154**	**32.0%**	**153,130**	**126.7%**
EXPENSES							
Personnel costs	69,123	63,425	47,225	5,698	9.0%	21,898	46.4%
Drugs and medical	43,104	35,400	25,181	7,704	21.8%	17,923	71.2%
Repair and maintenance	5,044	5,500	3,937	(456)	(8.3%)	1,107	28.1%
Purchased services	8,762	6,000	2,836	2,762	46.0%	5,926	209.0%
Minor equipment and instruments	598	500	290	98	19.6%	308	106.2%
Utilities	3,720	3,700	3,483	20	0.5%	237	6.8%
Non-medical supplies and expenses	4,247	4,000	3,939	247	6.2%	308	7.8%
Professional fees	250	300	420	(50)	(16.7%)	(170)	(40.5%)
Sales expense	796	1,000	702	(204)	(20.4%)	94	13.4%
Insurance	1,772	1,950	1,772	(178)	(9.1%)	0	0.0%
Provision for bad debts	6,783	8,220	5,332	(1,437)	(17.5%)	1,451	27.2%
Lease and rent expense	17,906	17,741	16,368	165	0.9%	1,538	9.4%
Non-income taxes	2,889	3,000	2,797	(111)	(3.7%)	92	3.3%
Total operating expenses	164,994	150,736	114,282	14,258	9.5%	50,712	44.4%
EBITDA	**108,055**	**55,159**	**5,637**	**52,896**	**95.9%**	**102,418**	**193.6%**
EBITDA %	**39.6%**	**26.8%**	**4.7%**	**78.8%**	**(294.0%)**	**66.9%**	**438.2%**
Depreciation expense	14,512	18,008	13,644	(3,496)	(19.4%)	868	6.4%
Interest expense	5,263	7,468	6,124	(2,205)	(29.5%)	(861)	(14.1%)
Total non-operating expenses	19,775	25,476	19,768	(5,701)	(22.4%)	7	0.0%
Pretax income (loss)	**$88,280**	**$29,683**	**($14,131)**	**$58,597**	**197.4%**	**$99,835**	**706.5%**
Ratio analysis:							
Gross patient revenue / case	$1,476	$1,485	$1,071	($9)	(0.6%)	$405	37.8%
Net revenue / case	$789	$698	$482	$91	13.1%	$308	63.9%
Salaries and benefits / case	$200	$215	$190	($15)	(7.1%)	$10	5.3%
D&M / case	$125	$120	$101	$5	3.8%	$23	23.2%
Other operating expense / case	$153	$176	$168	($23)	(13.3%)	($16)	(9.3%)
Total operating expense / case	$477	$511	$459	($34)	(6.7%)	$18	3.9%
EBITDA / case	$312	$187	$23	$125	67.0%	$290	1279.5%
Bad debt % of net revenue	2.5%	4.0%	4.4%	(1.5%)	(37.8%)	(2.0%)	(44.1%)

EBITDA: *Earnings before interest, taxes, depreciation and amortization is a key measure of profitability and cash flow*

Observations:

Volumes are ramping up nicely with current year cases 17% ahead of budget and 39% above prior year.

Gross revenue per case is right on budget and 38% ahead of prior year, which is primarily attributable to changes in specialty mix and/or complexity of cases performed consistent with what was planned.

Net revenue per case is 13% ahead of budget and 64% above prior year indicating an improved payor mix as well as more favorable contracts.

Personnel costs are above budget and prior year in total dollars due to the higher case volumes and complexity of cases, but are below budget on a per case basis indicating success in managing staffing levels and mix to actual case volumes. The per case increase of 5% over prior year is generally consistent with wage increases.

Drugs and medical expense per case are in line with budgeted levels but up significantly from prior year as a result of the increased complexity of cases.

Other operating expenses are generally consistent with budgeted amounts in total dollars but below budget and prior year on a per case basis reflecting the leverage potential of spreading these more fixed expenses over the higher case volumes that were achieved.

Bad debt expense as a % of net revenue is running lower than budget and prior year, which indicates good collection results.

Figure 10.2 A sample income statement.

of inventory by case in conjunction with the preference card utility discussed previously, using this for all supplies is typically not practical given the low dollar cost of routine supplies used in essentially all surgeries. The most simplistic approach to addressing this challenge is to record initial supply purchases to inventory and then expense any subsequent replenishment. However, this approach does not correctly reflect increases in inventory as volumes increase, nor properly account for more expensive supplies used in certain cases.

A hybrid approach is to expense routine supplies as purchased and track certain items such as implants or unique physician-requested items through inventory. Another, slightly more sophisticated, approach is to record all supply purchases to inventory and then record depletion of routine supplies on an average cost per case with implants or other specialty items expensed only as used. Regardless of the approach used to record inventory and expense supply costs, performing a physical count of supply items in inventory periodically is necessary in order to adjust the amount on the facility's balance sheet to reflect supplies actually on hand and to insure that any expired or damaged items are disposed of and recorded as expense. A complete count should be conducted at least annually with more frequent (quarterly if not monthly) counts of items more prone to waste as well as individually expensive items.

Significant monthly fluctuations in the amount of inventory reflected on the facility's balance sheet would indicate that the approach used for expensing supplies is not properly matching the expense with the revenue being generated by cases performed each month, which could yield misleading income statement results.

Accounts payable

Managing which bills are paid when can be a stressful aspect of managing the surgery center's business operations, particularly during the start-up phase. Entering invoices into the center's accounting system on a timely basis will insure that there is an accurate record of amounts payable and will facilitate use of the tools and reports provided by the system to manage payments effectively. Similar to the accounts receivable aging reports provided by the patient accounting system, the accounts payable module should provide an aging report of invoices and other items that are payable. Efficient use of the center's available cash will require balancing payment of invoices promptly enough so as not to jeopardize the center's credit history with the desire to maintain, and ultimately distribute, the center's cash.

Cash distributions

At the most basic level, the financial goal of the center will be to distribute sufficient cash to provide an attractive rate of return to the investors. Once the center begins collecting revenue from cases performed, there will probably be pressure from some of the investors to begin distributions quickly and, on an ongoing basis, pressure to keep those distributions as high as possible. However, commencing distributions too quickly or being overly aggressive with the amounts being distributed can lead to significant issues, including jeopardizing the facility's credit rating if it is unable to pay bills timely. Accordingly, the approach to determining reasonable distribution levels should be one that is fully vetted with the center's governing board, preferably with input from a financially disinterested business expert, probably either the center's outside accountant or a representative of the third-party management company. As a rule of thumb, once a facility has achieved somewhat stable volume levels, a minimum of 2 weeks' routine operating expenses should be maintained when making a cash distribution. Other considerations should include upcoming debt payments or other nonrecurring obligations as well as any potential cash reserves for new equipment purchases.

Satisfaction surveys

Monitoring and measuring the satisfaction levels of the center's "customers" will provide the management team and governing board with an assessment of how the center is perceived. The key groups to be surveyed include physicians, patients, and employees. Including a mix of questions or statements requiring objective responses or rankings with opportunities to provide narrative commentary provides the most actionable survey results. Maintaining some level of consistency in the survey items will facilitate tracking of results over time and evaluation of progress toward meeting and exceeding the expectations of all the constituent groups who will ultimately determine the long-term success of the surgery center.

References

1. R. D. Miller, L. I. Eriksson, L. A. Fleisher, J. P. Wiener-Kronish, W. L. Young. *Miller's Anesthesia*, 7th edn. New York: McGraw-Hill, 2008.

2. S. Springman. *Ambulatory Anesthesia: The Requisites in Anesthesiology*. New York: Mosby, 2006.

3. R. Frey. Ambulatory Surgery Centers. *Gale Encyclopedia of Surgery: A Guide for Patients and Caregivers*. 2004. Retrieved July 11, 2011 from Encyclopedia. com: www.encyclopedia.com/doc/1G2-34062 00021. html (last accessed May 10, 2012).

4. P. G. Barash, B. F. Cullen, R. K. Stoelting, M. Cahalan, M. C. Stock. *Clinical Anesthesia*, 6th edn. Baltimore, MD: Lippincott Williams & Wilkins, 2009.

5. C. Jahnle, K. A. Rebane. Ambulatory Surgery Centers – Fragmented Industry Poised for Consolidation. *Ambulatory Surgery Center Business Review*. Winter, 2003.

6. The History of ASCs. ASC Association and Ambulatory Surgery Foundation. www.ascassociation.org/ASCA/AboutUs/WhatisanASC/History/ (last accessed July 11, 2011).

Chapter

11

Preoperative evaluation and management

Alicia G. Kalamas MD

Components of comprehensive
preoperative risk assessment   121
Patient factors   121
Surgical factors   122
Anesthetic management   122
Aspects of the health-care delivery system   123
Various models for the delivery of
preoperative care   124
Preoperative clinics   124

Telephone interviews   125
Primary care providers   125
Day of surgery   125
Value of early remote triage   125
Nuts and bolts for starting a physician-
directed preoperative clinic   127
Economics of preoperative evaluation
and management   128
Embracing the preoperative clinic   129

Physician-directed preoperative clinics underpin the success of a patient's journey through the surgical continuum of care. These clinics not only allow for early identification and mitigation of perioperative risk [1–3], but also have been shown to: improve hospital resource utilization [4,5]; enhance patient satisfaction [6,7]; reduce duration of hospital stay [8–10]; and mitigate operating room (OR) delays and cancellations due to inadequate assessment or patient preparation [11,12].

In this chapter we will discuss six topics:

1. components of comprehensive preoperative risk assessment;
2. various models for the delivery of preoperative care;
3. value of early remote triage;
4. nuts and bolts for starting a preoperative clinic;
5. economics of preoperative evaluation and management;
6. embracing the preoperative clinic.

Components of comprehensive preoperative risk assessment

There is growing recognition that proper preoperative preparation goes well beyond the anesthesiologist's assessment of anesthetic risk. With the advent of new anesthesia techniques, innovative drugs, enhanced training, pulse oximetry, and capnography, the risks associated with anesthesia have declined sharply over the past 40 years. Contemporary estimates of mortality solely attributable to anesthesia are low (1 in 100 000) [13]. Conversely, all-cause 30-day surgical mortality for elective non-day surgery approaches 1 in 50 [14]. Understanding and identifying the factors that contribute to patient perioperative risks is the first step toward proper preoperative preparation.

Risks associated with surgical hospitalization can be divided into four categories: (1) patient factors; (2) surgical factors; (3) anesthetic management; and (4) aspects of the health-care delivery system. The overreaching goals of preoperative evaluation and management, therefore, are to: identify risk factors from within these categories; implement risk-mitigation strategies; and communicate information broadly to all members of the health-care team in a systematized fashion.

Patient factors

For several comorbid conditions, a robust literature exists to define the effect of a given patient risk factor on outcomes. For example, multiple risk indices have

Operating Room Leadership and Management, ed. Kaye A.D., Fox C.J. and Urman R.D. Published by Cambridge University Press. © Cambridge University Press 2012.

been developed to predict major adverse cardiac events (e.g., myocardial infarct; sudden cardiac death). One of the most widely used indices is the revised cardiac risk index (RCRI). The RCRI includes five patient risk factors with approximately equal prognostic importance: (1) coronary artery disease; (2) congestive heart failure; (3) history of cerebral vascular accident (stroke or transient ischemic attack); (4) diabetes; and (5) renal insufficiency. The presence of ≥2 of these factors has been shown to identify patients at moderate (7%) and high (11%) risk for postoperative cardiac complications. Furthermore, patients with at least three of these factors have an increased risk for cardiovascular complications during the ensuing 6 months, even if they do not experience major cardiac complications during their surgical hospitalization [15].

Tools such as the RCRI, therefore, not only allow for identification of candidates for whom further testing (e.g., stress tests) or other management strategies (e.g., perioperative beta blockade) may be beneficial, but also allow for identification of low-risk patients for whom additional evaluation or management is unlikely to be helpful (and may in fact be harmful).

Similarly, several patient-related factors such as chronic obstructive pulmonary disease, age older than 60 years, ASA class of II or higher, functional dependence, and congestive heart failure have been shown to increase the risk for postoperative pulmonary complications. Postoperative pulmonary complications play a significant role in overall morbidity and mortality in patients undergoing non-day surgery. Consequently, early identification of at-risk patients allows for targeted and timely implementation of evidence-based risk-reduction strategies, including incentive spirometry, deep breathing exercises, and neuroaxial blockade [16].

While documentation and optimization of existing medical conditions is paramount, equally important is identification of those previously unrecognized conditions that may impact a patient's perioperative course (e.g., obstructive sleep apnea [OSA]). This is not to suggest, however, that "routine" testing of all presurgical patients is justifiable, either medically or financially. Rather, a proper health history coupled with screening questionnaires such as those used for detecting OSA (e.g., STOP questionnaire) are valuable tools to help guide the appropriate ordering of diagnostic, rather than screening tests. Screening tests in presurgical patients are time-consuming and costly, and false-positive results expose patients to risky and unwarranted additional assessments [17–25].

Surgical factors

Although patient factors play a significant role in predicting postoperative complications, predictions of postoperative outcome must also take into account the invasiveness of the proposed surgical procedure. Every surgical procedure elicits a stress response, initiated by direct tissue injury, pain, and anxiety. This response sets off a predictable cascade of physiologic and metabolic events (tachycardia, hypertension, fever, immunosuppression, protein catabolism, and water retention) through direct activation of the sympathetic nervous system and hypothalamic–pituitary–adrenal (HPA) axis. The severity of this stress response, which begins with induction of anesthesia and peaks postoperatively, is directly related to the extent and duration of the surgical procedure.

The vast majority of surgical procedures can be considered safe (mortality risk of less than 1%). However, there is a >200-fold difference in the incidence of all-cause death between the highest and lowest risk surgeries, with the most invasive and lengthy procedures associated with the greatest risk of adverse outcome (e.g., vascular surgery adjusted adverse outcome incidence of 5.97% compared with only 0.07% for breast surgery). Hence for purposes of risk stratification, the traditional classification of surgical procedures as high or low risk appears inappropriate. Fortunately, a recently published observational population-based study of 3.7 million surgical procedures in the Netherlands provides a detailed and contemporary overview of postoperative mortality for the entire surgical spectrum [14]. The results of this study may eventually serve as a reference standard for surgical outcome in Western populations.

Anesthetic management

Morbidity and mortality are rarely attributable directly to anesthesia. However, there are several anesthesia-related factors beyond the choice of anesthetic agents that must be taken into consideration when safely preparing a patient for surgery. Both the safety of the anesthetizing location and selection of anesthetic provider are critical components of any perioperative risk-mitigation strategy.

The demand for anesthesia care in support of procedures performed outside the OR has dramatically increased in recent years. Although these procedures are relatively straightforward and often minimally invasive, the delivery of safe out-of-OR anesthesia is complicated by a variety of factors – cramped dark rooms, unfamiliar surroundings, and fewer supporting staff and resources relative to OR suites. All these factors can lead to delays in recognition and treatment of respiratory depression, offer poor access to the patient, and place patients at increased risk for catastrophic consequences. Data from the American Society of Anesthesiologists (ASA) Closed Claims Project demonstrate that monitored anesthesia care (MAC) in remote locations poses a sevenfold risk of oversedation and inadequate oxygenation/ventilation compared with the OR. Similarly, the severity of patient injury is greater in remote locations, with the proportion of death directly attributable to anesthesia almost double that seen in the OR [26].

Awareness and vigilance can minimize the risk of patient injury in these challenging settings. However, this requires careful identification of patients at highest risk for adverse events (e.g., those with OSA or morbidly obese, elderly, or debilitated patients). Unfortunately there is a frequent misperception that out-of-OR procedures are "benign" in nature. Additionally, there is often a failure to recognize that patients treated in remote locations tend to be older, sicker, and more likely to be in need of emergent care than patients receiving care in OR settings.

A specific out-of-OR location that warrants special consideration is the freestanding surgical center. Freestanding surgical centers are not connected to a hospital, and therefore access to both specialized medical resources and emergency care is limited. For these reasons certain patient populations are not suitable candidates for these surgical suites, as immediate access to *all* available health resources must be assured for even the most minor of procedures. Based on data collected through the National Survey of Ambulatory Surgery by the Centers for Disease Control, almost half of ambulatory surgery visits in the United States occur in freestanding centers each year [27].

As the obesity epidemic and aging US population expand, so too will the demand for surgical services in freestanding surgical centers and other remote locations. For both obese and aged patients, the presence of multiple chronic diseases demands heightened awareness of the location of, staffing models for, and resources available to out-of-OR care settings as part of any comprehensive perioperative risk-mitigation strategy.

Aspects of the health-care delivery system

The surgical episode of care is unfortunately highly fragmented. This is in large part the result of care provision via disparate services and providers. Consequently, information that originates with the patient subsequently flows along many pathways to physicians, nurses, pharmacists, and other care providers. Despite large investments in information technology, providing the correct information, when needed, to the appropriate care providers continues to be problematic. As a result, failures of information transfer and communication errors among care providers can lead to mistakes in care provision and patient harm [28]. To compound this issue, communication deficits are not discrete events; namely, information loss in one phase of care can potentially compromise safety in a downstream phase of patient care.

Although effective and standardized communication among health-care professionals during the perioperative period has been shown to facilitate surgical safety [29], few organizations have developed a systematized approach to insure that essential information is preserved. Integrated care pathways (ICPs) – also known as multidisciplinary pathways of care, care maps, and collaborative care pathways – offer one such approach for standardized communication. First introduced in the early 1990s in the UK, ICPs are structured, multidisciplinary plans of care for patients with similar diagnoses or symptoms [30]. The ICP specifies the interventions required for the patient to progress along the continuum of care. Additionally the ICP delineates these interventions against a time frame (measured in hours, days, or weeks) and/or patient care milestones designed to support clinical management. The ICPs are inherently "patient-focused," as they view the delivery of care in terms of the patient's journey through the system and place emphasis on the coordination of care across different disciplines and sectors.

In practical terms, the ICP can act as the single record of care, with each member of the multidisciplinary team required to record their input into the ICP document. The use of both process-based (i.e., the tasks to be performed) and outcome-based (i.e., the results to be achieved) documentation serves as a guide to decision making. This documentation also provides each health-care professional with information about the patient's condition over the course of therapy and beyond (e.g., referral back to the primary care physician [PCP]). A few large integrated health systems such as Intermountain Healthcare [31] and Geisinger [32] have successfully implemented care pathways with substantial clinical and financial benefit.

With regard to the surgical episode of care, the preoperative assessment is the natural point of entry into an ICP. Consider, for example, a patient on Coumadin for atrial fibrillation who requires perioperative use of bridging anticoagulation (e.g., Lovenox) to prevent thromboembolism. Proper management of this patient requires: (1) discontinuation of Coumadin preop; (2) initiation of Lovenox preop; (3) discontinuation of Lovenox 24 h prior to surgery; (4) lab draw day-of-surgery to verify that the international normalized ration (INR) is normalized; (5) reinitiation of therapeutic Lovenox *and* Coumadin 12–24 h postop; (6) daily INR measurements; (7) discontinuation of Lovenox when the patient is therapeutic on Coumadin; and (8) follow-up with the patient's PCP to insure the patient's INR is stable on the reinitiated Coumadin dose. Failure to initiate any one of the above-mentioned steps at the appropriate time point could have grave consequences.

The ICPs and their associated documentation are designed explicitly to insure that no step in a care continuum, such as the one described above, is missed. To accomplish this they codify the foreseeable clinical actions that represent best practice for most patients most of the time. They also include prompts for care providers to confirm critical steps have been completed at each appropriate point in the care continuum.

Development of comprehensive care pathways can be a daunting task, involving buy-in from several stakeholders (e.g., surgery, anesthesia, nursing, and hospital administration). Consequently, few organizations have developed and implemented ICPs. However, highly simplified care plans (i.e., checklists) can provide a reasonable alternative for capturing many of the important benefits of ICPs. Checklists can be developed with minimal effort, initiated during the preoperative assessment, and carried out in the absence of sophisticated electronic medical record (EMR) technology. They can increase the likelihood that critical information is preserved as a patient transitions from one phase of care to the next and can play a particularly important role in the surgical continuum of care [29]. Despite myriad documented benefits, checklists have unfairly been labeled "cookbook medicine." This moniker has inhibited their widespread adoption in the United States.

There is increasing appreciation that overall assessment of perioperative risk is a multifactorial process, only partly dependent on anesthesia. Unfortunately, comprehensive algorithmic risk scales that incorporate all potential sources of perioperative risk (i.e., patient, surgical, anesthetic, and system-related factors) do not exist. Therefore, proper preoperative evaluation and management relies heavily on astute clinical judgment.

Various models for the delivery of preoperative care

Surgical patients, even those with significant comorbidities, are seldom admitted to the hospital in advance of their procedure for preoperative care. Instead, preoperative assessment and risk management occur in the outpatient setting for the vast majority of patients. Four models for preoperative assessments exist: (1) the patient visits a preoperative clinic days in advance of their procedure; (2) a telephone interview is the sole basis for the evaluation; (3) the patient is seen by their PCP; or (4) an evaluation is performed at the bedside, on the day of surgery, in the preop holding area. Each of these approaches has merit for subsets of patients, but none is appropriate for all patients all of the time, given patient heterogeneity.

Preoperative clinics

Physician-directed preoperative clinics devoted exclusively to the preoperative evaluation of patients allow for comprehensive patient assessment. The focus of these clinics is to evaluate risk by taking into account the patient, the procedure, and anesthesia-related factors. In addition, these clinics typically have system-based processes in place to facilitate coordination of care across the entire surgical care continuum. That is, physician-directed preoperative clinics focus not only on identifying perioperative risk but also on implementing risk-mitigation strategies and communicating this information to the entire health-care team.

Not surprisingly, these clinics allow for early identification and mitigation of perioperative risk. Additionally, they have been shown to improve hospital resource utilization by: reducing unnecessary preoperative consults and laboratory tests; enhancing patient satisfaction; reducing duration of hospital stay; and mitigating OR delays and cancellations due to inadequate assessment or patient preparation. However, performing an exhaustive in-person evaluation for every patient prior to the day of surgery is cost-prohibitive and unnecessary.

Telephone interviews

The majority of hospitals and surgical centers do not have dedicated preoperative clinics because of the substantial costs associated with sizable staff and physical space requirements. Instead they rely upon telephone interviews typically conducted by registered nurses (RNs). This approach is less costly, but has several shortcomings: (1) overreliance on formulaic questionnaires that are not specific to the particular patient's situation; (2) failure to capture the breadth and depth of information required to properly assess risk; and (3) consumption of an unnecessary amount of time and clinical resources. Additionally, phone interviews typically occur the day before surgery, leaving little time to properly address perioperative risk. This model relies heavily on mid-level providers to merely *collect* information without adequate processes in place to order the appropriate diagnostic tests, follow through on risk management, optimize patient outcomes, and reduce adverse events.

Primary care providers

Primary care providers are often asked by surgeons to evaluate and "clear" a patient for surgery. The goal of this evaluation is to determine the risk of the proposed procedure to the patient and to optimize management of preexisting medical conditions. Primary care providers, however, are often ill-prepared to comment on several of the nonpatient-related risks that one may encounter during a surgical admission. A patient's primary medical provider may be well suited to assess and optimize that patient's medical conditions, but may be less familiar with the specifics of the procedure itself. These include anesthetic considerations and the systems-related issues that may pose risk to patients (e.g., monitoring on the wards for patients with OSA). Consequently, a dangerous misconception exists; namely, the belief that when a PCP has "cleared" a patient for surgery, the patient can automatically be assumed to be a good candidate for anesthesia, the surgical procedure, and all risks associated with the surgical episode of care.

To complicate matters, providers who are unsure of what is expected from them during this preoperative assessment often order myriad tests such as blood work, electrocardiograms, chest X-rays, and cardiac stress tests out of concern for "missing something." However, it is now appreciated that extensive routine testing is not justifiable, either medically or financially, and an excessively aggressive approach to preoperative testing may lead to specious, risky, and unwarranted assessments. This probably explains why medical consultation by physicians not specifically trained in perioperative evaluation is associated with increased length of hospital stay and increased postoperative mortality [33].

Day of surgery

Delaying the preoperative evaluation until the day of surgery creates a potentially dangerous situation; namely, an inherent bias to downplay perioperative risk factors such that surgery can proceed as planned. There are several reasons for this: a medical team that is intent on proceeding with their case; an OR suite and staff that have been mobilized; and a nervous patient who has mentally prepared for and made work and home-life arrangements to accommodate the surgery. Fortunately most health-care delivery systems within the United States recognize the inherent dangers and financial consequences of delaying preoperative assessment to the day of surgery. Consequently, this model is not commonly employed.

There is widespread disagreement regarding the best model for delivering preoperative care because none of the approaches described above optimizes for the individual needs of each patient. Collectively these approaches result in a subset of patients who are not appropriately evaluated for perioperative risk and another subset of patients who are unnecessarily subjected to exhaustive evaluations and diagnostic tests that are not indicated. The answer to optimal preoperative assessment for all patients lies in careful triage based on each patient's medical history. Such triage can identify those patients in need of aggressive preoperative management and those who can safely proceed to surgery with minimal management.

Value of early remote triage

Although there is no consensus on the optimal approach to preoperative assessments, there is widespread acceptance that certain patient populations are more likely than others to benefit from an in-person clinic visit and/or diagnostic testing. Healthy patients with no/low perioperative risk can be safely "fast-tracked" to the day of surgery with little hospital staff intervention. Patients with modifiable risk factors should ideally be identified far enough in advance (e.g., proximate to the time of surgical scheduling) to allow ample opportunity to intervene in a meaningful way. The challenge to date has been finding a system that allows for accurate triage of those presurgical patients who require intense preoperative clinical resources – lengthy phone calls, in-person visits, diagnostic testing – and those who do not.

To facilitate presurgical patient triage, many hospitals rely on RN-initiated phone-based interviews. These interviews use static preformulated questionnaires to elicit the patient's preoperative medical history. Unfortunately, the static nature of these questionnaires makes it difficult for the nurses administering them to capture the breadth and depth of information required for proper triage. Consequently, it is common that important elements of the patient's medical history are missed by RN phone triage and only identified upon further questioning on the day of surgery. Two studies have shown that nurses are better at "ruling out" patients who did not need additional assessment rather than "ruling in" patients who need to be seen [34,35]. Such omissions leave patients vulnerable to adverse events and day-of-surgery delays and cancelations.

To overcome some of the shortcomings inherent in the manual capture of patient medical histories by clinicians, Dr. Michael Roizen developed one of the first computer software programs for preoperative assessment, Health Quiz, in the early 1990s [36]. However, the slower-than-anticipated adoption of the EMR markedly inhibited the success of Health Quiz. Since that time many authors have validated the use of automated techniques to gather health histories and have found a low discrepancy when comparing the outputs generated by an automated questionnaire with those gathered via person-to-person interviews [37–39].

Building upon the Health Quiz concept, the Cleveland Clinic created HealthQuest in the late 1990s as a "home-grown" solution. HealthQuest is an outpatient preoperative evaluation computer program designed to triage presurgical patients. Patients are administered a computer-based questionnaire. Responses to questions are coded to create a HealthQuest score, using a scale of 1 (healthy) to 4 (multiple complex medical issues). The HealthQuest score is used to guide the timing and level of required preoperative evaluation. This triage system was tested over a 3-year period in 63 941 outpatient surgical patients. Of these, 22 744 (35.6%) did not require a visit with a health-care provider prior to the day of surgery, as guided by the computer-assigned HealthQuest score and surgical classification scheme. In addition, patient interview time, patient dissatisfaction with the preoperative process, and the average monthly surgical delay rate all decreased during the study period [1]. Although the Cleveland Clinic continues to reap enormous benefits from triaging their patients using HealthQuest, most institutions do not have the staff or surgical volume to support development and maintenance of such a sophisticated "home-grown" software solution.

Perhaps the two most important elements of a preoperative health history are a *current* medication list and a *current* review of systems. Data within EMRs, however, are highly perishable and therefore cannot be relied upon for making perioperative management decisions. Eliciting up-to-date information directly from the patient can be time-consuming. Although it is widely recognized that using mid-level providers as scribes is not an effective use of health-care resources, little emphasis has been placed on finding ways to directly engage patients in the process of clerical data entry. In fact, none of the commercially available hospital-wide EMRs has developed a patient portal capable of eliciting a *comprehensive* health history directly from the patient.

Unlike many other industries that have been revolutionized by the wave of self-service the Internet provides, medicine has lagged behind in its acceptance of the Web as a means for communication and, therefore, has been reluctant to enter the arena of Web-based applications. However, the Internet can be utilized as a telemedicine portal and there are a handful of commercially available Web-based preoperative assessment tools. Many of these products are offered either on a per-click basis or for a nominal annual licensing fee, thus eliminating the large upfront and ongoing maintenance costs typical of traditional hardware- and software-based information technology products.

One such product, BREEZE™ (MedSleuth, Inc.), is the focus of an NIH-funded clinical trial. MedSleuth's BREEZE™ software generates a unique questionnaire for each user of the system, based on the patient's medication profile and successive answers to questions. Branched-chain questionnaire systems have a significant advantage over standardized digitized paper questionnaires in being able to deal with a wide variety of medical problems while sparing patients the burden of answering scores of irrelevant questions. Initial results from clinical trials using the BREEZE™ product are favorable and consistent across a broad spectrum of patient populations. Patient ease of use and satisfaction with this Web-based approach to eliciting a medical history is >90%; median time to complete the questionnaire ranges from 16 to 22 min; and the output generated by the survey has been shown to be more accurate for purposes of assigning ASA classification than the output generated by health professionals using a standardized questionnaire [39,40,41]. Furthermore, use of early, remote Web-based triage has been shown to limit day-of-surgery cancelations due to a new or previously unrecognized medical condition to <1% [42]. These results indicate patient-centered Web-based preoperative assessment tools offer great promise in addressing the shortcomings of today's preoperative triage techniques.

Nuts and bolts for starting a physician-directed preoperative clinic

The first step in planning a preoperative clinic is to define the clinic's mission. In its most robust form, a preoperative clinic should be designed to identify and mitigate *all* risk factors that impact a patient's surgical hospitalization. In essence, a well-functioning preoperative clinic serves as the epicenter for the surgical episode of care. For this to occur, however, representatives from hospital administration, surgery, anesthesia, and nursing must explicitly define and agree to the operational goals (Table 11.1) of the clinic and implement a standardized system for communicating information between any and all providers who will interact with patients during the surgical continuum of care.

Once the goals of the clinic have been defined, the clinic structure can be developed and individual roles delineated. A Medical Director should be appointed. Ideally this person will have a background in both anesthesia and internal medicine. Hospitalists are well suited for this position as well. In situations where hospitalists are used to staff a preoperative clinic, however, there should be a plan in place for immediate access to an anesthesia consultant should questions arise regarding anesthetic options, appropriateness of anesthetizing location, and/or airway management.

The clinic Medical Director is responsible for developing protocols, guidelines, and care pathways in conjunction with their surgical, medicine, and anesthesia colleagues. The Medical Director should also educate the residents and mid-level providers who staff the clinic

day to day. Additionally, a Clinic Manager (typically an RN) should be appointed to insure there is adequate infrastructure and support for the administrative and nursing staff. Pre-registration, laboratory work, and electrocardiograms can either be performed within the clinic (one-stop-shop) or patients can be directed to other parts of the hospital for these services.

Appointments should be scheduled only after the patient has been triaged. This triage should occur proximate to the patient's initial visit in the surgeon's office, thereby allowing ample time for medical optimization, required testing, and/or subspecialty consultation. Triage should be performed by a highly experienced nurse practitioner (NP) or physician assistant (PA), who can determine if additional information is required prior to formal perioperative risk assessment. Failure to make the correct triage decision or to secure relevant health records *before* formal evaluation has potentially negative consequences downstream – adverse outcomes, low clinic throughput, high cost, low patient satisfaction. Thus it is imperative that a robust triage system be in place and that triage is conducted by a highly experienced member of the preoperative assessment team. Once triaged, patients can be scheduled for either a telephone consultation or in-person visit (where appointment duration is consistent with the complexity of the patient's care). When possible, patients should be evaluated a minimum of 7 days prior to their surgical date to insure ample time for medication management.

At the time of formal evaluation, the health history and all pertinent medical records are reviewed. Additional tests or subspecialty consultation can be arranged and a formal risk assessment takes places. Patients suitable for care pathways or protocols are identified (e.g., OSA, perioperative beta blockade) and special arrangements are made (e.g., move a diabetic to first case of the day; order stat potassium on the day of surgery for a dialysis patient). Personal communication between the clinic Medical Director, surgeons, PCPs, and the anesthesia consultant insures that any questions or concerns regarding the patient's condition and appropriateness for surgery are discussed. This avoids day-of-surgery delays and potential cancellations secondary to questionable patient suitability for surgery.

Once risk has been assessed and a plan devised, this information must be communicated to all members of the health-care team. This communication is often conducted via an EMR. Unfortunately, both progress notes and best practice alerts within EMRs are frequently overlooked. The alerts can result in a type of "fatigue"

Table 11.1 Operational goals of a physician-directed preoperative clinic

1. Triage all surgical patients proximate to their initial surgical consultation to determine need for in-person evaluation versus phone consultation

2. Retrieve all relevant health records (e.g. cardiac) *prior to* formal preoperative evaluation

3. Make contact with all surgical patients no less than 7 days prior to scheduled surgical date (to insure adequate time for medication management, etc.)

4. Perform a comprehensive risk assessment taking into account the four broad sources of risk

5. Determine need for further testing/subspecialty consultation

6. Develop a strategy aimed at optimizing patient's preexisting medical conditions/mitigating perioperative risk

7. Communicate findings with surgeon and primary care provider/agree upon plan that will carry patient through entire surgical hospitalization

8. Codify plan in the form of a document (checklist) that will follow patient throughout and beyond surgical hospitalization

9. Educate patient

whereby the provider, after receiving too many alerts, begins to ignore and/or override the alerts. Prolonged alert fatigue can negatively impact patient care, as important alerts may be ignored [43,44]. Introduction of checklists, on the other hand, has been associated with a significant decline in the rate of complications and death from surgery. Although the exact mechanism of improvement is not known when a checklist-based program is in place, the evidence of improvement in surgical outcomes is substantial [29]. Therefore, the development and consistent use of patient checklists should serve as the foundation for and communication of a patient's perioperative management plan.

Once established, the perioperative plan must be effectively communicated to the patient. Patients should receive explicit information on medication management and pertinent information concerning the surgical process, including anticipated length of stay and probable outcomes. For communication of preoperative information to be effective, the information should be available in many forms, such as visual, auditory, or face-to-face education. Preoperative teaching has several well-documented advantages, including decreased length of stay, less demand for analgesia postoperatively, and increased patient satisfaction [45,46]. Despite the known benefits of patient education, this component of preoperative preparation is unfortunately often overlooked.

Economics of preoperative evaluation and management

Given today's cost-conscious environment, there are concerns about appropriate resource use in nonrevenue-generating areas. Preoperative evaluation falls within this category for most hospital administrators. They view preoperative evaluation as a cost-intensive operation for which they receive no incremental reimbursement. That is, sending a patient through a preoperative clinic or phone-based preoperative evaluation is considered part of the surgical service provided by the hospital and therefore is bundled within the global reimbursement for the surgical fee. Consequently, the adoption of physician-directed preoperative clinics has been slow.

Physician-directed preoperative clinics, however, have consistently demonstrated value in excess of the cost of the evaluation itself via their impact on: patients' health status; improved resource utilization; and reduced day-of-surgery delays and cancellations. In fact, use of physicians to evaluate patients and order indicated tests was shown to have the potential for reducing preoperative testing costs by several billion dollars without negatively affecting patient care [4].

Furthermore, inadequate preoperative evaluation is a contributory factor in adverse operative outcomes. Of the first 6271 incidents reported to the Australian Incident Monitoring Study, 11% of the reports listed inadequate preoperative evaluation as a contributing factor. Well over half of the incidents were considered preventable. The investigators did not make an estimate of the economic impact of these adverse cases, but many of the adverse outcomes noted – case cancellation (5%), unexpected death (4%), prolonged hospitalization (7%), and use of intensive care facilities (9%) – are understood to rapidly consume resources [47].

In addition to realizing cost savings, proper preoperative preparation has the potential to generate incremental revenue for a hospital by justifying: (1) increased diagnosis-related group reimbursements for comorbidities that would otherwise have been overlooked; and (2) reimbursement for professional fees. "Usual preoperative care" as performed immediately prior to a procedure is not a billable service. However, physicians and physician extenders are entitled to separate reimbursement for professional fees if the service does not fall within the Medicare surgical global period. Additionally, the following requirements must be met: (1) the consultation is being performed at the request of another practitioner seeking advice regarding evaluation and/or management of a specific problem; (2) the request for the consultation and the reason for the request are recorded in the patient's medical record; and (3) after the consultation is provided the practitioner prepares a written report of their findings.

Finally, as patients take on more responsibility for their health-care decisions with the rise of consumerism, well-executed preoperative evaluation can serve as a competitive differentiator for surgical providers. Given that a patient's first encounter with a health-care facility is often during a preoperative evaluation, it is imperative that hospitals and surgical centers critically assess patient experience and satisfaction during the preoperative evaluation process. Length of waiting time and overall time spent in a preoperative clinic correlate inversely with patient satisfaction [48,49]. Long patient waiting times due to late start/finish of appointments are the result of poor triage, incomplete health information (most importantly up-to-date medication lists and external medical records) [50], suboptimal operational workflow, and poorly defined staff goals and incentives. Consequently, hospital administrators and preoperative clinic medical directors would be well served to mitigate these issues to insure a positive patient experience.

Embracing the preoperative clinic

In today's competitive surgical environment, efficiency, quality, and patient satisfaction are important criteria by which consumers and their insurers select health-care providers. Increasingly only those hospitals and surgical providers that deliver high-quality care and high patient satisfaction at an affordable price will maintain their financial viability. Consequently, there is growing appreciation for the health and economic benefits of proper perioperative evaluation and

management; yet hospitals and surgical providers continue to struggle with optimizing the flow of patients through the surgical episode of care. The solution to this dilemma lies in proper perioperative evaluation and management via physician-directed preoperative clinics.

Perioperative evaluation and management is complex and requires close coordination and cooperation between several members of a multidisciplinary team. Physician-directed preoperative clinics, when properly designed and managed, can achieve this coordination by serving as the epicenter for patients' surgical care, both inpatient and outpatient. The benefits that these comprehensive clinics can offer are well documented, yet their adoption has been inhibited by the substantial investment of capital and ongoing operating expense they require. Fortunately, the costs of starting and managing these clinics can be substantially reduced through the use of: best-practice workflow techniques; Web-based technologies to engage patients in remote triage; evidenced-based perioperative management; and well-managed reimbursement. As such they should be embraced by clinicians, administrators, and patients alike for the important benefits they can deliver to surgical care.

References

1. B. M. Parker, J. E. Tetzlaff, D. L. Litaker, W. G. Maurer. Redefining the preoperative evaluation process and the role of the anesthesiologist. *J Clin Anesth* 2000; **12**: 350–6.

2. P. Parsa, B. Sweitzer, S. D. Small. The contribution of a preoperative evaluation to patient safety in high-risk surgical patients: a pilot study (abstract). *Anesth Analg* 2004; **100**: S-147.

3. D. J. Correll, A. M. Bader, M. W. Hull, C. Hsu, L. C. Tsen, D. L. Hepner. Value of preoperative clinic visits in identifying issues with potential impact on operating room efficiency. *Anesthesiology* 2006; **105**: 1254–9.

4. S. P. Fischer. Development and effectiveness of an anesthesia preoperative evaluation clinic in a teaching hospital. *Anesthesiology* 1996; **85**: 190–206.

5. L. C. Tsen, S. Segal, M. Pothier, L. H. Hartley, A. M. Bader. The effect of alterations in a preoperative assessment clinic on reducing the number and improving the yield of cardiology consultations. *Anesth Analg* 2002; **95**: 1563–8.

6. D. L. Hepner, A. M. Bader, S. Hurwitz, M. Gustafson, L. C. Tsen. Patient satisfaction with preoperative assessment in a preoperative assessment testing clinic. *Anesth Analg* 2004; **98**: 1099–105.

7. C. E. Klopfenstein, A. Forster, E. Van Gessel. Anesthetic assessment in an outpatient consultation clinic reduces preoperative anxiety. *Can J Anaesth* 2000; **47**: 511–15.

8. T. M. Halaszynski, R. Juda, D. G. Silverman. Optimizing postoperative outcomes with efficient preoperative assessment and management. *Crit Care Med* 2004; **32**(suppl): S76–86.

9. N. Duminda. Wijeysundera preoperative consultations by anesthesiologists. *Curr Opin Anesthesiol* 2011, **24**: 326–30.

10. J. B. Pollard, P. Garnerin, R. L. Dalman. Use of outpatient preoperative evaluation to decrease length of stay for vascular surgery. *Anesth Analg* 1997; **85**: 1307–11.

11. W. A. Van Klei, K. G. Moons, C. L. Rutten, *et al.* The effect of outpatient preoperative evaluation of hospital inpatients on cancellation of surgery and length of hospital stay. *Anesth Analg* 2002; **94**: 644–9.

12. M. B. Ferschl, A. Tung, B. Sweitzer, D. Huo, D. B. Glick. Preoperative clinic visits reduce operating room cancellations and delays. *Anesthesiology* 2005; **103**: 855–9.

13. G. Li, M. Warner, B. H. Lang, L. Huang, L. S. Sun. Epidemiology of anesthesia-related mortality in the United States, 1999–2005 *Anesthesiology* 2009; **110**: 759–65.

14. P. G. Noordzij, D. Poldermans, O. Schouten, J. J. Bax, F. A. Schreiner, E. Boersma. Postoperative mortality in The Netherlands: a population-based analysis of surgery-specific risk in adults. *Anesthesiology* 2010; **112**: 1105–15.

15. T. H. Lee, E. R. Marcantonio, C. M. Manqione, *et al.* Derivation and prospective validation of a simple index for prediction of cardiac risk of major noncardiac surgery. *Circulation* 1999; **100**: 1043–9.

16. A. Qaseem, V. Snow, N. Fitterman, *et al.* Risk Assessment for and strategies to reduce perioperative pulmonary complications for patients undergoing noncardiothoracic surgery: a guideline from the American College of Physicians. *Ann Intern Med* 2006; **144**: 575–80.

17. G. L. Bryson, A. Wyand, P. R. Bragg. Preoperative testing is inconsistent with published guidelines and rarely changes management. *Can J Anaesth* 2006; **53**: 236–41.

18. F. Chung, H. Yuan, L. Yin, S. Vairavanathan, D. T. Wong. Elimination of preoperative testing in ambulatory surgery. *Anesth Analg* 2009; **108**: 467–75.

19. S. Mantha, M. F. Roizen, L. Madduri, Y. Rajender, K. Shanti Naidu, K. Gayatri. Usefulness of routine preoperative testing: a prospective single-observer study. *J Clin Anesth* 2005; **17**: 51–7.

20. E. B. Kaplan, L. B. Sheiner, A. J. Boeckmann, *et al.* The usefulness of preoperative laboratory screening. *JAMA* 1985; **253**: 3576–81.

21. J. M. Turnbull, C. Buck. The value of preoperative screening investigations in otherwise healthy individuals. *Arch Intern Med* 1987; **147**: 1101–5.

22. B. J. Narr, T. R. Hansen, M. A. Warner. Preoperative laboratory screening in healthy Mayo patients: cost-effective elimination of tests and unchanged outcomes. *Mayo Clin Proc* 1991; **66**: 155–9.

23. B. J. Narr, M. E. Warner, D. R. Schroeder, M. A. Warner. Outcomes of patients with no laboratory assessment before anesthesia and a surgical procedure. *Mayo Clin Proc* 1997; **72**: 505–9.

24. D. S. Macpherson, R. Snow, R. P. Lofgren. Preoperative screening: value of previous tests [see comments]. *Ann Intern Med* 1990; **113**: 969–73.

25. G. W. Smetana, D. S. Macpherson. The case against routine preoperative laboratory testing. *Med Clin North Am* 2003; **87**: 7–40.

26. J. I. Metzner. Risks of anesthesia at remote locations. *ASA Newsletter* 2010; **74**: 17–18.

27. National Survey of Ambulatory Surgery. Available online at: www.cdc.gov/nchs/nsas/about_nsas.htm. (last accessed May 10, 2012).

28. K. Naqpal, A. Vats, B. Lamb, *et al.* Information transfer and communication in surgery: a systematic review. *Ann Surg* 2010; **252**: 225–39.

29. A. B. Haynes, T. G. Weiser, W. R. Berry, *et al.* A surgical safety checklist to reduce morbidity and mortality in a global population. *N Engl J Med* 2009; **360**: 491–9.

30. S. Middleton, A. Roberts. *Integrated Care Pathways: A Practical Approach to Implementation*. Edinburgh: Butterworth Heinemann, 2000; pp 3–11.

31. C. Jimmerson., D. Weber, D. K. Sobek. "Reducing waste and errors: piloting lean principles at Intermountain Healthcare." *Jt Comm J Qual Patient Saf* 2005; **31**: 249–57.

32. R. A. Paulus, K. Davis, G. D. Steele. Continuous innovation in health care: implications of the Geisinger experience for health system reform. *Health Aff (Millwood)* 2008; **27**: 1235–45.

33. D. N. Wijeysundera, P. C. Austin, W. S. Beattie, J.E. Hux, A Laupacis. Outcomes and processes of care related to preoperative medical consultation. *Arch Intern Med* 2010; **170**: 1365–74.

34. H. Vaghadia, C. Fowler. Can nurses screen all outpatients? Performance of a nurse based model. *Can J Anaesth* 1999; **46**: 1117–21.

35. P. K. Barnes, P. A. Emerson, S. Hajnal, W. J. Radford, J. Congleton. Influence of an anaesthetist on nurse-led,

computer-based, pre-operative assessment. *Anaesthesia* 2000; **55**: 576–80.

36. R. E. Lutner. The automated interview versus the personal interview. Do patient responses to preoperative health questions differ? *Anesthesiology* 1991; **75**: 394–400.

37. R. E. Lutner, M. F. Roizen, C. B. Stocking, *et al.* The automated interview versus the personal interview: do patient responses to preoperative health questions differ? *Anesthesiology* 1991; **75**: 394–400.

38. E. G. VanDenKerkhof, D. H. Goldstein, W. C. Blaine, M. J. Rimmer. A comparison of paper with electronic patient-completed questionnaires in a preoperative clinic *Anesth Analg* 2005; **101**: 1075–80.

39. J. M. Ehrenfeld, P. Reynolds, S. Hersey, B. A. Campbell, W. S. Sandberg. *Pilot Implementation & Assessment of a Computerized Preanesthetic Assessment Tool.* Abstract A 851, Annual American Society of Anesthesiologists Meeting 2011, Chicago, USA.

40. A. Walia, R. Sierra-Anderson, A. Robertson. *Feasibility of Using a Web-based Patient Portal to Directly Elicit a Comprehensive Medical History from Veterans.* Abstract S-104, International Anesthesia Research Society, Annual Meeting 2011, Vancouver, Canada.

41. E. Lobo, J. Feiner, R. Cahlikova. *Web-based Mobile Health: Novel Ways to Engage Patients in Their Care and Reduce Healthcare Costs for Hospitals and Patients.* Abstract TO-P437, International Health Economics Association, Annual Meeting 2011, Toronto, Canada.

42. W. Shapiro, J. Feiner, E. Lobo. Impact of patient-centered remote triage on day of surgery cancellation rate 2011. (manuscript in preparation).

43. S. Kreimer. Quality & safety. Alarming: Joint Commission, FDA set to tackle alert fatigue. *Hosp Health Netw* 2011; **85**: 18–19.

44. T. Isaac, J. S. Weissman, R. B. Davis, *et al.* Overrides of medication alerts in ambulatory care. *Arch Intern Med* 2009; **169**: 305–11.

45. N. Kruzik. Benefits of preoperative education for adult elective surgery patients. *AORN J* 2009; **90**: 381–7.

46. A. Coulter, J. Ellins. Effectiveness of strategies for informing, educating, and involving patients. *BMJ* 2007; **335**: 24–7.

47. M. T. Kluger, E. J. Tham, N. A. Coleman, W. B. Runciman, M. F, Bullock. Inadequate pre-operative evaluation and preparation: a review of 197 reports from the Australian incident monitoring study. *Anaesthesia* 2000; **55**: 1173–8.

48. D. L. Hepner, A. M. Bader, S. Hurwitz, M, Gustafson, L. C. Tsen. Patient satisfaction with preoperative assessment in a preoperative assessment testing clinic. *Anesth Analg* 2004; **98**: 1099–105.

49. M. J. Harnett, D. J. Correll, S. Hurwitz, *et al.* Improving efficiency and patient satisfaction in a tertiary teaching hospital preoperative clinic. *Anesthesiology* 2010; **112**: 66–72.

50. F. Dexter. Design of appointment systems for preanesthesia evaluation clinics to minimize patient waiting times: a review of computer simulation and patient survey studies. *Anesth Analg* 1999; **89**: 925–31.

Chapter

A surgeon's perspective
Perioperative standards, quality, and consents

Frank G. Opelka MD, FACS

Perioperative standards   132
Quality in perioperative care   133

Informed consent   136

The disciplines of anesthesia, surgery, and perioperative nursing care have a long track record with setting standards, improving quality, and assuring that patients are informed about the entire operative experience. From a surgeon's perspective, quality and standards in perioperative care began when the American College of Surgeons first formed the Minimum Standards for Hospitals in 1917 at the urging of a Massachusetts surgeon, Ernest Codman, MD. It was back in 1910 when Dr. Codman defined the "end results" as the perioperative goal for patients [1,2]. It took nearly half a century before this initial effort ultimately led to the formation of the Joint Commission in 1951. The Joint Commission sets standards of care throughout the acute care setting of the hospitals it certifies. The Joint Commission now has expanded its key role in defining care in and beyond hospitals with standards that insure that patients receive care in a safe and appropriate environment. In addition, over 100 years after Codman's call for accountability, the recent United States Congress has taken significant legislative actions on quality and value in health care with the passage of several new laws. These national legislative efforts are bringing about change from the status quo. Codman's "end results" are referred to in modern health-care performance jargon by the title of clinical outcomes. His efforts are now merged into health-care law and delivery system credentials.

The perioperative clinical disciplines of anesthesia, surgery, nursing, and pharmacy are joining together to leverage the work each group has accomplished over the last century to define the new setting of care to insure the best measurable clinical outcomes. This

chapter highlights further expansions in perioperative standards, quality, and the informed patient to coincide with the changes coming forth in health care.

Perioperative standards

The perioperative standards are designed to protect patients and providers in the complex environment surrounding surgery. The standards are the foundation for assuring patient safety and reducing errors and near misses, with the hope of limiting patient harm. The attention to perioperative standards intensified when the Institute of Medicine (IOM) released *To Err is Human* in 1999. This report extrapolated an estimate of 44 000 to 98 000 patient deaths in the United States as a direct result of medical errors [3]. Continued scientific advances in anesthesia, nursing care, and surgical care have led to expansion of the complexity surrounding the patient in the operating room (OR) environment. Thus, the operating experience is a highly concentrated and complex treatment experience that exposes patients to great risks, and demonstrated errors demand rigid standards and team-based approaches to best protect patients.

It is only through a fully transparent, system-based approach, including an activated and engaged patient and family, that we can best provide care and protect the patient from unintended harm. Surgeons rely on the system and the entire team to provide the best environment for the care of the patient. One way of considering perioperative standards draws comparisons from other management resources. The aviation industry is in many ways similar to the surgical experience. Using

Operating Room Leadership and Management, ed. Kaye A.D., Fox C.J. and Urman R.D. Published by Cambridge University Press. © Cambridge University Press 2012.

the aviation management standards in crew resource management (CRM) empowers the entire team to accomplish the objective in the safest manner [4]. Crew resource management promotes preoperative briefings for the operating team and the patients. The focus is on communication and open team involvement, in particularly when the team departs from the expected plan.

McCafferty and Polk discussed other perioperative types of errors for standards to address that relate to the surgeon's level of experience [5]. Surgeons once graduated from their residencies and "hung their shingle" to begin their clinical work. Now, the complexities of surgical care and technical skills have created a need for appreciating the level of expertise and performance after residency. Lifelong learning has become a part of a surgeon's career. McCafferty and Polk highlight some key differences in patient safety related to the surgeon's level of experience. Junior surgeons should be identified and have resources for mentorship when newly challenged by novel or complex clinical scenarios. Senior surgeons can create errors related to complacency tied to years of success in how they have routinely performed surgery. Appropriate means must exist within standards that address all types of errors, including errors related to a surgeon's level of experience.

Standards involve a list of focus areas in the perioperative environment. Those focus areas in the broadest sense across all disciplines of surgery rely on standards for anesthesia, medication standards, controls and regulations for medical gases, structure and protocols for antispesis, environmental sanitation, surgical instrument sterilization, perioperative assessment, specimen management, medical equipment management, and more. Anesthesia has long been a leader in recognizing safety issues in the perioperative experience [6]. Anesthesia-related deaths are now at 1/200 000 to 300 000.

It is beyond the scope of this chapter to review each aspect and each standard in the perioperative experience for every aspect in every discipline of surgery. Two challenging examples of current interest to the public include wrong-site surgery (WSS) and surgical site infection (SSI). These represent potential avoidable harms. Wrong-site surgery is a component of the Joint Commission's Sentinel Event Database [7]. The Joint Commission reported 5901 events from 1995 through 2008, a rate of 13% in the reporting hospitals. The data are not complete or perfect, but they do reflect an opportunity for better, safer care. With regards to WSS,

frequent areas involve orthopedic surgery, urology, general surgery, and neurosurgery. It is a rare but devastating event in perioperative care, and standards that limit it serve in protecting patients. Surgical site infection is a far more common condition that creates complicated harm and has proven costly to the delivery of care. In both WSS and SSI, applied standards used by the entire OR team greatly increase the chance for success and improved outcomes for patients.

Recent perioperative standards have focused on tools such as the universal protocol and surgical checklists. Even with standards in place we face challenges in protecting patients. Despite the perioperative universal protocols for assuring that the correct patient had the correct procedure performed on the correct side, we continue to have errors in surgery, with increasing occurrence of WSS. The Joint Commission reported several key drivers that lead to WSS. These include root cause analyses that demonstrate risks for WSS when an operation involves more than one surgeon involved in the care, more than one procedure on a patient, and unusual time pressures surrounding the procedure [7]. Fixing the problems with WSS involves setting standards and assuring that those standards are met. Prevention of WSS has several crucial processes. These processes begin with scheduling of the patient. The patient details must be verified and reconciled at time of scheduling and on the day of surgery. Site marking and surgical "time outs" are additional crucial processes that occur in the preoperative area before surgery. Once in the OR, staff turnovers must have hand-off protocols that include avoidance of WSS. Organizational culture that insures safe surgery and protects against WSS is important. Organizations should include education and prevention and tracking of WSS and other sentinel events on a regular basis. Open communication and targets that track results help focus the entire organization on the patient. It is important to recognize the patient's voice as well. Patients should be encouraged to participate in assuring success.

Quality in perioperative care

"… (o)utcomes are cues that prompt and motivate the assessment of process and structure in a search for causes that can be remedied" [8].

Why are health systems around the globe engaging in conversation about surgical quality? Since the IOM report of 1999, *To Err is Human*, the follow-on report, *Crossing the Quality Chasm* [9], brought tighter focus on performance measurement and quality. It is thought that quality of care plays a critical role in controlling costs. For example, lower SSIs translate into lower patient morbidity and mortality and also cost avoidance in treating the infection, with hospitalization or reoperation adding to the care. *Crossing the Quality Chasm* detailed a path forward in defining ways to measure quality. These two IOM reports have brought attention to new areas of health care that reach beyond the traditional clinical and biological sciences into the realm of performance measurement and improvement. Furthermore, the Dartmouth Atlas began shining a light on the regional variations in care and demonstrated tremendous opportunities for improvement [10].

Health-care delivery systems have become aware of performance measurements, of quality, and of defining value through payment and policy levers. Care delivery and payment also focus the public transparency in quality reports and eventual value-based payment systems as key drivers in quality. By the end of 2017, up to nine percent or more of Medicare hospital revenues will be linked to quality and performance. These changes will have tremendous impact on anesthesia, surgery, and perioperative care. How do health systems provide a framework for discussing surgical quality? What must health systems do to assess quality and drive towards improvement? What will high-performing, high-value health-care systems look like in the coming years?

Over time, anesthesia and surgery have made great strides in clinical sciences with new and improved therapeutics and technological advances that are unparalleled in history. Patients have benefited from these medical advances. Patient lives have greatly changed because of the advances in medicine. At the same time, the Dartmouth Atlas has demonstrated how much variation has developed in the actual delivery of care. The variation noted has also generated variable outcomes in quality. At the same time, the population has aged and, as a result of medical successes, is living with more complex chronic conditions. In Medicare, for example, the age of the average patient had increased to 76 years by 2008, with more people suffering from multiple chronic conditions and typically having overlong medication lists. During this same period of medical advancement little has changed in the model for the delivery of care. We still have a primary physician and hospital-centric system, in which care is delivered in hospitals, ambulatory centers, or in offices. Cost pressures are now demanding that health-care delivery

systems match the advances in clinical science and technology. In a patient-centric format, surgery and anesthesia must join efforts in using evidence-based care and appropriate use of guidelines. Performance measurement, public reporting and aligned payment systems and the value delivered in care are bringing modern delivery systems into the advanced world of clinical science and surgical technology. Surgeons and anesthesiologists will have to lead patients through a new format within more integrated and coordinated delivery systems.

Performance measurement involves quality, safety, resource use, and patient experience of care and care coordination. In a patient-centric format, patients will have publicly reported performance measures and must learn to judge the value of the services offered. Patients will select care from institutions that have high value. Health plans (insurers) and purchasers of health insurance want patients to focus more on the value of services provided and use patient levers such as co-pays and deductibles as a way to attract patients to become more engaged consumers. In addition, health plans and health insurance purchasers are designing benefits that create health care that encourages new payment systems that link performance measures and outcomes to the value of the services.

What does all of this mean to the individual surgeon or anesthesiologist? It means that the health-care changes will affect payment systems in ways that will move closer to bundling payment aligned with the quality of care an entire team delivers to the patient. The high-performing teams will receive greater incentives and rewards. Greater quality, safer care, and improved patient experience at lower costs will receive the rewards of more payment and more patients. Surgeons, anesthesiologists, and hospitals may wish to combine efforts to accept risk and share services in a prearranged bundled of care. Tied to the bundled care are performance measures that insure the patient is receiving high-value care.

Bundles of surgical care can be constructed in several ways. Two common ways to construct bundles are procedure-specific bundles and condition-specific bundles of care. Procedure-specific bundles are typically related to groups of procedures such as all the Current Procedure Codes for all the colectomies. The procedure itself would serve as a trigger event to identify the actual bundle, such as the scheduling of the colectomy. The start date for the bundle could begin several days before the actual procedure and would define all the services to be included in the bundle. The procedure bundle would also have an end point such as 90 days. The procedural bundle would consist of the surgeon and the hospital as a minimum. The bundle participants could expand the acceptance of risk to include anesthesia services, anatomic and laboratory pathology, and imaging services. The larger the bundle, the greater the risk shared across the participants and the greater the opportunity for savings. A colectomy procedural bundle would also have performance measures assigned to the bundle to capture quality, safety, resource use, and patient experience of care. The performance measures would include measures attributed to the anesthesia care, the hospital care, and the surgeon. These measures would address quality measures of process and outcomes. The measures would consider resource use or appropriateness of care consistent with evidence-based guidelines. These measures would also capture the patient experience of care.

Condition-specific bundles differ from procedural bundles. Condition-specific bundles reflect a trigger event or condition that the patient may have, such as a colon cancer. In this instance, the trigger event is linked to the diagnostic procedure that identified the cancer, which could be a colonoscopy. The time interval for a condition may reflect longer care episodes, perhaps 12–18 months in the instance of a colon cancer. The participants in the bundle would include many more services, such as a list that includes the endoscopist, the surgeon, anesthesia services, pathologic services, imaging, oncologic services, and perhaps radiation therapy. The facilities in the condition bundle could expand also to include the hospital, the endoscopy suite, and the oncology infusion center. Condition-specific bundles are more complex and difficult to administer. Integrated delivery systems already have the infrastructure and health information technology to manage these complex conditions.

In procedure- or condition-specific bundles, performance and risk assumption are key components. The focus on the individual services shifts to a more team-based approach for care. The team begins with optimizing the patient's health and chronic care with the primary care physician or the patient-centered medical home. Anesthesia and surgery serve key leadership roles in optimizing the preoperative care and coordinating that care with the pre-anesthesia services such as cardiology, pulmonology, or nephrology. Success comes from a well-constructed team that insures that evidence-based guidelines drive optimal

care and push for the best outcomes. It is the shared risk and reward wrapped into a performance measurement system that brings more of a team-based performance to the forefront. Nonperformers will have to adapt or face consequences from the public reporting of the system-level performance.

Value comes from judgment applied to the care delivered from the perspective of many stakeholders. Certainly purchasers and payers of health insurance seek to define value. Patients, too, seek value in the care delivered. Health care has become too complex for patients, purchasers, and payers to easily assign value to the health-care services that people receive.

Defining a value judgment begins with performance assessment, transparent comparisons, and accountability. Establishing performance assessment is no simple task. Performance measures include measures of quality, safety, patient experience of care, appropriateness, and resource use. Quality is often framed by the Donebedian principles of structure, process, and outcomes measures [11]. Safety relates to avoiding preventable harms to patients. Appropriateness attempts to define that the highest quality and safest care delivered was necessary and consistent with the best available evidence. Patient experience of care insures that the patient's voice is a central part of the perioperative decisions and measures the value of the care. Finally, in a time of serious concern over health-care expenditures and resource limitations, performance measurement seeks to focus on the highest quality and safety in care with the most prudent use of the resources available.

A value-based system has brought many industrial sciences to health care, and sharing across industries has driven much of the opportunity. Performance measurement science has taught health care how to define numerators and denominators. Implementation science has shown health care how other industries aggregate data, analyze the information, and create dashboards to inform the end users. Statistics has brought focus on reliability and validity so that what we measure has more meaning and ultimate use. Finally, improvement sciences have shown health care the many tools it can use to drive improvement.

All of the changes in performance measurement and in new payment alternatives will drive changes in the care of the patient. In surgery, the changes will increase the dependence of the hospital, the nursing staff, anesthesiologists, and surgeons to work collaboratively. It is success for the patient that will prove the most important focus for the business model. Once the perioperative experience is redesigned, the natural expansion from procedure-specific bundles to more longitudinal condition-specific bundles of care will create care coordination across the continuum. The perioperative team will expand to include care that begins before surgery and extends well beyond the time in hospital.

To redesign a perioperative delivery system for a patient rather than a provider will measure the patient level of quality, safety, appropriateness, resource use, and the experience of care for the entire team. The perioperative care of the twentieth century focused on the health-care providers and optimizing their contributions to the patient more than it focused on the overall patient care. The twenty-first century will leverage all that we learned from the experiences in our individual silos of care and remix our delivery within a new framework. Surgeons once focused on the surgical procedures, the techniques, and the many emerging surgical technologies. Anesthesia focused on the explicit perioperative anesthesia experiences for the patients. Both disciplines of perioperative health-care services have made major advances within our individual domains and patients have benefited greatly from these efforts.

We have begun to see the initial phases of tearing down the silos and building a new foundation for perioperative clinical delivery of care. The first few performance measures that linked the perioperative experience began with the Universal Protocol, the Surgical Care Improvement Project (SCIP) measures, and the surgical checklists. These measures, although basic, demonstrated wide variation in performance. We still have episodes of WSS or retained foreign bodies. Perfect performance of SCIP measures has had little influence on reducing SSIs. Yet, these initial efforts have taken down the silos of care and created communication streams across the perioperative system.

An important aspect of delivery system redesign will include restructuring the age-old clinical departments. Institutions such as the Cleveland Clinic [12] and MD Anderson [13] have created new multidisciplinary teams that are patient-condition-specific and focused on delivery of high-value health care. Surgical morbidity and mortality conferences would need to change from a strong focus on the technical aspects of surgical care to a more longitudinal view of driving safety, quality, outcomes, appropriateness, resource use, and patient experience of care across a continuum in the delivery system that included primary care, medical specialties, anesthesiologists, surgeons,

intensive-care-unit teams, perioperative teams, nurses, pharmacists, and more.

Building the infrastructure and the data systems needed to provide the clinical experts with a patient continuum of information will emerge. The federal program to invest in electronic health records for clinicians is the first step towards building the information infrastructure. The electronic health record will serve as a clinical repository for derivatives that will provide clinical dashboards for reporting on clinical care. The care delivery system is just scratching at the surface of the emerging clinical integration. Much of health care still remains in silos and lacks information technology. Over the next decade, more will come as payment and performance measurement merge around a new patient goal.

Informed consent

Informed consent is a process that reflects communication from the physician and understanding for the patient, who decides whether or not to consent to treatment. It is best to use a structured document to insure that all the elements of informed consent are completed and documented. In surgery, informed consent addresses the patient's understanding and consent for the proposed operation or procedure. Informed consents have found common use more broadly in complex care plans and in support of patient decisions beyond the OR. Informed consent has found its way into several aspects of the health-care delivery system. For these purposes, informed consent is a vital part of the perioperative engagement of surgical patients. The intent of informed consent provides a structured document that reasonably insures patients understand their condition, their treatment options, goals of therapy, and the common risks related to the proposed intervention or treatment.

The history of informed consent took a structured path in 1914 when Judge Cardozo rendered a landmark opinion in the case of Schloendorff v The Society of New York Hospital [14]. In this legal opinion, the patient had consented to an exam under ether for assessment of a uterine fibroid. When the surgeon found the lesion to be malignant, he removed the tumor without patient consent. Judge Cardozo opined, "Every human being of adult years and sound mind has a right to determine what shall be done with his own body; and a surgeon who performs an operation without his patient's consent commits an assault for which he is liable in damages. This is true except in cases of emergency where the patient is unconscious and where it is necessary to operate before consent can be obtained."

Jumping forward in time across the century, over the last half of the twentieth century, the common-law standards for informed consent developed physician-oriented standards of disclosure that consist of three details an experienced physician would communicate to a patient. These three components involve informing the patient about their condition, discussing the alternatives to treatment, and discussing the risks and benefits of all the options. The physician-centered approach was subsequently replaced after case law shifted the emphasis onto patients. Informed consent focuses on the patient's rights to understand and decide to accept or reject the care offered to them. Patients have a right to be given material information, and the legal standards have moved from a physician-oriented standard to a patient-oriented standard. The patient-centric standard is referred to as the "reasonable person standard" [15]. The standards for informed consent have become focused on a "reasonable" patient, not the particular patient being informed. The standards seek to inform a reasonable person about what they would need to know to make a meaningful decision. The consent represents the voluntary agreement of the patient to accept the care under consideration.

In order to be fully informed, the consent generally contains several key elements. These elements are: (1) disclosure; (2) patient understanding; and (3) patient decision to accept or reject the consent [16]. In the disclosure element, informed consents typically begin with a description of the patient's condition or disease and the nature of a proposed procedure. In addition to the proposed procedure, informed consent should relate to reasonable alternatives, including the option for no further care or to receive supportive care only. Informed consent outlines the attendant risks of the proposed procedure as well as the risks and benefits of the alternatives. When uncertainties in outcomes are important for a reasonable person to evaluate in the treatment considerations, these uncertainties are also highlighted in the consent process.

For patient understanding, informed consent should demonstrate, with written words and terms a reasonable patient would use, the condition and the procedure proposed for treatment. Often patients are bombarded with medical jargon and are reluctant to interpret the clinical dialog surrounding informed consent to ask for clarity. In order to best capture a patient's understanding of the proposed care, and time

permitting, patients should describe the key elements included in their consent. A patient should begin by stating their disease or condition; next they should describe the treatment and its common risks; finally, they should state their understanding of the alternative care or options. When all these elements are combined into a reasonable patient informed consent, the patient should next establish the expected outcome or goal of the therapy. In order to insure a valid consent, the patient must be considered to be competent to understand and make the decisions and they must voluntarily agree to the consent. When patients are thought to have impaired competency, family members or legal guardians may represent the patient.

For patients undergoing any operation or procedure, the health-care delivery system may seem intimidating and leave patients exposed or vulnerable. Physicians and nurses engaged directly in perioperative care must be cognizant of the patient's level of health literacy and their comfort in asking about their care. To encourage patient activation, the physician can make clear to the patient that she/he is participating in a decision, not merely signing a form.

The decision process of informed consent involves patient selection bias. Most patients have already considered the necessity of surgical therapy in taking the necessary steps to seek a surgeon's evaluation. It is important to provide the patient with an appreciation for their present condition and a glimpse at the projected outcomes. When patients have entrusted the decision to their surgeon, the surgeon should nonetheless provide a fully informed consent. Patients are encouraged to make value judgments about the benefits and the risks of the procedure. These value judgments are difficult for even a reasonable patient, as most patients have little experience with the risks related to surgery. To assist patients in their value judgments, surgeons may elect to ask patients to describe what their treatment goals are and to express their understanding of the risks.

Every surgeon will experience a patient who may be undecided or refuse surgery. In that instance, patients may properly postpone a decision or elect alternative therapy. Supporting and respecting the patient's decision is important. At the same time, the surgeon needs to be assured that all the aspects of a reasonable patient informed consent standard have been met. The patient must demonstrate that they understand their condition, the postponed or denied treatment and the reason for their decision. The surgeon must assess that the patient's decision appeared to represent a thoughtful and competent action.

When patients cannot comprehend the informed consent process through poor understanding or a lack of decision-making capacity, the surgeon may need to seek action through a surrogate. Statutes in several states allow for family members to serve as surrogates for patients. In this instance, the family member has to protect the patient's interests and not the interests of the family. If the surgeon believes the patient is not adequately represented by a family member as any reasonable patient, the surgeon may petition the court to appoint the surrogate [17].

References

1. D. Neuhauser. Ernest Amory Codman MD. *Qual Saf Health Care* 2002; **11**: 104–5.

2. M. L. Millenson. *Trust me, I'm a doctor. In: Demanding medical excellence*. Chicago: University of Chicago Press, 1985. p. 141–7.

3. L. T. Kohn, J. M. Corrigan, M. S. Donaldson, eds. *To err is human*. Washington DC. National Academy Press, 1999.

4. J. McGreevy, T. Otten, M. Poggi, *et al*. The challenges of changing roles and improving surgical care now: crew resource management approach. *Am Surg* 2006; **72**: 1082–7.

5. M. H. McCafferty, H. C. Polk. Patient safety and quality in surgery. *Surg Clin N Am* 2007; **87**: 867–81.

6. W. Lanier. A three decade perspective on anesthesia safety. *Am Surg* 2006; **72**: 985–9.

7. N. Knight, J. Aucar. Use of an anatomic marking form as an alternative to the universal protocol for preventing wrong site, wrong procedure and wrong person surgery. *Am J Surg* 2010, **200**: 803–9.

8. J. M. Corrigan, M. S. Donaldson, L. T. Kohn, eds. *Crossing the Quality Chasm*, Washington DC, National Academy Press, 2001.

9. J. E. Wennberg, A. Gittelsohn. Health Care Delivery in Maine I: Patterns of use of common surgical procedures. *J Maine Medical Assoc* 1975; **66**: 123–30, 149.

10. A. Donabedian. Evaluating the quality of medical care. *Milbank Mem Fund Q* 1966; **44**(Suppl): 166–206.

11. K. E. Hammermeister, R. Johnson, G. Marshall, *et al*. Continuous assessment and improvement in quality of care. A model from the Department of Veterans Affairs cardiac surgery. *Ann Surg* 1994; **219**: 281–90.

12. M. E. Porter, E. O. Tiesberg. The Cleveland Clinic: Growth Strategy 2008. Case Report. Harvard Business School, 9–709–743, February 2009.

13. M. E. Porter, S. H. Jain. The University of Texas MD Anderson Cancer Center: Interdisciplinary Cancer Care. Case Report. Harvard Business School, 9–708–487, November 2009.

14. Schloendorff v Society of New York Hospital, 211 NY 125, 126, 105 NE 92, (1914).

15. Canterbury v Spense, 464 F2d 772, 785 (DC Cir 1972).

16. J. W. Jones, L. B. McCullough, B. W. Richman. A comprehensive primer of surgical informed consent. *Surg Clin N Am* 2007; **87**: 903–18.

17. A. Buchannan, D. Brock. *Deciding for others: the ethics of surrogate decision-making*, New York: Cambridge University Press; 1989.

Chapter

13

Anesthesia practice management
Core principles

Sonya Pease MD
Barbara Harris RN, MHA

Introduction   139
Anesthesia practice structure   139
The anesthesia care team model   140
Contracting   141
Recruiting   142
Scheduling   142
Marketing   143

Billing   143
Compliance and benchmarking   144
Evaluating the anesthesia practice   145
Evaluating the anesthesia department   145
Reforming an underperforming practice   147
Leveraging the partnership   149
Summary   149

Introduction

Managing a successful medical practice in today's complex health-care environment requires educated and talented physician and nonphysician leaders to insure excellence in patient care and to provide management services that support client satisfaction, promote efficiency, and insure regulatory compliance. For the anesthesia practice, there are other unique considerations. And although practice management skills are typically underemphasized in most residency programs, mastery of these skills may impact an anesthesia physician's career just as significantly as his or her clinical skills.

The Accreditation Council for Graduate Medical Education (ACGME) requires residency programs to address such issues as operating room (OR) management, practice structure, job acquisition, financial planning, contract negotiations, billing arrangements, professional liability, and legislative and regulatory issues. Few of these practice-management-related questions, if any, are covered in either written or oral board exams. As a result, many anesthesiologists are forced to attain their functional knowledge of effective anesthesia practice management on the job.

The success of the anesthesia practice is likewise important to the partners with which it contracts. Anesthesiology, with the exception of pure pain management, is predominantly practiced in a hospital or other health-care setting. As regulatory and financial pressures increase, hospital leaders increasingly seek anesthesia providers to act as true collaborative partners. Effective practice management positions the anesthesia provider to optimize opportunities for partnerships that maximize practice efficiencies, improve reportable measures, insure quality care, and increase patient satisfaction.

Anesthesia practice structure

Structure of the practice is a critical driving force in anesthesia practice management. There are numerous ways to provide anesthesia services, ranging from independent or group providers to full employment by a hospital, staffing company, or professionally managed practices. Within each structure various care-delivery models, including all-physician, all certified registered nurse anesthetist (CRNA), and blended care team models, also exist. Each structure and model offers distinct advantages and disadvantages. Just as providers make patient care decisions based on risks and benefits, anesthesia providers must make business decisions based on the needs of its hospital or other health-care provider partner, the financial risks and liabilities of each structure in a particular practice setting, and the preferences of the principals in the group.

Operating Room Leadership and Management, ed. Kaye A.D., Fox C.J. and Urman R.D. Published by Cambridge University Press. © Cambridge University Press 2012.

Independent practice

In an independent practice, the individual provider acts as a sole proprietorship or single-member corporation, often contracting services directly to specific facilities or surgeons. Although independent practice offers the physician or CRNA the highest level of professional independence, the economic challenge of covering practice overhead coupled with the increasing difficulty of meeting hospital administrative demands make long-term sustainability of single-provider practices, or even a coalition of multiple single providers, difficult to sustain.

Group practice

Group practice remains the prevalent anesthesia practice structure in the United States, with small practices of 10 physicians or less and medium practice groups of 11 to 50 physicians representing the largest population in the 2011 Medical Group Management Association (MGMA) survey. The private practice group model offers a high level of independence and autonomy, while also facilitating options for structured work hours, standardized call rotation, and group collaboration to share knowledge, experience, and expenses to an extent that is not possible in individual provider practices. Although the potential to realize these group-practice benefits certainly exists, the absence of strong practice leadership and the variance in individual work ethics, personalities, and practice preferences can divide the practice and threaten its viability.

Larger groups consisting of more than 50 physicians continue to gain market share, both as anesthesia-only and multi-specialty practices. These larger entities offer less autonomy and professional independence than their smaller counterparts, but can provide greater opportunity for sharing administrative workload, thus positively impacting quality of life for practice members. Large groups may also offer benefits such as internal continuing medical education (CME) activities, online resources, and career advancement opportunities within the group. In addition, large group practices typically maintain a lower operating cost per physician owing to greater economies of scale, which may in turn improve margins and related physician compensation. Large groups may also be better positioned to employ or contract professional management services to improve financial outcomes while reducing internal disagreements over management philosophy.

Provider employment

An increasingly common choice for many anesthesia providers is to enter into an employment agreement with a health-care facility or large practice, either privately owned or managed by a professional management company. These employers offer numerous advantages over the self-dependence of private practice (an environment in which providers must, as the industry saying goes, often depend upon eating only what they kill). Large employees typically offer compensation packages that include some level of financial security in the form of a guaranteed base salary somewhat immune to fluctuations in practice volumes or payer mix. They also offer economies of scale that leverage more favorable payer contracts and often significant reductions in overhead costs. Most also offer expanded benefit packages with structured retirement plans, choice of insurance packages, paid CME, and broader access to state and federal employee benefits such as family medical leave.

The anesthesia care team model

Once group structure is determined, the choice of care delivery model remains. Both all-physician (and all-CRNA) and care team model practices offer unique benefits and disadvantages. Almost all anesthesia care is provided either personally by an anesthesiologist or by a nonphysician anesthesia provider such as an anesthesiologist assistant (AA) or CRNA. Nonphysician providers function most often under the direction or supervision of a licensed physician – typically an anesthesiologist, although in some circumstances a proceduralist such as a surgeon or cardiologist may supervise the delivery of anesthesia care.

In the anesthesia care team model, anesthesia care is delivered by nonphysician providers directed by an anesthesiologist. Under this model, monitoring and perioperative tasks are delegated to nonphysician providers, whereas the anesthesiologist remains responsible for the overall care and safety of the patient.

The anesthesia care team model typically consists of one or more anesthesiologists directing nonphysician providers at physician to CRNA/AA ratio ranging from 1:1 to 1:4. Although the ratio of physicians to nonphysicians may fluctuate depending upon the geographic layout of the facility and the acuity of patient care provided, payers – particularly Centers for

Medicare & Medicaid Services (CMS) – often have very specific guidelines for billing under the medical direction model.

The care team staffing model has been shown to improve access to anesthesia services by expanding the number of anesthetizing locations, increasing opportunities for parallel processing so work that was once done in a linear fashion can occur concurrently, thereby freeing physician providers for rapid access to areas of greatest clinical need.

State regulatory bodies license nonphysician anesthesia providers and set the conditions under which they can work. These parameters may vary profoundly by state. Some states, for example, require physician supervision of CRNAs, whereas others allow CRNAs to work independently of physician supervision. Anesthesia assistants always function within an anesthesia care team model and are always directed by an anesthesiologist. In addition to the consideration given to the level of physician supervision desired by the facility and its medical staff in the delivery of anesthesia services, developing an intimate familiarity with the state requirements for supervision of nonphysician anesthesia providers for the state and Medicare region is imperative in determining the practice model.

Contracting

When negotiating a contract for delivery of anesthesia services, both the anesthesia practice and the health-care facility must establish and clearly define mutual goals and desired outcomes to insure success for all parties. Health-care organizations generally seek to partner with anesthesia groups that are willing to build and structure a team that supports the culture and needs of the health-care organization. Likewise, the organization and its key stakeholders must be willing to consider and adapt to recommendations for a practice model and structure that allows the anesthesia group to optimize clinical outcomes while maintaining the highest degree of financial independence.

Hospitals and health-care facilities seeking an anesthesia partner typically issue a request for proposal (RFP), in which the facility issues a formal invitation to multiple anesthesia groups to submit a proposal.

The RFP process for both the anesthesia group and the health-care facility starts with a very detailed and thoughtful analysis of the anesthesia needs of the organization. This analysis helps insure facility leadership has developed an understanding of the exact

services required and the optimal manner in which they may be provided. A well-structured RFP provides sufficient information for anesthesia practices not only to determine the services being sought but also to obtain critical insight into the environment in which those services will be provided. If not present in the RFP, anesthesia practice leaders should request the following information before submitting their response.

1. Facility demographics, including location, size, classifications (community, trauma, for-profit, not-for-profit, etc.), governance structure, and leadership.

2. Status of current anesthesia services, including group structure (independent providers, group, etc.), model (all-physician, care team, etc.), number of each type of provider, and contract expiration date.

3. Detailed listing of anesthetizing locations, including number of locations staffed by client personnel at different times of the day for each day of the week. This should include expectations for workflow support that may require additional providers, such as extra rooms used to flip cases in procedural areas, expectations for staffing variation by shift, and depth and intensity of call coverage.

4. Information about caseloads, including: service lines; frequently performed procedures; case/patient volumes, including surgery, deliveries, and C-section rate; and ancillary services such as endoscopy, cardiac catheterization lab, and interventional radiology. The percentage of ancillary volumes supported by anesthesia should be indicated, including the same type of day-of-week and hour-of-day detail provided for surgery volumes and any available information about volume trends by procedure area and service line.

5. Expectations and requirements for anesthesia provider specialty training and skills, such as pain, cardiothoracic, and pediatric fellowship training or transesophageal echocardiography (TEE) anesthesia and regional pain management skills.

6. Patient demographics (age, gender) for procedure areas and the facility as a whole.

7. Payer mix information for the procedure areas and for the facility as a whole, including trends in payer mix and reimbursement by payer.

8. Information about organizational governance of the medical staff and where anesthesia fits into the model, including specific bylaws or relationships

with other facilities or parent organizations that may impact the anesthesia management structure.

9. Clearly defined service expectations details; for example, in-house 24×7 coverage of the labor and delivery unit, participation in hospital quality or service initiatives such as HealthGrades, reduction in emergency room to OR times for trauma patients, or presurgical phone calls to patients.

10. Details about any strategies in the five-year business plan of the facility that will impact provision of anesthesia services through increased or decreased volumes, major changes in payer mix, loss or acquisition of major service lines or medical staff providers, and facility expansion plans.

The RFP process should provide the opportunity for serious candidates to tour the anesthetizing locations to observe existing patient flow, physical plant, and anesthesia equipment. It should also require all parties to keep confidential any information disclosed by either the health-care organization or practices submitting proposals. Otherwise, the parties may be reluctant to release detailed information about their internal business plans and performance, making it difficult to align proposed goals and services with those of the facility accurately.

Once a facility has identified a potentially suitable anesthesia practice to be its business partner, it is critical that all the appropriate stakeholders engage in discussions, including the facility's C-suite members with administrative oversight of the procedural areas; chief financial officer; key medical staff members (including chiefs of surgery, obstetrics, and cardiology); and departmental leaders in perioperative services, obstetrics, and other anesthetizing locations.

Recruiting

Recruiting and retaining talented anesthesia providers is a critical function of anesthesia leadership, secondary only to maintenance of clinical excellence. The costs associated with recruitment of a single anesthesiologist may range from $25 000 to $50 000 and even reach $100 000 for high-demand subspecialists with advanced training and skills. Successful recruiting requires detailed knowledge of the hospital or health-care facility work environment, including case mix and surgeon/proceduralist expectations.

Once candidates are identified, the practice should gather information that includes credentials related to: education, certifications, and licensure; work history;

personal goals and attributes; and references. As the interview process necessarily exposes the candidate to the facility, it is critical that practice leadership perform full due diligence before any on-site visits.

The information gathering phase should include requests to candidates to explain employment gaps, past and current malpractice, litigation, and/or disciplinary actions, and other details about education and employment history. Sufficient time should be allowed to follow up on any questionable items before the interview. Ideally, at least two members of the practice should conduct a preliminary interview with the candidate by phone, exploring any areas that have been at the root of past issues for the practice with former group members as well as areas recognized as highly desirable in the work environments of the practice.

Only candidates who pass the initial background review and are found to be probable matches in the initial phase of the selection process should advance to an on-site interview. On site, candidates should have the opportunity to interact with numerous members of the practice, facility leadership, and key members of the medical staff. Interview questions should focus on areas not covered by the curriculum vitae and be designed to gain insight into the candidate's opinions and ideas, and knowledge and experience, as well as work style, interpersonal skills, and leadership capabilities. For instance, the interviewer may ask the candidate to provide extemporaneous examples of work experiences that expose his or her strengths and weaknesses, team skills, and interpersonal relationship style.

Special care is advised when vetting PRN (as-needed) or locum tenens (temporary) staff. Although they may step in to fill the position of a permanent staff member for an extended period of time, their goals and work habits may not be fully aligned with those of the practice and the facility. Many practices make the critical mistake of assuming exemplary clinical skills are sufficient to be a successful member of the practice when, in fact, clinical skills are a minimal qualification for success. Consult with a human resource specialist to gain information about material that cannot be discussed in the hiring process to avoid risk of equal employment violations.

Scheduling

Scheduling coverage for the practice is a complex task that goes well beyond the simple task of assigning staff to shifts and rooms. Effective scheduling begins with determining the true needs of each anesthetizing location. Rarely are anesthesia coverage needs static throughout the day or throughout the week. In high-volume, complex departments such as surgery, work with department leadership to use data from the surgery information system to determine actual capacity demands by hour of day and day of week. Smaller departments use manual scheduling logs or review patient records assessed over several weeks or months. This extra effort will help avoid gaps in coverage during busy periods and wasted resources during downtimes.

Any scheduling methodology must take into consideration not only staff preferences but also shift equity, fair distribution of responsibilities, limits on consecutive work hours, numbers of day and night shifts, on-call needs, weekend off requests, and absences for personal time off. Also of vital importance is the employment status of staff members. In practices where nonphysician providers and support personnel (CRNAs, AAs, and anesthesia technicians) are salaried, the added expense of overtime can be avoided if the typical workload remains reasonable. However, if the work week consistently runs past 40 h or the personnel works on an hourly basis, use historical caseload data to staff the practice with adequate staff to work late hours.

Consider creating a long-range schedule with vacations, weekend call, and weeknight call occurring in a consistently repeating rotation. This type of schedule offers the greatest predictability for planning one's personal life in advance, as call commitments are predictable and occur with consistent repetition. The rotating schedule also offers the easiest option for covering post-call days off and/or days with spikes in volume. Staff members who need a particular day or series of days off can then swap with assigned teammates as needed. Conversely, staff members can make scheduling requests in advance, and the schedule can be built around those personal preferences.

Marketing

Marketing activities by the anesthesia practice, like other health-care providers, must be conducted in a manner that insures compliance with legal and regulatory restrictions on such activities. With the exception of pain-management practices that need to generate patient volumes, most anesthesia practices are hospital based and are therefore not the primary patient driver in choice of a health-care facility. Thus marketing of the anesthesia department usually involves collaboration with the health-care facility to spotlight specific service lines such as acute regional pain management programs or subspecialty programs such as pediatric services, cardiac services, or obstetric specialty services.

Acute regional pain management services provided by the anesthesia department can be huge patient satisfiers in terms of excellence in pain management as well as decreasing patient length of hospital stay and early physical therapy interventions. In this situation some of the most effective marketing comes from the surgeons who utilize these modalities to calm patient fears of the procedure and build volumes by being affiliated with these services.

Almost all health-care facilities have public relations resources that can be tapped into. Highlighting specific physician services or programs in community mailers or audiovisual communications such as radio and billboard advertisements can be a good place to start. Anesthesia departments may also want to develop a practice website and create practice brochures and direct mailers that assist in educating both the professional and patient communities as to the scope of practice and subspecialty programs offered by the practice.

Billing

Reimbursement for anesthesia services is unique from all other medical specialties. At one time, hospitals paid anesthesiologists directly for their services. This practice was replaced by a fee-for-service structure based on a percentage of the surgeon's fee. Today, anesthesia transaction code sets determine how electronic claims are submitted to payers. Increasingly, these new standards require anesthesiologists to provide the surgical code in addition to the anesthesia code on claims. Several key resources are therefore vital for the billing function of the anesthesia practice.

For the past 40 years, the *Relative Value Guide* (RVG) published by the American Society of Anesthesiologists (ASA) has linked the relative value of anesthesia services to the American Medical Association (AMA) catalog of *Current Procedure Terminology* (CPT). The CPT catalog provides widely accepted medical nomenclature and the associated numeric codes used to report medical procedures and services under public and private health insurance plans. The RVG contains the most up-to-date CPT codes with full descriptors for anesthesia services and provides a valuation of the work performed, called a base unit value.

A third tool, the ASA *CROSSWALK*, provides the CPT anesthesia code that most specifically describes the anesthesia service for a particular diagnostic or therapeutic CPT procedure code.

Typically, anesthesia codes are site-specific, whereas a single surgical or procedural code could apply to multiple anatomical sites. Accurate identification of site, therefore, becomes critical to selection of the correct anesthesia code.

Once a code is assigned, a base unit value is calculated that includes all anesthesia services associated with that particular procedure in that specific anatomical location, including pre- and postoperative assessments, fluid administration, and interpretation of basic anesthesia monitoring data. Units of time, typically measured in 10-min or 15-min increments, are then added to base units.

Modifiers such as physical status of the patient, unusual anesthesia circumstances, anesthesia services beyond those associated with the base code, complex positioning, or multiple procedures are then applied to arrive at the final valuation for the services provided.

The anesthesia practice bills for its services by combining base units from the CPT and *CROSSWALK* codes, time units, and modifier codes. Note that the RVG and *CROSSWALK* are guides only. The anesthesia practice may also bill some services as flat fee codes, which are negotiated for particular procedures with individual payers. These flat fee codes are all inclusive of base units, time units, and any applicable modifier codes.

Care team model billing

Billing for professional anesthesia services takes on additional complexity in the care team model. In addition to the coding process previously described, additional modifier codes are added to indicate the type of provider involved in delivery of care and the level of supervision provided. Examples of these codes are shown in Table 13.1.

The CMS has outlined specific anesthesia guidelines for the delivery of anesthesia services that delineate rules and regulation for health-care facilities to maintain their conditions of participation (CoP). These rules outline how anesthesia services are furnished within a facility and the survey procedures used to evaluate delivery of services. Failure to function and code within these guidelines can result in both financial and regulatory risk to the practice.

Table 13.1 Examples of codes for billing for professional anesthesia services

AA	Services provided personally by the anesthesiologist
AD	Services delivered by nonphysicians under the medical supervision of a physician who has more than four concurrent anesthesia procedures under supervision at the same time
QK	Services provided by a nonphysician, but medically directed by a physician who has two to four procedures under medical direction at the same time
QX	Service provided by a CRNA with medical direction by a physician
QY	Indicates an anesthesiologist medically directing only one CRNA
QZ	Service provided by a CRNA without medical direction by a physician

It is vital that anesthesia leadership become intimately familiar the requirements for compliant coding and billing as well as the requirements for compliance with CMS regulations and work with their billing service to insure that those requirements are met.

Compliance and benchmarking

Medical quality assurance is every provider's job, but there are specific areas in which an engaged anesthesia service partnering with effective hospital leadership can have a profound impact on reportable measures such as core measures and surgical care improvement project (SCIP) measures – SCIP is a national campaign, launched in 2005, to substantially reduce surgical mortality and morbidity through collaborative efforts.

The anesthesia practice should insure that each provider's ongoing professional practice evaluation includes performance on anesthesia-relevant SCIP quality measures, which typically include:

- SCIP-Inf 1a: prophylactic antibiotic received within 1 h prior to surgical incision, overall rate;
- SCIP-Inf-2: prophylactic antibiotic selection for surgical patients, overall rate;
- SCIP-Inf-10: surgical patients with perioperative temperature management;
- SCIP-Card 2: surgery patients on beta-blocker therapy prior to arrival who received a beta-blocker during the perioperative period.

In addition to these specific quality measures, maximizing the full value of anesthesia services requires physicians to participate and report on specific measures for the Physician Quality Reporting System (PQRS). From 2008 to 2010, anesthesia providers could report on specific quality measures for covered services for Medicare beneficiaries and receive an incentive payment of up to 2% at the group practice level. Proposed changes to the PQRS initiative underscore the importance of staying on top of both specific measures of quality, including their reporting requirements, and their impact on the practice financially if not reported properly.

For instance, proposed changes to the PQRS on the horizon at the time of the writing of this text mean failure to meet reporting requirements can result in a potential loss of revenue for specific patient populations. Certain measures have been or may be designated for potential incentive payments that can impact those payments if not properly reported including:

- measure #76: prevention of catheter-related bloodstream infections;
- measure #30: perioperative care – timing of prophylactic antibiotics by the administering physician;
- measure #193: perioperative temperature management.

Many health-care facilities do not understand the complexities of anesthesia services and the lost revenue opportunities that result when anesthesia services fail to report these measures. It is the responsibility of anesthesia leadership, therefore, to insure optimal performance for these reporting requirements.

Evaluating the anesthesia practice

It was traditionally simple for a facility to assess the performance of its anesthesia provider relative to their expectations for service. Expectations were so consistent that they were easily defined as "the four A's": ability, availability, affordability, and affability. This meant: provide quality care, be on time, remain financially independent from the organization, and act in a professional manner. Today, the expectations of health-care organizations have grown to also encompass accountability and outcomes. Together, these attributes can be defined by the following "six A's."

Ability – provision of consistent, high-quality patient care that optimizes patient outcomes, avoids patient complications, and demonstrates excellence in evidence-based standards of anesthesia care. The providers and the services they provide demonstrate the art and science of good medicine.

Availability – perioperative program management to include maintenance of workflow dynamics and proper pairing of anesthesia resources with nursing resources to optimize perioperative systems, improving throughput and efficiency. Practice resources are expected to flex as necessary to adapt to dynamic caseloads in multiple departments and geographic locations.

Affordability – providing anesthesia program services that are cost-effective to both the facility and the patient population; this includes service outreach to facilitate optimal utilization of client resources (time, staff, space, equipment, and supplies) as well as risk-sharing in development of new service lines.

Affability – delivery of a client-centric service that supports the hospital, surgeon, and patient as valued customers. Going beyond service with a smile, providers are expected to anticipate the needs of the customer and to actively support achievement of their goals.

Accountability – assuming primary responsibility for and leading quality initiatives as well as measuring and meeting mutually agreed-upon metrics for quality, service, and satisfaction.

Answerability – linking of provider compensation to fulfillment of each of these components of anesthesia services.

Evaluating the anesthesia department

As a wise hospital chief executive once put it, "I don't know exactly what makes a great anesthesia department, but I sure do know one when I see it." Many involved in procedural care environments would agree with this statement.

A great anesthesia department operates almost seamlessly, and the lack of disruptions in its daily patient flow and the results of satisfaction surveys from patients and surgeons speak for themselves. The evaluation of the following objective criteria, however, will help facilitate proper evaluation of the anesthesia department.

Look at the data

The delivery of anesthesia services can either facilitate throughput and performance in procedural care areas or hinder it. Review key performance indicators, including patient throughput, day-of-procedure cancellations, and case turnover times. Once identified, these performance indicators can be tied to performance benchmarks. Throughput indicators such as on-time starts, turnover times, and case delays cause and frequency are a measure of the group's responsiveness to the daily operational needs of the client. Day-of-procedure cancellations and timeliness of pre- and post-anesthesia assessment are indicative of the quality of the pre-anesthesia clearance process and attention to patient outcomes. Great practices will have access to and proactively deploy proven tools for improving performance in these areas, including access to perioperative management specialists, lean manufacturing techniques, and ongoing quality improvement cycles.

Review quality outcomes

Quality management is a regulatory requirement for anesthesia departments. This includes insuring that case reviews are completed, effective peer review is in place, and effective remediation for quality issues is deployed. Great anesthesia groups develop strong relationships with the health-care facility's quality assurance/quality management and risk and regulatory compliance departments. They also have their own internal audit process and routinely have their quality outcomes, documentation compliance, and regulatory performance reviewed by an objective, knowledgeable outside source with programs in place to insure benchmark performance on all measures. In addition, they actively support and provide required focused provider performance reviews on new providers and ongoing provider performance reviews on active members of the practice. Great practices maintain their anesthesia policies and procedures in current compliance with ASA standards as well as those of the health-care facility's specific accreditation partner – typically The Joint Commission or Healthcare Facilities Accreditation Program.

Evaluate the leadership

Effective anesthesia physician leadership and organizational governance are key to running a great practice. Lack of effective leadership triggers problems both internally and externally as the cohesiveness of the group decays, commitment to standards declines, and support of the health-care facility's interests take second chair. Effectiveness as a group leader depends less on tenure or years of experience and more upon possession of key leadership skills. The anesthesia leader must either possess or have immediate access

to current evidence-based knowledge on effective perioperative management and clearly understand how the department of anesthesia impacts the day-to-day effectiveness of the procedural care area. The leader must possess the interpersonal skills to build relationships with and engender trust from even the most recalcitrant member of the medical staff. It is not necessary that the leader have active clinical experience in all specialty areas served, but superior knowledge in anesthesia fundamentals is imperative. The leader must also commit to devoting adequate time to maintaining up-to-date expertise in anesthesia quality and compliance standards and to monitoring and assessing the performance of the anesthesia staff relative to those standards.

Examine the credentials of the providers

Although there are numerous highly qualified providers who practice anesthesia without board certification and specialty certifications, the presence of these credentials is an outward measure of the group's overall clinical qualifications. At a minimum, physician members should be board-eligible and actively pursuing certification. Mid-level nonphysician providers should be actively licensed with no restrictions. The great anesthesia practice will insure that all its members meet these requirements. If specialty services are offered, such as cardiothoracic anesthesia, pain management, and neonatal, all providers who participate in the service should be experienced and qualified and at least one member should hold active fellowship-level training in the discipline. Policies and protocols for specialty services should be clearly delineated and all providers serving the specialty should have mentored introduction to the service.

Assess the group's financial strength and stability

Financial sustainability has a profound effect on both the members of the practice and its health-care facility partner. In assessing financial strength and stability, determine if the practice has internal or external resources to provide expertise in managing payer relations and billing. A great anesthesia practice will be a good steward of its financial potential, contracting favorable terms with payers, carefully documenting patient care to support optimal billing, and coding in full compliance with regulatory guidelines. Failure in any of these pursuits could lead to inadequate cash flow, which could cause the practice to become dependent upon financial support from the health-care facility, even in markets with a favorable payer mix. Obviously, not all health-care markets can sustain an independent anesthesia practice, but even in those difficult markets, a great anesthesia practice will accurately forecast any shortfalls and actively work to reduce any financial support. Financial performance should be assessed regularly through structured meetings in which transparency is assured and mutual goals are aligned.

Evaluate the ability of the group to respond and adapt

The optimal anesthesia partner is well versed in the challenges that face its partner health-care facility in the areas of health-care reform. These challenges include new provisions for pay-for-performance and transformation funding in which more integrated systems of care linked with improved outcomes insure optimal global payments that encompass the entire patient episode of care. In addition, procedural services – particularly in the perioperative environment – are typically the largest single source of revenue for health-care organizations. Inefficient OR scheduling and patient throughput or poor staffing utilization, therefore, can have significant financial impact on the organization. As a major stakeholder in the perioperative department, the great anesthesia practice should have well-developed programs to help insure the health-care facility's financial success as well as its own.

Reforming an underperforming practice

When evaluation of the anesthesia practice identifies gaps in performance, creating an action plan for improvement is imperative. This may require practice leadership to share results with the health-care facility's leadership to develop a plan to improve performance. Just the act of voluntarily sharing performance data with the health-care facility partner can increase its confidence in the anesthesia practice, as members of the health-care facility have most likely already been assessing the data.

Reengineering an existing practice is a daunting task for even the most experienced leader. The ongoing demands of providing anesthesia services to an active caseload demand time and attention, and the practice

may simply lack the skill set required to accomplish the required transformation. In these instances, practice leaders may want to consider seeking outside management support.

To turn around an existing practice, consider the following guidance to address some of the most fundamental practice issues.

Poor performance

When benchmarks and goals are not being met, performance improvement plans must be put in place. As suggested earlier, a meeting between practice and health-care facility leaders may help prioritize efforts. Then begin by attacking one metric at a time. Although initiating an analysis of the entire preoperative process may be the initial inclination, the department is likely to be overwhelmed by the scope of this exercise. In place or in conjunction with a full assessment, choose a component easily controlled to start, such as ensuring charts on all elective cases are reviewed, anesthesia admission orders are written, and a tentative anesthesia plan developed.

Many issues are not problems of process but rather problems of communication or interpersonal conflict. The anesthesia provider interacts with professionals at all levels of the health-care organization and is therefore in a unique position to improve communication and change paradigms. Bring the anesthesia team together to utilize the goodwill and political capital it holds as perioperative leaders to affect behavioral changes in health-care peers.

Quality deficiencies

Meeting quality metrics begins with a shared commitment to improvement. A thorough assessment of each provider in the practice may reveal that some do not understand the metric, do not understand the importance of meeting the requirements, are not committed to fulfilling their responsibility to meet the goal, or a combination of all these factors. Anesthesia leaders must clearly communicate the importance of meeting quality metrics and follow through to insure all providers are compliant with established standards. Establish a system of effective peer review to identify individual providers who perform below benchmarks or whose clinical practice does not represent the highest level of patient care. Use any variance from expected performance as a learning opportunity for the whole team.

Ineffective leadership

Ineffective leadership in the anesthesia practice presents a difficult challenge for both members of the group and health-care facility leaders. The failure of a group to discipline internally or to create a culture of citizenship built on professionalism, effective communication, and accountability can create an environment of conflict. The measure of a leader in the clinical environment, particularly a close-knit environment like anesthesia, is the ability to foster this culture and to apply effective professional discipline when the culture is breached. Underperforming providers decrease the productivity of the entire group, and an effective leader will quickly progress these individuals through a performance improvement plan, culminating with removal from the group, if required. Both members of the anesthesia group and facility leadership should not confuse being well liked or having clinical expertise with being an effective leader. Unfortunately, the leader may be the underperformer. In this case, facility medical staff leadership may be called upon to help effect a change. This may best be accomplished by bringing in a management consultant or by encouraging the members of the group to move the practice under the management of a larger anesthesia management group.

Underperforming or under-qualified providers

The anesthesia group is no better than the sum of its parts. As anesthesia practice, even in groups, involves periodic solo practice – while on call, for example – even one poor performer can impact the entire group. Poor clinical practice is actually the easiest issue to address. Providers with deficiencies should be offered immediate remedial training. Clinical performance is a base expectation for overall performance, so if performance does not improve to benchmark or above, the provider should be removed.

The situation becomes more complex when providers are clinically competent – perhaps even exceptional – yet lack the certifications required by medical staff, such as anesthesia boards or cardiac fellowship. Some deficiencies can be overcome with structured study assignments, workshops, and CME offerings, but if medical staff bylaws or the contract with the facility requires all providers to be board-eligible or certified, group leadership has no option but to require this of its providers.

Even more challenging is dealing with the problem provider who meets all clinical, credentialing, and regulatory standards, yet fails to blend with practice or client personnel as a team. Others may meet all expectations, including those required for effective teamwork, but commit some transgression, such as drug diversion or inappropriate behavior with a member of the staff. The optimal way to deal with these situations is to have in place a zero-tolerance policy for any behavior detrimental or counter to the best interests of the facility partner. Tolerance by members of the practice, which may stem from a desire to buy forbearance for their own behaviors, will likely be viewed as lack of commitment to the facility and its patients and will, over time, decrease the stability of the contract and the practice.

The solution to each of these issues is straightforward: set a standard, measure performance, execute a performance improvement plan – if appropriate – and remove those who do not comply.

Financial instability

Anesthesia has a fiduciary responsibility to the members of the group and the health-care facility partner to maintain the highest possible level of financial integrity and independence. Payer contracting and billing is complex and time-consuming, and it may be tempting for anesthesia leadership to seek support from the health-care organization rather than to apply the necessary resources needed to optimize the group's own reimbursement. A sufficient proportion of anesthesia proceeds must be allocated to high-quality financial management of the group's business concerns. To facilitate financial independence, the health-care organization must work in partnership with the anesthesia group to create efficiencies in the procedural care areas to conserve resources. Financial success and independence can also be fostered by allowing the anesthesia provider latitude in negotiating favorable payment terms with payers rather than expecting it to fall in lock-step with facility contracts.

Anesthesia practices often sabotage their own success by cutting corners to reduce costs associated with contract management, coding, and billing. A high-quality practice management firm, or even an anesthesia-specific billing firm, may dramatically improve receipts, reducing dependence on the health-care organization and increasing the stability of the contract. Processes should be in place to automate patient eligibility verification, track and pattern denials, provide automated concurrency tracking and billing, and speed payment postings. The health-care organization should require annual evidence of these and other advanced financial practices to insure contracted providers optimize their own financial support. If the practice is performing all possible due diligence for financial management and is still unable to meet contracted expectations, then the parties should perform additional, more extensive analysis to determine possible causes for anesthesia financial shortfalls and explore costly inefficiencies in resource utilization that may need to be better allocated.

Leveraging the partnership

The goal of anesthesia practice managers should be to establish a program that is high quality, efficient, compliant, service-oriented, and client-centric. Even a practice successfully meeting all of these goals should seek further opportunities to leverage the relationship between the practice and the health-care facility. In the wake of health-care reform, collaboration to create integrated systems of care within the health-care facility will help better contain costs and improve patient outcomes.

Value-based purchasing (VBP) presents one such opportunity for collaboration. Under CMS guidelines, beginning in October 2012, noncritical access facilities will be rated on their performance on defined clinical metrics, and that performance will impact the level of reimbursement for Medicare and Medicaid services. This is a historic shift, as reimbursement will be based on quality, not quantity of services provided, and facilities that fall short on these quality goals will lose funding. Value-based purchasing links pay to performance, with quality outcomes driving 70% of reimbursement and patient satisfaction driving the other 30% of reimbursement. This creates an opportunity for anesthesia to support optimal outcomes on clinical measures in the procedural environment. And, with the frequent interaction between anesthesia provider and patient in the continuum of care, anesthesia is also perfectly positioned to drive patient satisfaction. The "great" anesthesia practice will not have to be forced into this role but, rather, will embrace it as a way to insure the mutual success of the practice and its health-care facility partner.

Summary

Any discussion of anesthesia practice management must end where it began, with mention of the necessary components of success: quality patient care that optimizes outcomes, patient and health-care facility satisfaction, regulatory compliance, and efficient use of both provider and facility resources. Whether in concert with other members of a group, as an employee of a larger organization, or in solo practice, those involved in the delivery of anesthesia services must remain focused on delivering each of these prerequisites to the patients and health-care partners they serve. Oddly enough, they must abandon one of the key pursuits of those who seek practice in specialty – independence – and instead subrogate their own interests and those of the members of the practice to focus first on the needs of their health-care partner. By aligning goals and attending to the success of the surgeon, the nurse leader, the administrator, the patient, and the hospital, they insure fulfillment of their own success.

Suggested reading

ACGME Program Requirements for Graduate Medical Education in Anesthesiology. Available online at: www.acgme.org/acWebsite/downloads/RRC_progReq/040_anesthesiology_07012008_u03102008.pdf (last accessed May 10, 2012).

K. E. Becker, N. H. Cohen, Committee on Economics. Update on alternate payment methodologies workgroup. *ASA Newsletter* 2007; **71**, number 11.

K. Bierstein. Pros and cons of exclusive contracts. *ASA Newsletter*, 2006; **70**: 36–7.

C. G. Chute, S. A. Beck, T. B. Fisk, D. N. Mohr. The Enterprise Data Trust at Mayo Clinic: a semantically integrated warehouse of biomedical data. *J Am Med Inform Assoc* 2010; **17**: 131–5.

Compilation of Patient Protection and Affordable Care Act, US Government. Available online at: http://docs.house.gov/energycommerce/ppacacon.pdf (last accessed May 10, 2012).

Department of Health and Human Services, 42 CFR Parts 422 and 480 Medicare Program; Hospital Inpatient Value-Based Purchasing Program found at: http://healthreformgps.org/wp-content/uploads/iwpfile1.pdf (last accessed May 16, 2012).

C. J. Donovan, K. A. Whitmore. Enterprise business intelligence: Part I of II. Presented at American Medical Group Association Annual meeting, March 2009, Las Vegas.

A. M. Harrison, A. W. Proctor. Enterprise business intelligence: Part II of II. Presented at American Medical Group Association Annual Meeting, March 2009, Las Vegas.

Mass Health Law, Insurance, MA Medicaid waiver approved through June 2014, December 20, 2011, Chelsea Conaboy. Available online at: www.boston.com/Boston/whitecoatnotes/2011/12/deal-extends-medicaid-funding-mass/uYekJKAgdfc8KtQaLrZdQP/story.html (last accessed May 16, 2012).

Medical Group Management Association. *Cost for Anesthesia and Pain Management Practices 2011 Report Based on 2010 Data Print Edition.* 2011.

B. Parker. Managing Hospital and O.R. Throughput. *ASA Newsletter* 2010; **74**,: number 1.

J. D. Judith Jurin Semo. When the Going Gets Tough: Hospital Contract Negotiations, Round Two. ASA 2008 Conference on Practice Management, January 25–27, 2008.

J. B. Sexton, M. A. Makary, A. R. Tersigni, *et al.* Teamwork in the operating room: frontline perspectives among hospitals and operating room personnel *Anesthesiology* 2006; **105**: 877–84. Clinical Investigations

Chapter

14

Anesthesia staffing models, productivity measurement, and incentive plans

Ashish Dabas MD
Dipty Mangla MD
Asa C. Lockhart MD, MBA
George Mychaskiw II DO, FAAP, FACOP

Anesthesia staffing models   151
Challenges affecting anesthesia-staffing models   152
Supply and demand of anesthesia providers   152
Regulatory issues   152
Management change   152
Assessment of staffing needs   153
Staffing model choices   153
Productivity and compensation   154

Factors complicating productivity measurements   155
Individual productivity   155
Measures of individual productivity   155
Academic productivity   156
Measures of productivity in an academic setting   156
Incentive plans   156
Ancilliary personnel   157
Union and labor law considerations   158
Summary   158

Anesthesia staffing models

One of the most important issues in perioperative care is the anesthesia staffing model. That is, what is the best and most efficient use of anesthesia personnel to provide safe and contemporary care? Although this may appear to be a relatively straightforward calculation of personnel allotment as permitted by federal, state, and local regulations, it is, in reality, perhaps the most vexing problem facing the perioperative care manager. Questions regarding scope of practice, a lack of convincing objective data, and cultural expectations of physician-directed health care all contribute to make this decision extraordinarily complex and controversial. At one extreme, there is the opinion that anesthesia care is a technical function that never requires physician involvement. At the other is the opinion of anesthesia as the practice of medicine that must always be administered by physicians only. Between these two points lies the care team model, which constitutes the majority of US anesthesia practice, wherein certified registered nurse anesthetists (CRNAs) (or anesthesiologist

assistants [AAs]) are medically directed by a physician anesthesiologist (or other physician, in the case of CRNAs in some locales). These are not questions that will be resolved in the foreseeable future and certainly not in this text.

Anesthesia-related costs are estimated to represent 3 to 5% of the total health-care expenditure in the United States [1]. Most of these costs involve personnel. However, revenue from anesthesia services has been decreasing for the last two decades, forcing hospitals and health systems to subsidize their anesthesia departments [2]. In fact, 78% of anesthesia groups are receiving financial support, as of the time of this writing [3]. Since personnel constitute the largest share of expenditure by an anesthesia group, the staffing model is one of the key considerations that affect the size of subsidy a group receives. Therefore every anesthesia group ideally requires the correct staffing model to improve efficiencies, add revenue streams, decrease costs, and support excellence in clinical quality [4].

Operating Room Leadership and Management, ed. Kaye A.D., Fox C.J. and Urman R.D. Published by Cambridge University Press. © Cambridge University Press 2012.

Challenges affecting anesthesia-staffing models

There are intrinsic and extrinsic influences that affect that anesthesia staffing for a facility. Staffing analysis must take into account the following [4]:

- current and future supply and demand;
- state regulations and scope of practice of mid-level providers;
- management change and transition issues.

Supply and demand of anesthesia providers

There are around 40 000 anesthesiologists (ANs) – including anesthesia residents – and 39 000 licensed CRNAs and student CRNAs in the United States who provide most of the anesthesia services. A RAND corporation survey in 2010 (an analysis of the labor market for anesthesiologists) concluded that there is a shortage of ANs and CRNAs at the national level, with 54% of the states having an AN shortage and 60% having a shortage of CRNAs. The survey also projected a continued shortage of ANs and an excess supply of CRNAs by 2020 [5].

Along with a shortage of anesthesia providers, there has been increase in demand for anesthesia services as a result of growth in ambulatory surgeries. Changes in the demographic profile of the population over the coming decades are also expected to increase demands for anesthesia services. By 2050, it is expected that 88.5 million of the US population (nearly 20% of the total population) will be 65 years of age or older [6].

This imbalance between demand and supply make it challenging for hospitals to provide high-quality anesthesia services at a reasonable cost.

Regulatory issues

In selection of any staffing model, a clear understanding of state regulations and guidelines from the Center for Medicare and Medicaid Services (CMS) should be sought, especially regarding CRNA scope of practice. Hospital bylaws may further affect the staffing model.

Physician supervision

In the November 2001 Federal Registry, the CMS published a final ruling that provided states with an option to "opt out" of a federal requirement for physician supervision of CRNAs. As of October 2010, 16 states have done so. The states are Iowa, Nebraska, Idaho, Minnesota, New Hampshire, New Mexico, Kansas, North Dakota, Washington, Alaska, Oregon, Montana, South Dakota, Wisconsin, California, and Colorado.

In these states, the CRNAs can perform anesthesia services independently without supervision from an anesthesiologist or other physician. New CMS guidelines also allow CRNAs to administer epidural analgesia for labor and delivery without physician supervision.

One anesthesia service

The new CMS guidelines require the organizing of all hospital anesthesia and analgesia services, including on-site and off-site surgical services, under the direction of a qualified physician. The requirements include the integration of anesthesia services with the hospital's quality improvement program.

Immediate availability

The physician supervising the CRNAs must be physically present within the same area, such as in the same operative suite. In addition, the physician should not be occupied in a manner that would prevent immediate intervention. Unfortunately, CMS regulations tend to be somewhat vague regarding the specific definition of immediate availability, and many groups are unclear on whether this is some sort of geographic definition, response time definition, or some combination thereof. Firm decisions regarding these questions are frequently the result of local opinion or ruling from a particular state and the reader is advised to query their local CMS administrative authority for clarification.

Pre- and postanesthesia evaluation

The anesthesia provider must perform an evaluation within 48 h of anesthesia administration. A postanesthesia evaluation must also be performed no later than 48 h after surgery for all patients.

Management change

Changing anesthesia staffing affecting models may affect surgeons who want stable, consistent anesthesia coverage in the operating room (OR). Similarly, in physician-only anesthesia practice, a change to a team care staffing model threatens anesthesiologists, who fear loss of clinical sovereignty and anesthesia reimbursement. Change, although inevitable, is seldom easy.

A new staffing model must consider all stakeholders for it to be successful.

Assessment of staffing needs

The OR is an inherently interdependent environment and demands a four-way conversation to develop an optimal staffing configuration. Surgeons, anesthesiologists, and hospital administrative and OR nursing representatives should develop the staffing grid in a conference/consensus so that there are no missing stakeholders and no misunderstandings of the coverage expectations. All sites that require anesthesia must be included in the staffing grid to determine the number of anesthesiologists and anesthetist full-time equivalents (FTEs) needed to provide optimum coverage. The grid should be specific about the duration of coverage needed, including hours to be covered and the number of days in a week. The grid should also specify personnel configuration for each potential location. In addition, there must be appropriate administrative, vacation, illness, and day-after-call allowances (when locally appropriate). All potential anesthetizing locations should also be categorized into dedicated, cross (or best efforts) coverage, flip rooms, and closed rooms.

- Best efforts coverage is the coverage that is not included in the budget or guaranteed contractually but may be provided with slack capacity or day-after-call personnel.
- A flip location is a second dedicated clean room that would permit a rapid turnover for a surgeon, but would not duplicate anesthesia personnel. Presence of duplicated personnel would require two locations on the staffing grid.
- A closed location is a room that lacks necessary equipment and is not functionally available at any time. A room can also be closed for a defined period (hours or days) with no assigned personnel.

Staffing model choices

A health-care facility can choose from the following anesthesia staffing models:

1. physician only;
2. physician–CRNA/AA mix;
3. CRNA only;
4. academic setup – residents, student nurse anesthetists (SRNAs).

The appropriate staffing model for a facility depends upon numerous factors, including regulatory issues, patient population profile, surgical procedures performed, comfort level of the surgeons and anesthesia care team, and number of ORs.

Physician-only model

In this model an anesthesiologist personally provides anesthesia services to a single patient at any one time and there is no hands-on care to another patient. As an anesthesiologist can only perform anesthesia in one room, this is the most expensive (and some would argue most inefficient) staffing model.

This model is more appropriate for a small suite with less than three ORs. Some facilities use this model in selected subspecialties (e.g., cardiothoracic surgeries), where there is a larger proportion of high-risk patients undergoing complicated surgeries. Regional cultural norms also influence the choice of this model and physician-only anesthesia staffing is more frequently found in the Western and Southwestern US, especially in urban areas, where AN supply is plentiful.

Physician–CRNA/AA mix

In this model anesthesia is administered by a team of physicians and CRNAs/AAs. The ratio of physician to CRNAs/AAs depends on state regulations and hospital bylaws. An anesthesiologist usually oversees a group of CRNAs, and the number of CRNAs depends upon whether the physician is performing medical direction or medical supervision. The AA is analogous to the physician assistant and must always be medically directed by an anesthesiologist – AAs are a relatively recent development and are not licensed in all states. When they are available, they are medically directed in ratios similar to CRNAs; however, medical supervision/independent practice is not an option with AAs.

"Medical direction" and "medical supervision" are terms used to describe the physician work required to oversee, manage, and guide both residents and nonphysician anesthesia providers in the anesthesia care team. Although these terms are often used interchangeably, they have different implications for billing and the way anesthesiologists oversee CRNAs.

Medical direction

Medical direction occurs when an anesthesiologist is involved in two, three, or four concurrent anesthesia procedures or a single anesthesia procedure with a qualified anesthetist. The CMS has established rules for medical direction by an anesthesiologist. These state that for each anesthesia procedure, the anesthesiologist must meet the following seven requirements:

- perform a pre-anesthetic examination and evaluation;
- prescribe the anesthesia plan;
- personally participate in the most demanding procedures of the anesthesia plan, including, if applicable, induction and emergence;
- insure that any procedure in the anesthesia plan that he or she does not perform are performed by a qualified anesthetist;
- monitor the course of anesthesia administration at frequent intervals;
- remain physically present and available for immediate diagnosis and treatment of emergencies;
- provide the indicated postanesthesia care.

If one or more of the above services are not performed by the anesthesiologist, the service is not considered medical direction.

Medical supervision

Medical supervision occurs when an anesthesiologist is involved in five or more concurrent anesthesia procedures. Medical supervision also occurs when the seven required services under medical direction are not performed by an anesthesiologist, which might occur in cases when the anesthesiologist left the immediate area of the operating suite for more than a short duration. A supervising physician does not have to be present during critical points in the procedure and available for immediate diagnosis and treatment of an emergency.

Medicare reimbursement for anesthesia services is different for medical supervision and medical direction. For medically directed cases, the CRNA and the physician is each paid 50% of the case bill. For a medically supervised case, the CRNA is paid 50%, and the supervising physician is allowed reimbursement at a rate of three base units per procedure [7]. There is some variation in this with regard to insurance carrier and local regulation. For example, because of the complexity of medical direction, some anesthesia groups routinely only bill for medical supervision or solo CRNA, whereas some insurance carriers do not reimburse for any coverage less than medical direction.

The physician–CRNA model is less expensive than the physician-only model and is appropriate for facilities having high volumes of complicated cases.

The CRNA-only model

In this model anesthesia services are provided by CRNAs independently without any supervision by anesthesiologists or surgeons. In 16 states, which have opted out of federal requirement for physician supervision of anesthetists, CRNAs can work with the same scope and functions as anesthesiologists. This is a common model in rural areas, where there are shortages of physician anesthesiologists, or some office practices, such as gastrointestinal/endoscopy facilities, where a physician anesthesiologist is cost-prohibitive. This model is analogous to the physician-only model in terms of efficiency, albeit at a somewhat lower cost. In states requiring physician medical direction of CRNAs, the operating physician practitioner is considered to be the physician providing medical direction. As noted previously, AAs always require anesthesiologist medical direction and cannot practice in an AA-only model.

Academic setup – residents, SRNAs

Academic facilities usually have residents, SRNAs, and CRNAs working along with anesthesiologists. Medical direction of residents in an academic setup is governed by both CMS and Accreditation Council for Graduate Medical Education (ACGME) guidelines, which restrict the concurrent direction by a physician to maximum of two locations when a trainee (resident or SRNA) is involved in one or both sites (ACGME requirement for GME in anesthesiology).

Medical direction of SRNAs is likely to be governed by hospital bylaws as well and may or may not require concurrent CRNA involvement.

Productivity and compensation

Strategic planning of private and academic anesthesiology groups requires meaningful measures of productivity. Measuring clinical productivity in the discipline of anesthesiology poses unique challenges because of the different billing system (i.e., base units plus time), the need to staff ORs independently of workload, differences in concurrency and non-anesthesia factors (length of surgery, type of surgery, and obstetric units) [1]. Quantification of clinical productivity is further complicated by the need to have different measures for individual and departmental productivity. Abouleish *et al.* reported that "clinical days worked" is the most meaningful measurement of individual productivity [8]. For departmental productivity, the only industrial measures available are total American Society of Anesthesiologists (ASA) units per FTE. However, because of concurrency differences between groups (i.e., anesthesia care delivered personally by anesthesiologists versus direction of variable numbers of residents, nurse anesthetists, or AAs), measuring units per FTE is insufficient to permit meaningful comparisons.

Factors complicating productivity measurements

1. Staffing needs and workload: unlike most clinical specialties, in which physicians see a particular number of patients, the number of sites and number of patients in each site vary from day to day for anesthesiology. To complicate matters further, the number of people required at each particular time of day differs. The other determinants for staffing needs include requirement of a second evening shift and number of people on call and post call.
2. Existence of a different billing system: the relative value unit (RVU) is used for billing in all medical care (as per Medicare reimbursement part B) except for anesthesiology. Relative value unit is calculated by summing three relative value components: physician work, practice overhead, and professional liability for a given procedure and multiplying the sum with a particular conversion factor. However, in anesthesiology, the unit of measurement for billing is variable (i.e., fixed ASA units multiplied by variable time units) [9,10,11]. The RVUs include work, overheads, and malpractice, unlike ASA units, which include only work.
3. Varied FTEs: FTEs, the percentage of times a full-time physician provides clinical care, are used commonly for time commitments in clinical specialties. However, FTEs do not account for time consumed in research and educational and administrative activities.
4. Confounding factors (non-anesthesia-related factors): factors such as duration of surgery, turnover times, and type of surgery, OR suites, and downtime also affect anesthesia billing and thus make measurement of productivity difficult.

Individual productivity

As individual responsibilities vary from one anesthesia group to another, it is prudent to compare individual productivity within a group. Before measuring individual productivity, a group should decide what measure is appropriate for that particular group. The right measurement index is the one that will value the group's services, make the group successful, and fulfill clinical obligations. When implementing any system of rewards and penalties, one must recognize that this will lead to behavior modification. It is imperative to understand what "behavior" the measurement system values and devalues before implementing a system. When this is not done, the law of unintended consequences will make itself painfully apparent.

Measures of individual productivity

Individual productivity measures can be categorized into three groups: total ASA units, time-based units, or availability measurements (see Table 14.1).

1. Total ASA units: anesthesia care is billed using ASA units that include both base units and time units. Non-anesthesiologists have viewed total ASA units as measures of productivity equivalent to work-relative value units used for other departments. However, total ASA units may not accurately reflect the needs of an anesthesiology department for anesthesiologists to perform required work. As noted above, it is confounded by anesthesiologist-independent factors and differences in concurrency, and does not reflect activities that cannot be billed.
2. Time-based units: this involves using days worked in a clinical setting as a productivity measure. The major advantage of using time units is the elimination of base units from the calculation of productivity. This system works best if all the anesthesiologists in the group rotate equally through surgeries with higher base units. However, if the group is large and caters to different subspecialties, time-based units are not a good measure of clinical productivity. The major disadvantage of using time units is the issue of concurrency. If concurrency is not controlled, then individuals cannot be compared. Also, obstetric anesthesia practice, in which the actual availability of an anesthesiologist is different from billed hours, remains a challenge with this system.

Table 14.1 Summary of individual clinical productivity measures and services valued and devalued

	Services valued	Services devalued
tASA/OR FTE	Only billed sites, total charges billed, specialty care, shorter cases, medical direction, higher concurrency	Nonbilled sites, nonbillable care, cases performed by anesthesiologists, low ASA unit-generating sites, downtime
TU/OR FTE	Only ASA-billed sites, long cases, medical direction, higher concurrency	Not all clinical sites, anesthesiologist-performed cases, specialty care, ambulatory setting, downtime, low ASA unit-generating sites
CD/FTE	Measures availability, all clinical sites, days worked	Specialty care, longer work days, billable charges

3. Availability measurements: measurement in this category is full clinical days worked per FTE (CD/FTE). "Clinical day" is the working day irrespective of billed units. The advantage of using this as a measure is that all services provided by anesthesiologists get valued. However, specialty care is valued. Thus, a person who is available from the morning receives the maximum number of productivity points. Another advantage of using this system is a lack of confounding factors such as duration of surgery, type of surgery, and downtime.

Academic productivity

Academic anesthesia departments in the United States have clinical, educational, research, and administrative responsibilities. The usual expectation from an academic group is to excel in all four, irrespective of financial compensation, even though funding is from clinical activities [9]. Recommendations of improving productivity and increasingly providing financial bonus payments to faculty instead of salary are examples of restructuring academic departments of many specialties in response to managed care. Total ASA units may not accurately reflect the needs of an anesthesiology department for anesthesiologists to perform required work. Confounding factors include the facts that: (1) anesthesiologist-independent factors influence the number of ASA units charged per billing period (e.g., the number of room sites that must be assigned, the number of cases posted per site, the surgeon's speed, the type of surgery); (2) total ASA units do not necessarily reflect increased reimbursement (different concurrency issues); (3) not all clinical activities of the department are billed using ASA units (e.g., intensive care, pain management, anesthesiology preoperative clinic); and (4) staffing requirements of some clinical

sites do not vary with workload (e.g., obstetric anesthesia, in-hospital night call). In 2000, Abouleish et al. analyzed different methods of measuring productivity in academic groups retrospectively [8]. The advantages and disadvantages of using units of time/day worked, clinical days worked, and/or cumulated numbers of ASA units earned were thoroughly and extensively described. However, the retrospective nature of their analysis prevented them from determining whether the method of measuring productivity would influence faculty behavior. Abouleish et al. concluded that the normalized clinical days per year (NCY) approach was the most helpful measure of productivity [8].

Measures of productivity in an academic setting

Measures of productivity in an academic setting can be categorized into groups (see Table 14.2):

1. Normalized clinical days worked per fiscal year: clinical days reflect the individual anesthesiologist's contribution to the clinical mission of the department. It can be applied to all clinical work irrespective of the setting and billing practices.
2. Operating room FTE: to avoid the non-billable sites (in terms of ASA units) it would be appropriate to use OR equivalent time instead of ASA units.

Incentive plans

Abouleish et al. conducted a survey in 2005 to study the prevalence and characteristics of incentive plans in various anesthesiology departments in the United States [12]. According to this, only 40% of the 88 programs responding to the survey had complete incentive plans that included regular hours and after hours. Another 30% provided some additional compensation

Table 14.2 Summary of measures of productivity in academic groups

	Measure	Services valued	Services devalued
1	Normalized clinical days/year (nCD/yr)	All clinical sites measured Includes non-anesthesiology measures	Specialty anesthesia care Longer work days or higher workload clinical sites
2	Time units/OR day (TU/OR day)	Only clinical sites that bill in ASA units measured Time providing billable anesthesia care Medical direction Higher concurrency	Not all clinical sites measured Non billable anesthesia care: preoperative evaluation, postop care Personally performed cases Specialty anesthesia care Low ASA generating sites Short and fast cases
3	Total ASA units/OR day (tASA/OR day)	Only clinical sites that bill using ASA units measured Total charges billed Medical direction, concurrency and specialty anesthesia care	Not all clinical sites measured Nonbillable anesthesia care Personally performed cases Low ASA generating sites
4	Normalized time units/year	nCD/yr × TU/OR day	Combination of 1 and 2
5	Normalized total ASA units/year	nCD/year × tASA/OR day	Combination of 2 and 3

for late rooms or on call. Anesthesiology departments have been facing increasing pressure from hospital administration to implement incentive plans. The reasoning behind this could be the increased number of surgeries or more grants to anesthesiology departments from medical schools. It is not clear that incentive plans can increase the number of cases, although incentive plans have been shown to better align compensation with clinical activity [13]. Incentive plans can also influence compensation as total faculty numbers change. If faculty numbers decrease, either productivity decreases or the remaining faculty increases individual productivity to achieve the same output. Compared with a straight salary system, clinical incentives allow compensations to vary. As per Abouleish *et al.*, larger practice groups used productivity-based compensation more than smaller groups. In most anesthesiology groups, incentive is less than 25% of total compensation. However, in equal share compensation, which is most often used in private practice anesthesiology, 100% of compensation is variable and no base salary is used for partners. Academic departments' base salary partly covers nonclinical responsibilities. For both academic and private-practice anesthesiology groups, the important factor in designing or evaluating an incentive plan is

to determine the goals that the department considers essential to success, including nonclinical goals. In a more recent survey, Mets and Galford reported that 95% of responding departments used incentives [13]. However, few departments reported use of all four parameters (clinical productivity, revenue, points, and academic productivity). A few others also reported inclusion of criteria such as citizenship and teamwork.

Ancillary personnel

Teamwork is important in running ORs efficiently. As mentioned earlier, efficiency in anesthesiology is dependent on ancillary personnel such as nurses, OR technicians, and other OR and anesthesia personnel. Nurses form an important part of the OR team. Nursing usually aims for predictable hours and standardization of cases. Nurses must have the OR and equipment ready for each case before the patient is brought to the room. Similarly, the anesthesia technicians should have equipment ready before each case. Housekeeping staff must clean the OR floors and wipe down all equipment, including the OR table. Thus, as can be seen above, apart from surgeons and anesthesiologists, the start and turnover times in the OR depend on a variety of OR personnel.

Union and labor law considerations

Labor unions in the health-care industry have been much in the news of late, particularly the emergence of large and well-funded nursing unions. There is a sense of urgency among nursing unions to organize nurses in large numbers, as well as an increased push to organize other groups of health-care workers. In 1967 the National Labor Relations Board recognized the right of health-care workers to join unions for the first time [14]. With the current health-care reforms, fundamental changes in health-care facilities will occur, and such facilities will probably be dealing with unions instead of individuals. The unions' interest is in all the employees collectively, rather than each individual employee. Instead of individual agreements with each employee there is one contract that applies to all. The disciplinary system of the health-care facility that has been unionized is the subject of mandatory collective bargaining. Likewise, the law requires management and unions to bargain over a grievance process, which nearly always results in a formal grievance procedure being included in the collective bargaining agreement [15]. With respect to discipline of employees, the union will grieve disciplinary action taken against an employee if the union believes it is a violation of the collective bargaining agreement. In a union setting it is important for human resources to have good relations with the union.

Summary

Operating room anesthesia staffing and compensation models are a continuing subject of vociferous debate. Given the tremendous number of internal and external variables influencing perioperative services (e.g., federal regulations, population demographics, provider supply and demand, etc.) the only certainty is that any conclusions agreed upon are likely to change. In the next 50 years, the US health-care system is going to encounter heretofore unseen stresses, as a record number of elderly patients live longer with multiple comorbidities and demand for medical intervention increases, coupled with the economic pressures of domestic and foreign commitments in a struggling economy. Additionally, technological advances are also changing the nature and potential risk and safety of anesthesia care. Ultimately, it is important for the perioperative manager to be able to respond to these demands and maintain an attitude of flexibility and ability to change in response to these undefined, but formidable challenges. Patient care, safety, outcomes and efficiency are the most critical measures and decisions regarding staffing, and compensation should be based on objective data, rather than prevailing cultural norms and expectations. "This is how we've always done it," or "this works well for us" are (at best) relics of the past and (at worst) millstones around the neck of efficient perioperative care.

References

1. J. D. Klein. When will managed care come to anesthesia? *J Health Care Finance* 1997; **23**: 62–86.

2. M. Koch, D. B. Calder. 4 Decisions That Can Affect Your Anesthesia Subsidy. Available online at: www.hfma.org/Templates/Print.aspx?id=25894 (last accessed May 16, 2012).

3. K. Beirstein. Anesthesiology Practice Costs, Revenues, and Production Survey Data. *American Society of Anesthesiologists Newsletter*, April 2007.

4. Somnia Anesthesia. Anesthesia Staffing Models that Drive Value and Improve Quality. 2010. Available online at: http://simplystatedbusiness.com/wp-content/uploads/2011/02/WhitepaperSample1.pdf (last accessed May 11, 2012).

5. L. Daugherty, R. Fonseca, K. B. Kumar, P. C. Michaud. *Technical Report – An analysis of the Labor Markets for Anesthesiology*. RAND Health, 2010.

6. Population division, US Census Bureau. Available online at: www.census.gov/newsroom/releases/archives/facts_for_features_special_editions/cb11-ff08.html (last accessed May 10, 2012).

7. NHIC corp. Centers for Medicare & Medicaid Services – Anesthesia Billing Guide Oct 2010.

8. A. E. Abouleish, M. H. Zornew, J. Abate, D. S. Prough. Measurement of individual clinical productivity in an academic anesthesiology department. *Anesthesiology* 2000; **93**; 1509–16.

9. R. M. D'Alessandri, P. Albertsen, B. F. Atkinson, *et al.* Measuring contributions to clinical mission of medical schools and teaching hospitals. *Acad Med* 2000; **75**: 1231–7.

10. A. Garson, Jr, K. E. Strifert, J. R. Beck, *et al.* Metric process: Baylor's development of a "report card" for faculty and departments. *Acad Med* 1999; **74**: 861–8.

11. S. J. Barker. Lord or vassal? Academic anesthesiology finances in 2000. *Anesth Analg* 2001; **93**: 294–300.

12. A. E. Abouleish, J. L. Apfelbaum, D. S. Prough, *et al.* The prevalence and characteristics of incentive plans for clinical productivity among anesthesiology programs. *Anesth Analg* 2005; **100**: 493–501.

13. B. Mets, J. A. Galford. Leadership and management of academic anesthesiology departments in the United States. *J Clin Anesth* 2009; **21**: 83–93.

14. 29 USC 158.

15. US Gypsum Ca; 94 NLRB 112 29 LRRM 1015 (1951).

Compensation for anesthesia services

Asa C. Lockhart MD, MBA

Staffing   161
Evaluate the data   161
Data to information – information
to knowledge   163

Utilization   165
Strategic planning   166
Develop and execute your story   166
Summary   167

In this chapter, we will discuss why it is important to develop a strategy for the compensation of services provided. This involves understanding how to assess accurately the monetary and labor cost of anesthesia services, such as obstetric (OB) or trauma coverage requested by a health-care institution. It is also critical to understand how to successfully negotiate a financially viable contract with a health-care institution for delivery of anesthesia services. The anesthesia provider needs to be more adept in addressing practical and political issues related to the contractual delivery of anesthesia services in situations in which remuneration from patient billing alone is unlikely to adequately cover the cost of service delivery and in which the institution may be reluctant or unwilling to provide compensatory support or modification of the coverage expectations.

Stable anesthesia groups have a good payer mix, efficiently run operating rooms (ORs), an equitable compensation model, and a sound internal professional and business infrastructure. Although severe problems can overwhelm a group with a strong infrastructure, relatively minor issues can engulf a group that has not invested in strategic and business planning. If any of the above elements are missing or diminished, the initial warning signs of retention and recruiting instability brought on by below-market compensation and lack of patient access to surgical services can quickly erode a practice. These confounding factors justify compensation for service (CFS) arrangements between anesthesia groups and hospitals; however, the days of merely

asking hospital administrators to stabilize an anesthesia group by giving them an unsubstantiated "stipend" are gone. Therefore, your need to reframe the negotiation process from a simple request for money into a concept that more accurately reflects the driving force – compensation for the desired level of anesthesia services requested by the hospital but not supported by the revenue generated from clinical activities owing to poor OR efficiency, surgeon practice patterns, utilization, and/or payer mix. If the group determines that a CFS is required, you must develop a strategy for a successful negotiation. You cannot manage what you cannot measure. To have a winning strategy, one must define the stakeholders and their expectations, evaluate the data, convert the data to information, convert the information to knowledge, and develop a fact-based story. The internal and external stakeholders include patients, surgeons, anesthesiologists, proceduralists, obstetricians, perioperative staff members, and hospital administrators. A benefit, either real or perceived, must exist to motivate the various stakeholders who require, use, or provide anesthesia services to take action. Each stakeholder group has its own goals and deliverables that may or may not conflict, and which other stakeholders may or may not understand. Most anesthesia groups want to maximize efficiency, whereas most surgeons, proceduralists, obstetricians, and administrators want to maximize access and market share. As stated above, patient access to surgical services is the basic justification for a CFS agreement. If there is a threat to access owing to anesthesia recruitment and

Operating Room Leadership and Management, ed. Kaye A.D., Fox C.J. and Urman R.D. Published by Cambridge University Press. © Cambridge University Press 2012.

retention deficiencies, there will be a greater sense of urgency from multiple stakeholders for a successful CFS negotiation. It is also important to evaluate the practice patterns and customer service philosophies of all of the anesthesiologists and their employees to determine whether there will be pushback from external stakeholders if the hospital agrees to a fair market value (FMV) CFS agreement. When preparing a strategy for a contract negotiation that requires a CFS, it is important to include the following steps: (1) identify the appropriate staffing using a staffing grid; (2) evaluate operational and practice performance against national benchmarks; (3) quantify the OR utilization metrics; and (4) embrace strategic planning concepts. The goal is to develop a logical sequence of events that results in a story of why the group cannot provide the desired level of access of anesthesia services with its native revenue stream.

Staffing

The OR is an inherently interdependent environment and demands a four-way conversation to develop an optimal staffing configuration. Surgeons/proceduralists, anesthesiologists, and hospital administrative and OR nursing representatives should develop the staffing grid in conference, so that there are no misunderstandings of the coverage expectations; two-way conversations may not reflect the needs of the missing stakeholders, resulting in a patchwork or inadequate plan. This process permits the adjudication of conflicts in real time. The ability to perform a surgical procedure requires a functional and synchronized unit – a surgeon/proceduralist/obstetrician, patient, anesthesiologist/anesthetist, nursing staff, and an OR – otherwise someone is wasting resources. The proceduralists and obstetricians are included because out-of-OR sites are the fastest growing service lines requiring anesthesia, and these services are often not represented on the OR committee. All sites requiring anesthesia must be included in the staffing grid to determine the number of anesthesiologist and anesthetist full-time equivalents (FTEs) needed. There should be a consensus among all stakeholders that the grid is a "just-say-yes" document. If the hours are listed, anesthesia services will be available and reflected in the budget. The grid should specify the hours per day, number of days per week, and personnel configuration for each potential location. In addition, there must be appropriate administrative, vacation, and day-after-call allowances. All potential anesthetizing locations should reflect either dedicated, cross- (or

best-efforts) coverage, flip rooms, and closed rooms. Best-efforts coverage is coverage that is not included in the budget or guaranteed contractually but may be provided with slack capacity or day-after-call personnel. A flip location is a second dedicated clean room that would permit a rapid turnover for a surgeon, but would not duplicate anesthesia personnel; duplicated personnel would require two locations on the staffing grid. A closed location is a room: (1) that lacks the necessary equipment and is not functionally available at any time; or (2) one closed for a defined period (hours or days) with no assigned personnel (Figure 15.1).

Evaluate the data

In preparation for CFS negotiations, it is important to see where the group fits in the local and national marketplace. Remember that you are not asking for an undefined amount of money, you are developing a strategy with concrete data to present to the hospital administration. For operational trending purposes, 3 years or 2 years plus year-to-date performance data will provide staffing, collection, business cost, and productivity metrics. The basic benchmark data used in this process are charges, contractual adjustments/allowances/refunds, revenue, cases, full-rate or undiscounted conversion factor (CF), and physician/anesthetist FTEs. Adjustments include contractual allowances and refunds. The contractual allowances represent the difference between the full charge and the allowable charge (i.e., Medicare or managed care). Charges should be at the full undiscounted rate, or they may later understate the relative performance of the group compared with benchmarks (Figure 15.2). The question of what represents an FTE varies greatly by group. For fractional FTEs, the measure might be a relative percentage of days worked or hours worked, or a relative percentage of compensation compared with full-time personnel. The Medical Group Management Association (MGMA) represents business managers for all specialties, and the Anesthesia Administration Assembly (AAA) represents anesthesia and pain management practices. The MGMA produces a number of publications, including those formulated by the AAA, which are useful in benchmarking your practice. Other organizations produce salary surveys; however, most of their surveys do not distinguish between the salary of a new hire and a partner. Also, some of their sample sizes are not statistically significant relative to the number of anesthesia personnel represented in a survey that may have more than 1000 responses for all physicians and

STAFF GRID - CAMELOT MEDICAL CENTER

LOCATION		LOCATIONS AND HOURS OF COVERAAGE (coverage notes)	STAFF MD #	STAFF CRNA #	CRNA HRS	MD HRS	DAYS/WEEK	CRNA HRS/WK	CRNA FTEs	MD HRS/WK	MD FTEs
MAIN	OR 1	(2)	1			16	5	0	0.0	80.0	1.6
	OR 2	MD / (1)	2	1	10	12	5	50	1.3	60.0	1.2
	OR 3		2	2	10		5	50	1.3	0.0	0.0
	OR 4	CV	2	3	10		5	50	1.3	0.0	0.0
	OR 5	CV / (1)	3			10	5	0	0.0	50.0	1.0
	OR 6		2	4	8		5	40	1.0	0.0	0.0
	OR 7	FLIP-SAME CREW / CROSS COVERED				0		0	0.0	0.0	0.0
SURGICENTER	OR 1		4	5	9	10	5	45	1.1	50.0	1.0
	OR 2		4	8	8		5	40	1.0	0.0	0.0
	OR 3		4	7	8		5	40	1.0	0.0	0.0
	OR 4	FLIP-DIFFERENT CREW	4	8	8		5	40	1.0	0.0	0.0
	OR 5		5	2		8	5	0	0.0	40.0	0.8
OB	OB 1		6			24	5	0	0.0	120.0	2.4
	OB 2	CROSS COVERED				0	5	0	0.0	0.0	0.0
OOOR (Out of OR)	GI	CROSS COVERED	7			8	5	0	0.0	40.0	0.8
	MRI	T-T	8			8	2	0	0.0	16.0	0.3
	EP	M-W-F	8			8	3	0	0.0	24.0	0.5
	AIRWAY	CROSS COVERED						0	0.0	0.0	0.0
Float	FLOAT	T-W-T	4			2	3	0	0.0	6.0	0.1
	Float	(12)		9	8		5	40	1.0	0.0	0.0
WEEKEND	SAT 1	BU CALL / (1)				12	1	0	0.0	12.0	0.2
	SAT 2					1	1	0	0.0	1.0	0.0
	SAT OB					24	1	0	0.0	24.0	0.5
	SUN 1	BU CALL				7	1	0	0.0	7.0	0.1
	SUN 2	(1)				1	1	0	0.0	1.0	0.0
	SUN OB					24	1	0	0.0	24.0	0.5
DAC	MD										1
	CRNA								0		
VACATION	MD										2.4
	CRNA								1.4		
ADMIN	ADMIN								0.2		0.2

	CRNA HRS/WK	CRNA FTEs	MD HRS/WK	MD FTEs
TOTAL COVERAGE HRS	395	9.875	531	10.6
MANDATED BY HOURS		11.3		14.2
MANDATED BY DAY SLOTS		10.4		11.5

TOTAL STAFFING

Total Hrs per Wk-EmpCRNAs	395	Total OR Hrs/Wk	531
# CRNAs Working	9.88	# MDs Working	10.6
Avg Hrs/EmpCRNA/wk	40.0	Avg Hrs/MD/wk	50.0

Figure 15.1 Staffing grid example. Key points: (1) identify all potential anesthetizing sites, specify dedicated or cross (slack) coverage; (2) identify average hours per day for each location in the facility; and (3) designate call and late-stay hours on actual time in the facility; full credit for in-house call. Reprinted with permission from Golden Caduceus Consultants © 2010.

physician extenders. Executive search firms produce some of the surveys and tend to have lower numbers; this is not surprising given their population, which occasionally makes them a popular resource during negotiations, even though they may not reflect the true market value for services rendered. There is statistically significant compensation survey data for the United States as a whole and by geographic sections in the annual MGMA Compensation and Productivity Survey. The geographic sections are Eastern, Midwest, Southern, and Western. On the disk version only, there are minor regions as well. They are Northeast, North Atlantic, Mid-Atlantic, California-Alaska-Hawaii, Eastern Midwest, Lower Midwest, Northwest, Rocky Mountain, Southeast, and Upper Midwest. The relevant markets often extend beyond the minor regions; therefore, most clients use either the geographic sections or national data points. Although not present in the printed 2009 survey, the data previously permitted the calculation of demographic and multispecialty differentials. The compensation categories are anesthesiologists, pediatric anesthesiologists, pain medicine, and anesthetists (including nurse anesthetists and anesthesia assistants). Because anesthesiologists historically average 44 weeks of productivity per year, this translates into 8 weeks of vacation and continuing medical education. By calculating an adjustment/vacation modifier if the group takes a different time than the benchmark, neither the group nor the hospital is penalized for the variation. Most groups fall between a 6-week and 10-week range. Most anesthetists are around 6 weeks, with a much smaller variation. By factoring in these variables, the calculation will reflect similar practice comparables. Trending and confounding factor explanations build an even more compelling story.

Data to information – information to knowledge

Tabulate the basic and derived data and convert them to information with the derivation of other key performance indicator (KPI) metrics. The derived data provide the basis for calculations that yield information but do not provide a context for determining FMV. These include average charge per case, average revenue per case, average units per case, cases per FTE, FTEs per 1000 cases, average charges per physician, compensation to gross charges ratio, average or aggregate CF, total group units generated, and per-FTE average.

However, from an administrative viewpoint, the most important KPI metrics are the net collection percentage, bad debt percentage based on total charges or revenues, benefit costs, units per physician FTE, and billing and administrative costs. In addition, to demonstrate the billing and revenue cycle management efficiency, evaluate the accounts receivable (A/R). It may be necessary to evaluate the A/R with adjustments for accounts that are greater than 180 days old, because many practices roll those accounts into bad debt or suspended accounts (e.g., auto accident, where the account may not be adjudicated for several years). It is also important to know whether accounts have been re-aged; the desired methodology is not to re-age the accounts. One can better evaluate A/R performance based on date of service or date of posting rather than date of payment. Date of insurance payment is important in evaluating prompt pay from the insurance company. However, except for the group inserting language into their contracts and enforcing the provision, practice managers have little control over this metric. The calculation of an aggregate or average CF demonstrates the group's economic potential and may be useful in evaluating the billing performance. Another major determinant for a viable practice is the public payer mix (i.e., Medicare, Medicaid, Worker's Comp, and Tri-Care). Owing to the disproportionate impact of Medicare and Medicaid relative to other specialties and facilities, the public payer mix is a key factor in an anesthesia group's economic potential, making the aggregate CF benchmark determination an important part of the story (Figure 15.3). This will allow the administration to appreciate the performance trends of the practice. As one compares the practice information to benchmarks, there is a transformation from information to knowledge. With benchmarks in anesthesia, it is important to know when to use "All Respondents" data and when to use "mode of practice" data. If the mode of practice is material to the metric, use the "By Staffing Model" section; otherwise, use the "All Respondents" section, because it will have a higher number of responses. Full charges and revenue per unit, A/R, and payer mix are examples that are appropriate for "All Respondents" metrics. The productivity per FTE will vary significantly between practice modes such as personally provided, anesthetist-to-physician ratio of less than 1:1, and anesthetist-to-physician ratio greater than 1:1. Avoid using the "All Respondents" data for productivity-related metrics, because it does not accurately portray any of the specific practice modes, and the billing/

	ANESTHESIOLOGY ASSOCIATES		CURRENT MGMA SURVEY
YEAR	2011	2012 EST	25th-Median-75th-90th
CHARGES	$36,454,900	$40,226,052	
ADJUSTMENTS	$22,987,573	$24,926,156	
REFUNDS	$233,127	$95,096	*Table references from:*
COLLECTIONS	$12,999,672	$11,210,202	
CASES	30,495	29,560	
FULL RATE	$88	$93	
# MDs	18.0	20.0	
# CRNAs	44.0	56.0	
NET COLLECTION %	96.5%	73.3%	
GROSS COLLECTION%	35.7%	27.9%	
UNITS PER HOUR:	4	4	4

PRODUCTIVITY		
Adjusted for split billing duplications		
	2011	2012 EST
AVG CHARGE PER CASE	$1,195	$1,361
AVG REIMBURSMENT PER CASE	$426	$379
AVG UNIT PER CASE	13.6	14.6
CASES PER FTE	1,694	1,478
FTES PER 1000	2.03	2.57
AVG CHARGE PER MD	$2,025,272	$2,011,303
Comp/Gross Charges Ratio	21,232	20,894
MAIN OR		2,186
OB		1,198
OOOR	5,568	5,282
ASC	30,495	29,560
AVERAGE CF	$34.02	$30.09
GROUP UNITS	414,564	432,444
AVG UNITS PER FTE	21,227	18,627
BAD DEBT %	4.1%	2.1%

Figure 15.2 Example of relative productivity display. Values on right column to be taken from Medical Group Management Association (MGMA) publications. (FTE, full-time equivalent; OOOR, outside of OR; ASC, ambulatory surgery center; CF, conversion factor.) Reprinted with permission from Golden Caduceus Consultants © 2010.

administrative overhead is very sensitive to practice mode (Figure 15.3). Having calculated the above data, benchmarking against national databases will build the group's story. The development of a budget summary sheet based on projected revenues and expenses will display the financial impact of the group-facility relationship. Unless a substantial change is expected, the previous year's revenues are the basis for the following year's revenue projection; as one passes midyear, year-to-date calculations may be used. However, one must be careful to avoid extrapolating data points that do or do not include unusual or one-time events (e.g., lump sum adjudication from previous year accounts or lump sum professional liability premiums and/or retirement contributions paid at the end of the year). The expenses will be the number of anesthesiologists and anesthetists required, multiplied by the salary and benefit costs, billing and administrative costs, and other professional overheads. The other professional overhead represents cost that is not discretionary, which includes federal payroll (FICA) tax, Medicare tax, various unemployment taxes, professional liability insurance, dues and subscriptions, continuing medical education allowances, business and occupational taxes, and miscellaneous items. Other than continuing medical education, these costs are essential

CALCULATION OF ANESTHESIOLOGY ASSOCIATES AGGREGATE CONVERSION FACTOR -(CF)						
PAYOR	MARKET SHARE	CF	Contribution	MGMA MEAN-MEDIAN	2007 MGMA: 25th-Median-75th-90th	GCP MAXIMUM
Self Pay	3.61%	$4.97	$0.18			
BC	13.53%	$55.89	$7.56			
Commercial	1.81%	$80.00	$1.45			93.0% TARGET
United HMO/PPO	12.90%	$61.00	$7.87			
Workers Comp	4.63%	$44.87	$2.08			ACTUAL
Medicare	22.41%	$20.44	$4.58			
Medicaid	15.81%	$16.00	$2.53			Avg Natl Potential CF 2011
Cigna	2.37%	$72.00	$1.71			
Humana	0.00%	$0.00	$0.00			
AETNA	3.00%	$67.00	$2.01			2010
Tricare/Other gvt payers	7.50%	$20.23	$1.52			
Other: MultiPlan	7.58%	$54.50	$4.13			2009
Other: StateIndigent	2.67%	$4.97	$0.13			
Other: DirectContract	0.51%	$80.00	$0.41			2008
Other: Hospital Plan	1.33%	$54.50	$0.72			
Total companies/ <1% market share	0.00%	$0.00	$0.00			IMPUTED GROUP Actual Aggregate CF $34.02
TOTAL	99.7%	POTENTIAL CF	$36.88			
Actual to Predicted Ratio ---►			92.26%	Historical Norm -94.5%	GROUP Reported Units	CALCULATED GROUP Actual Aggregate CF $31.36
Benchmark of 93.0% yields an expected CF of --►➚			$34.30	$34.85	382,078	
GROUP Est Aggregate CF			➚$34.02	$34.02		
Actual CF to Benchmark CF Differential			$0.27	➘ ($0.83)		
Financial Impact of Differential			($104,197)	($316,940)		

Figure 15.3 Example of aggregate conversion factor (CF) calculation. Values on right column to be taken from Medical Group Management Association (MGMA) publications. Reprinted with permission from Golden Caduceus Consultants © 2010.

professional overhead categories that are non-negotiable and mandatory. The net income of revenue less expenses may justify a CFS if it is negative and the hospital is requesting a level of coverage not supported by the net income (Figure 15.4). Once there is a validation of sound business practices, assess whether the practice is above, at, or below market, because a CFS can only be justified if a practice is materially below market. Two common methods for determining CFS are net income guarantees pegged to a commonly accepted benchmark such as the MGMA Compensation Survey, and guaranteed units per location per day that result in a targeted income. As stated above, these levels will vary with clinical acuity (e.g., neonates, Level 1 trauma, in-house call), geographic location (Eastern, Southern, Midwest, and Western), number of vacation/continuing medical education weeks, and demographic category. Anesthesia departments within multispecialty clinics require further adjustments. One basis for selecting the appropriate compensation survey percentile (25th, 50th, 75th, and 90th) is the relative practice acuity; however, it may also reflect local/regional competitors to avoid defections in a retention-based strategy. Some consultants will use an average of several performance metrics. These metrics may include information such as call frequency and acuity that are material considerations, but they may not carry equal

weight with potential recruits. This method may skew the fair market value if one of the metrics is unusually low and one is averaging only a handful of numbers. The FMV must ultimately reflect the percentage of the workforce that is able to meet the clinical expectations and willing to make the lifestyle sacrifice required by the position.

Utilization

The nationally accepted utilization benchmarks are 70% without turnover time and 80% with turnover time. Suboptimal utilization of ORs can be attributed to a silo culture, preadmission testing strategies, block posting policies without discipline, high cancellation rates, and physician referral patterns. By far, the major opportunity for stabilization is block posting – if there are consequences for poor citizenship. An anesthesia group cannot sustain itself if the surgeons and proceduralists follow operating patterns that leave large blocks of time in the daily schedule and then insist on adding patients to the evening schedule. Even though it is clear that utilization is the key to a self-sufficient anesthesia group, many administrators are not willing to eat the political fire by telling the surgeons they must be more efficient, which may be a legitimate strategic consideration to retain market share in very competitive markets. That business decision is another reason

GROUP @ 50th PERCENTILE-INITIAL MODEL							2009	2011 EST	2011 EST
REVENUE							ACTUAL	PROJECTED	MONTHLY
GROUP REVENUE							$11,210,202	$12,999,672	$1,083,306
ADJUSTMENTS									
XYZ JV ASC							$2,369,411	$2,369,411	$0
GEN CFS							$5,488,000	$0	$0
BILLING SERVICES REVENUE							$325,788	$325,788	$0
PROJECTED REVENUE							$19,393,401	$15,694,871	$1,307,906
	# FTEs								
PROFESSIONAL COMPONENT	BY GRID	CURRENT	SALARY	BENEFITS		TOTAL COMP/FTE			
PHYSICIAN PARTNERS	13.0	9.0	$468,549	$59,566		$528,115	$7,662,105	$6,885,495	$638,509
PHYSICIAN-ASSOCIATES	0.0	3.1	$260,000	$48,166		$308,166	$0	$0	$0
CRNAS-Call	52.3	51.3	$140,542	$25,000		$165,542	$8,180,883	$8,657,885	$881,740
OTHER	0	0	$0	$0		$0	$0	$0	$0
LOCUMS	0	2	$230,000	$0		$230,000	$1,052,106	$0	$87,676
OVERHEAD									
BILLING AND ADMINISTRATIVE							$1,294,511	$1,294,511	$107,876
RECRUITING EXPENSE	0		$25,000				$0	$0	$0
OTHER PROFESSIONAL OVERHEAD							$1,203,796	$1,203,796	$100,316
					INCREMENT FOR		$19,393,401	($18,021,657)	$1,616,117
					ADDITIONAL OR		OPTION A	($2,326,786)	($193,899)
					($3,861,608)		OPTION B	($6,188,394)	($515,700)

Figure 15.4 Budget display example. Key point: Do not build the projected compensation for service (CFS) on the base year (GEN CFS) but do allow continuing revenue streams outside of the CFS negotiation (XYZ ASC and BILLING SERVICE REVENUE). Reprinted with permission from Golden Caduceus Consultants © 2010.

for a CFS agreement. In the post-health-system-reform world, these considerations will become even more significant.

Strategic planning

The cornerstones of strategic planning are a SWOT (strengths, weaknesses, opportunities, and threats) analysis and a business plan that includes an action plan. The planning process is most successful when using a survey instrument that is enhanced through group discussion after the results have been tabulated. Running a medical practice like a business is not only helpful internally; it strengthens the group's position with the hospital if there is a "partnership" element to the negotiations. Deliverables might include improved on-time starts, group discipline, and champions for improved utilization and perioperative redesign. The focus is to determine what issues enhance or diminish utility. The goal is to develop a "win–win" scenario in which both organizations reinforce their relative strategic plans in a mutually beneficial relationship on a functionally unified balance sheet.

Develop and execute your story

An anesthesia group's success will depend upon its ability to convert information into knowledge in an impactful, organized manner. In addition, it is crucial that a decision-making committee and negotiating team be empowered to effect change to assess the achievable goals and implement them to the benefit of the anesthesia group and/or various stakeholders. Mere discussion and vetting of the issues does not achieve the goal of correcting the underlying factors that led to the stated difficulties. There must be an alignment of incentives with a clear understanding that CFS is not the same as pay for performance, nor is it an annuity. It is essential that the practice data be in the same format as the benchmark (i.e., the number of time units per hour) and presented in a tabular, trended format to optimize the visual impact. Benchmark the KPI against the MGMA Anesthesia Cost Survey results, published every other year, to assess the relative efficiency and productivity of your organization. As noted earlier, one must be cautious in using the generic MGMA Cost Survey that is produced annually and cannot be used for data points impacted by mode of practice. Because failure to implement the required changes is the most common reason for a failed result, adequate time and resources should be devoted to this aspect of the process. Once a consensus is reached, the formal implementation phase should begin immediately. Although the appropriate plan will give the stakeholders a sense of well-being, it is the implementation, and not the plan itself, that ultimately solves the problems and meets expectations. Persistence is the key. Although the numbers tell the story, they tend to be arcane and confusing to hospital administrators and their consultants if they lack anesthesia experience. The goal is to develop an easy to follow story using a logical sequence of information that explains outliers and anticipates potential flashpoints. For instance, assigning revenue and expenses to a responsibility center such as OB may explain why

OB places undue pressure on a group, as fully staffed in-house OB coverage may easily consume 40% of the gross revenues of a small anesthesia practice. Another example would be a primary care practitioner who sits on a hospital board. This physician would have to be educated in advance regarding anesthesiologist and anesthetist salaries because primary care pay tends to be unfairly low and could result in a disruptive or subversive position in closed door board of directors' meetings. Anesthesiologist salaries do not surprise them, but many are justifiably incensed that a nurse outearns them. Depending on the level of trust and market knowledge of the key stakeholders, it is important not to create a perception that this exercise is only to guarantee high levels of income to the anesthesiologists. There is a greater chance of success if framed in the context of stabilizing the anesthesia platform when it is requested to provide a level of service that is not supported by the revenue stream generated. Recruitment, retention, and stability are the desired goals. Your presentation/story should flow in a logical and believable manner that demonstrates an alignment of incentives between the group, hospital, and community and that provides the desired level of access. Assess the political timing before scheduling the first hospital meeting to make sure this is the right moment to raise the question. It must pass the "smell test" internally before being presented externally. If the objective assessment is that there is not a satisfactory answer to these issues/questions, then the negotiation is not ready for prime time. Lastly, it is important to determine the group or organization's best alternative to no (or negotiated) agreement. Pre-agreed consensus should drive leadership on when to walk away from the negotiation, and group members must be intellectually honest in determining what they are willing to accept or not accept. You should never walk out of the room unless you are willing to stay out until the other party blinks. Be cautious in asking the consultant what he or she would do; they are not the one who has to relocate if things do not work out to the group's preference! If the hospital administration senses a weakness in the group's resolve, they will make the most of it because that is their fiduciary responsibility to their organization. Our economic system is built on a price–quantity combination between two willing parties – nothing mandates that both, or either, are happy with the outcome. The best plan in the world is worthless unless implemented. Once the strategic analysis indicates that the presentation is ready for prime time, execute it.

Summary

Determine the critical success and critical failure factors, objectively assess the group's reasonable needs, assets, and liabilities, and then synchronize your requests with the institutional objectives and your mutual key stakeholders. The result should be a fair market value proposition that truly benefits the community by providing a stable and sustainable anesthesia platform. Persistence is the key!

Reprinted with permission from the American Society of Anesthesiologists.

Suggested reading

Medical Group Management Association. Physician Compensation and Productivity Survey. Published annually.

Medical Group Management Association. Cost Survey for Anesthesia and Pain Management Practices. Published every other year.

Medical Group Management Association. Medical Directorship and On-Call Compensation Survey. Published annually.

P. M. Senge. *The Fifth Discipline. The Art and Practice of the Learning Organization.* London: Random House, 1990.

R. Fisher, W. L. Ury, B. Patton. *Getting to Yes: Negotiating Agreement Without Giving In.* New York, NY: Penguin Group USA, Inc, 2011.

Chapter

16

Basics of billing, coding, and compliance

Deborah Farmer CPC, ACS-AN
Devona Slater CHC, CMCP

Overview of coding systems   168
Evaluation and management services   170
Billing for surgical services   171
Billing for anesthesia services   172
Key documentation elements   174
Concurrency   174
Important documentation factors for
anesthesia billing   175

Ancillary services for anesthesiologists   176
Acute pain management   178
Obstetric anesthesia   178
Physician Quality Reporting System   179
Measurement of key billing
benchmarks   179
Compliance   180
Summary   182

Overview of coding systems

Providers are required to use a variety of coding systems to translate services into reimbursement. Understanding these systems is critical, not only for correct reimbursement but also for compliance and maintaining your medical license.

Coding is defined as the process of translating a service, a supply, or a patient condition into a numeric or alphanumeric code, using only those codes in a mandated code set so that a third party can understand what happened to the patient and why. For a code to be considered correct it must be supported in the official medical record and legally accurate – that is to say that it will not mislead the recipient into a false belief about the services performed.

Many confuse the difference between correct coding and reimbursement rules. Although both are extremely important to providers, correct coding rules establish how a service must be represented so that it is properly understood. It incorporates interpretations from the American Medical Association (AMA) and the National Correct Coding Initiative (NCCI) to properly report services. Reimbursement rules, however, establish whether the service reported, which is correctly coded, is covered and payable under

an insurance benefit contract. A service may be correctly coded yet not paid because of insurance coverage policies.

The first set of codes providers need to become familiar with is the Current Procedural Terminology (CPT) codes. The AMA established the physicians' CPT coding as a consistent method of describing services performed by providers. The CPT codes are updated annually, with new codes added and established codes reviewed for revisions or deletions to reflect the ongoing changes in medical technology. The CPT lists descriptive terms and assigns numerical codes to the most commonly performed diagnostic and therapeutic procedures. Included with CPT codes is the concept of modifiers that help explain additional circumstances that may occur with the code. Examples of modifiers may include increased services, separate and distinct services, or – in the case of anesthesia – physical status. It is important to understand that not all payers recognize CPT modifiers.

The second set of codes providers must be aware of is the International Classification of Diseases (ICD). The World Health Organization (WHO) established the ICD to aid in the collection of morbidity statistics. The ICD-9 (ICD-10) codes refer to specific diagnoses

Operating Room Leadership and Management, ed. Kaye A.D., Fox C.J. and Urman R.D. Published by Cambridge University Press. © Cambridge University Press 2012.

of the condition for which the patient is receiving treatment. These codes must be linked appropriately to the CPT code to establish the medical necessity for the services provided. Thus, each provider is responsible for reporting why they are seeing or treating the patient. Reimbursement may hinge on whether or not medical necessity is established based on the ICD-9 (ICD-10) code(s) selected.

The Healthcare Common Procedure Coding System (HCPCS) is the third published code set that is universally used to identify drugs, supplies, special procedures, and products that may be covered by insurance. These codes are easily identified because they begin with an alpha character followed by four numerical digits. The codes primarily represent items and nonphysician services used in the office or ambulatory surgery center/outpatient facility. The HCPCS codes also contain modifiers, which are two-position codes and descriptors that alter the original code by some specific circumstance but do not change the definition of the code. Again, the goal in using HCPCS codes is uniform reporting of supplies, products, and services within the office or ambulatory surgery center/outpatient setting.

Some additional systems that providers must be familiar with to understand coding and reimbursement systems are those that have been generated by the federal government. The Resource-Based Relative Value Scale (RBRVS), implemented in 1992 by Medicare, is the most widely used standardized system for reimbursement of physician services. Simply put, payment for services is determined by the resource costs needed to provide a service. In the RBRVS the cost of providing each service is divided into three components: physician work, practice expense, and professional liability insurance. Reimbursement is calculated by multiplying the combined costs of the service by a conversion factor (which is adjusted by geographic region of the country). Annual updates are mandated and involve the AMA and national medical specialty societies known as the RVS Update Committee (RUC). Every CPT code must be reevaluated every 5 years.

The NCCI was developed by the Health Care Finance Administration (HCFA) in 1996 as part of an effort to reduce coding errors and the inappropriate payments resulting from those errors. The NCCI edits focus on what is known as "unbundling of procedures" by providing definition of the anesthesia and global surgery rules. These rules define all procedures/services necessary to accomplish a given procedure

to be included (bundled) in the description of that procedure. The edits are two tables that coders must consider in appropriate code selection: the mutually exclusive table, which matches codes for services that cannot reasonably be performed together based on code definitions or anatomic considerations, and the comprehensive/component table, which identifies component parts of a CPT code. The component code reflects the integral procedure or service when reported with another code. The integral code in certain circumstances can be separately billed with a modifier; the modifier would signify the component code is separate and distinct or performed at a different time in order for the procedure not to be included with the primary (comprehensive) service. NCCI edits change quarterly and coders should check the complete listing from the CMS web site before assigning codes.

The final system anesthesia providers must be familiar with is the American Society of Anesthesiologists (ASA) *Relative Value Guide* (RVG) and the ASA *CROSSWALK* for anesthesia coding. Published by the ASA, these publications are not intended to suggest any monetary value; they are designed and nationally recognized as a uniform fee schedule for anesthesia services. The RVG is best used in conjunction with the *CROSSWALK*, which links each surgical CPT code to an appropriate anesthesia code. Alternate anesthesia codes are given for certain circumstances in which the RVG may need to be consulted. Both guides are updated annually by the ASA, and providers should only use the most current edition when assigning codes.

In today's medical environment, understanding coding systems is as important as documenting the services that are delivered. Basic principles of documentation and the appropriate coding of services lay the foundation for reimbursement. Accurate coding provides a picture of the "work" that was performed. Many debate whether coding should be done by a coding professional or by the provider themselves. It is important to keep in mind that even if a professional coder performs the assignment of codes for the services performed, it is the provider that is held responsible for any coding errors. Coding must be assigned based on the written, legible, documentation that exists in the patient's medical record. The goal of correct coding is twofold: (1) to insure proper payment from government and third-party payers; and (2) to reduce the provider's chance of an audit.

Evaluation and management services

In the introduction of the evaluation and management chapter in the CPT-4 book there are specific instructions that define coding guidelines. In addition, the Centers for Medicare & Medicaid Services (CMS) has specific coding guidelines published on their website that give instructions on the appropriate assignment of levels to the coding of evaluation and management services. Both of these references should be consulted for more specific instructions, and only an overview of what is needed for coding for these services is given below.

There are two important underlying principles that specifically apply to documentation that a provider should always keep in mind. First, if the medical care is not documented in the medical record, it is treated as if it had not been performed. The second is that all services must be medically necessary. This medical necessity requirement specifically applies to evaluation and management services. In order for correct coding to occur, services must be evaluated based on the nature of the presenting problem and the medical decisions made during the visit. While it is possible to document a medical history and a physical examination that would meet the required elements of level 4 or 5 services, if the patient presents with only a minor problem, such as a rash, and the medical decision making is straightforward in nature, the lower level codes would be more compliant for billing regardless of the amount of documentation provided in the medical history and physical examination because only the lower level of care is really medically necessary for treating the problem.

Evaluation and management coding have seven components: history, examination, medical decision making, counseling, coordination of care, nature of the presenting problem, and time. The first three are considered the key components and will be the ones focused on in this section.

The documentation of each patient encounter should include:

- the reason for the encounter and relevant history;
- physical examination findings and review of prior diagnostic test results;
- assessment, clinical impression, or diagnosis;
- plan for care;
- date and legible identity of the provider.

New patient encounters require documentation of all three key components (i.e., history, examination,

Table 16.1 The body systems that are recognized in a review of systems

Constitutional symptoms (e.g., fever, weight loss)	Musculoskeletal
Eyes	Integumentary
Ears, Nose, Mouth, Throat	Neurological
Cardiovascular	Psychiatric
Respiratory	Endocrine
Gastrointestinal	Hematologic/Lymphatic
Genitourinary	Allergic/Immunologic

and medical decision making) and should meet or exceed the stated requirement to qualify for a particular level of evaluation and management (E/M) service. Established patient visits require documentation of only two of the three key components to qualify for a particular level.

All medical records should begin with the patient's chief complaint. This should be a brief statement about why the patient is seeing the physician and is usually stated in the patient's own words. The second component of the history portion of an E/M service is the history of present illness. This involves a chronological description of the development of the patient's present illness and should describe the location, quality, severity, timing, context, modifying factors, and associated signs and symptoms significantly related to the presenting problem.

A review of systems is an inventory of body systems obtained through a series of questions seeking to identify signs and/or symptoms that the patient may be experiencing or has experienced. Table 16.1 shows the systems that are recognized.

The review of systems helps define the problem, clarify the differential diagnosis, and identify the necessary testing, or serves as baseline data on other systems that might be affected by any possible management options.

A review of the patient's past medical history (e.g., prior major illnesses, operations, medications, etc.), family history (health status/cause of death of parents, siblings, etc.), and social history (marital status, employment, use of drugs, alcohol and tobacco, etc.) completes the history portion of the E/M service.

The required examination documentation guidelines set forth by CMS for each E/M level are complicated and very specific. Physicians have two options

Table 16.2 The four levels of exam in the general multisystem examination

Problem focused – a limited exam of the affected body area or organ system

Expanded problem focused – a limited exam of the affected body areas or organ system and any other symptomatic or related body area(s) or organ system(s)

Detailed – an extended exam of the affected body area(s) or organ system(s) and any other symptomatic or related body area(s) or organ system(s)

Comprehensive – a general multisystem exam or a complete exam of a single organ system and other symptomatic or related body area(s) or organ system(s)

from which they may choose. The 1995 guidelines outline the general multisystem examination. The 1997 guidelines detail single organ system examinations. Table 16.2 shows the four levels of examination.

For all examinations, the number of elements/body systems that must be examined increases with the level of E/M service provided. The type of exam and the content of the exam should be based on the provider's clinical judgment, the patient's history, and the nature of the presenting problem. Medical necessity for the amount of detail performed during the examination is dictated by the nature of the presenting problem.

Medical decision making refers to the complexity of establishing a diagnosis or selecting management options measured by: (1) the number of possible diagnoses and/or management options that must be considered before completing the plan of care; (2) the amount and/or complexity of medical records, diagnostic tests, or other information that must be obtained, reviewed, and analyzed; and (3) the risk of significant complications, morbidity, and mortality, as well as comorbidities associated with the patient's presenting problem, the diagnostic procedure, or possible management options. The higher levels of medical decision making include an abrupt change in neurological status, acute or chronic injury that poses a threat to life or bodily function, or chronic illnesses that have a documented exacerbation or progression, or side effects from treatment.

The CPT book includes time in the definitions of the specific levels of E/M services. The specific times expressed in the CPT visit code descriptors are averages, and therefore represent a range of times that may be higher or lower depending on actual clinical circumstances. For coding purposes, face-to-face time for these services is defined as only the time that the physician spends face to face with the patient and/or family. This includes the time in which the physician performs such tasks as obtaining a history, performing an examination, and counseling the patient.

When counseling and/or coordination of care dominates (more than 50%) the physician/patient and/or family encounter (face-to-face time in the office or other outpatient setting), the time may be considered the key or controlling factor to qualify for a particular level of E/M service. The provider should document the nature of the counseling and/or coordination of care, the actual amount of time spent counseling the patient, and the total time of the patient encounter.

Billing for surgical services

As stated, the most important aspect of coding is the documentation itself. Without proper documentation, it is impossible to perform coding and be paid appropriately for services. In general surgical coding there are four basic steps that coding professionals follow.

First the coder must identify the appropriate anatomical site and locate the applicable section in the CPT-4 book. It is best to code directly from the operative/procedure note dictated by the surgeon. Second is to determine the level of service which should be assigned. The CPT-4 book is divided into anatomical sections, with subcategories, in which the procedures are listed from the simplest to the most complex. It is important to review the entire section when coding to insure that the services performed relate directly to the code assigned. The operative note will indicate whether the surgical service was simple, complex, closed, open, and so forth. It is important to note that if specific documentation does not exist, coders are instructed to bill for the minimal service for that procedure.

The third step evaluates whether the code selected is inclusive of all services that were provided. It is important to have the most recent version of the NCCI edits available for reference when coding. This document lists CPT codes that are considered a component of another service. This is often referred to as bundled services. Providers are to remember that services that are incidental to the primary procedure are not separately billable.

The final step is assigning a code for a surgical service is to review the code for any applicable modifiers that may need to be assigned. Modifiers help to explain circumstances that may have occurred during the surgical service. For example, when procedures are performed bilaterally during the same operative session, it would be appropriate to append modifier -50 to the service. This explains to the carrier that one procedure was performed bilaterally. This does have payment implications, in that bilateral payment rules reimburse at 150% of the unilateral rate. Modifier codes are usually a two-digit code that attaches to the original CPT-4 code. Table 16.3 is a listing of some of the current modifiers that may be used and their definitions. This is not an all-inclusive list, and providers and coders should consult the current CPT-4 book before assigning a modifier.

Every procedural service must be supported by a diagnosis. The primary diagnosis is the reason for that service. The diagnosis should always be assigned to the highest level of specificity as known at the time of service. Additional diagnoses may be added for each service to explain the medical necessity of why a particular service was justified or the underlying conditions of a patient that factored into the medical decision making of the service.

Billing for anesthesia services

Anesthesia services include all types of sedation. Typically there is no separate payment for local/topical anesthetic. It is included in the surgeon's global fee and cannot be charged separately.

The next level of services is moderate (conscious) sedation. Sedation services are billed with CPT codes 99143–99150 depending on whether the surgeon is overseeing a trained third-party observer (99143–99145) or whether a separate physician is providing moderate sedation (99148–99150). Moderate (conscious) sedation is a drug-induced state of consciousness in which patients can respond purposefully to verbal commands, either alone or by light stimulation. Interventions are not required to maintain a patent airway and spontaneous ventilation is adequate. It requires the recording of intra-service time, which is

Table 16.3 Some of the current modifier codes

Modifier	Description
22	Unusual procedure services – services that go beyond the scope of the normal CPT description
50	Bilateral procedure services – identical services performed bilaterally that are not specified in the CPT description itself
52	Reduced services – services provided are partially reduced or eliminated but do not compromise the identification of the basic service
53	Discontinued procedure – when a procedure is terminated prior to its completion
59	Distinct procedural service – services that are distinct from other procedures performed during the same operative session
62	Two surgeons – when two surgeons work together to perform one primary procedure
78	Return to the operating room for a related procedure during the postoperative period
79	Return to the operating room for an unrelated procedure during the postoperative period
80	Assistant surgeon – when a surgical assistant is required to perform a given surgical service

defined as continuous face-to-face attendance with start time defined as indicating administration of the sedation and end time defined as the conclusion of the personal service of the physician providing or overseeing the sedation. One cannot discuss moderate sedation without noting Appendix G in the CPT book, which is a list of codes that include moderate sedation as a component of the code. Providers are not allowed to bill moderate sedation in addition to codes listed in Appendix G according to CPT guidelines.

Monitored anesthesia care (MAC) is a billable anesthesia service and involves intraoperative monitoring by a physician or qualified anesthesia professional. While MAC may or may not include the administration of drugs, it differs from moderate sedation in that the anesthesia provider must be prepared and qualified to convert to a general anesthetic when necessary.

Although payment for MAC is equal to that of a general or regional anesthetic and requires all the same level of documentation, specific modifiers are required when filing claim forms for MAC services. The following modifiers denote MAC services for Medicare claims:

QS – designates monitored anesthesia care;

G8 – designates the monitored anesthesia care services are necessary because the procedure is noted as deep, complex, complicated, or markedly invasive;

G9 – designates the monitored anesthesia care services are necessary because the patient has a personal history of cardiopulmonary disease.

Other third-party payers may or may not require the above modifiers for the identification of MAC services. Payer policies should be closely reviewed before appending modifiers.

The importance of the anesthesia pre-evaluation cannot be overemphasized to support MAC. Many carriers have requirements for payment that reference specific diagnosis to support the medical necessity for an anesthesia provider. Documenting physical conditions and comorbidities that place the patient at risk are to be explained on the claim form with supplemental diagnosis.

Regional anesthesia care includes many types of blocks. The main purpose of a regional technique is to anesthetize only one area of the body, such as an arm, leg, or lower extremities in order to perform an operation. Regional anesthesia care is compensated in exactly the same way as a general anesthetic, and unlike MAC services does not require any special modifiers to denote the service. It requires all of the same elements in documentation such as the pre-anesthesia evaluation, administration of anesthesia agents, and monitoring intraoperatively and postanesthesia care.

General anesthesia is the final level of anesthesia compensated. General anesthesia is a state of unconsciousness in which the patient loses protective reflexes as a result of the administration of drugs. A physician, a certified registered nurse anesthetist (CRNA), or an anesthesiologist assistant (AA) under the medical direction of an anesthesiologist may be reimbursed for anesthesia services.

Billing for all types of anesthesia services must take into consideration base units, time units, physical status, and qualifying circumstances. The base unit is defined by the ASA RVG. Base units take into account the complexity, risk, and skill required to perform the service. The base units include all of the value for normal and usual anesthesia services except for time factors and what is known as modifying factors. The base value specifically includes the anesthesia pre-evaluation service in which the physician must document an evaluation, a physical examination, an anesthesia plan, and discuss the risks of the anesthetic plan with the patient. It also includes the administration of fluids and blood products that may be incidental to the anesthesia care as well as any noninvasive monitoring. The final element included in the base unit value is the postoperative visits. Anesthesia billing is different from other specialties in that only one anesthesia code is reported no matter how many procedures are performed. When multiple procedures are performed during a single anesthetic encounter, only report the anesthesia code with the highest base unit value.

Added to base units are time units. Anesthesia time is defined as the period of time that an anesthesia practitioner is present with the patient. It begins when the anesthesia provider begins to prepare the patient for anesthesia services in the operating room or an equivalent area and ends when the anesthesia provider safely places the patient with postoperative care personnel. Anesthesia time is a continuous time period. Medicare does recognize the concept of discontinuous anesthesia time, in which a provider may add blocks of time around a break in anesthesia time as long as the provider is furnishing continuous anesthesia care within the time periods around the interruption. An easy example of discontinuous time occurs in regional anesthesia techniques. As the regional block is the mode of anesthesia for the case, the anesthesia time could start while the provider is placing the block. The first recorded time is the amount of time it takes to place the block. Recognizing that it may take several minutes for the block to take effect, the anesthesia provider may step away from the patient, and during that time the documentation indicates a break in anesthesia care. The time starts again when the patient is rolled into the operating room for the surgery. Although the ASA states that time units may be calculated according to what is customary in the local area, most carriers pay in exact minutes or 15-min blocks of time to equal one unit.

Modifying units come in two specific categories. First we have physical status modifiers, which are designed with the initial P followed by a single digit. These modifiers distinguish between different levels of complexity of anesthesia service provided, depending on the patient's circumstances, and are consistent with the ASA ranking of the patient's physical status. Carriers may or may not pay for physical status modifiers based on payment policies. The second category of modifying units is qualifying circumstances (99100–99140). These are conditions that significantly impact the anesthetic service provided. Again, these are separate line item charges that are added to the anesthesia service. Qualifying circumstance codes may or may not be covered, based on payer reimbursement policies.

Key documentation elements

Documentation is the cornerstone for billing. As the saying goes, if it is not documented, it did not happen. Only written entries in the official medical record can be used in the coding and billing process. Many practices use a charge ticket to summarize billing information, but the actual documentation of the service must be supported in the medical record because the charge ticket is not part of the medical record and cannot be relied upon for support in an audit situation.

There are key items that are reviewed for documentation in billing anesthesia services. The anesthesia pre-evaluation is the first item reviewed. From a billing viewpoint, the preoperative evaluation would include an appropriate anesthesia evaluation and examination, discussion of risk with the patient, and an anesthesia plan. From the pre-evaluation, billing personnel look for justification of the ASA physical status and monitored anesthesia care to add diagnosis for support in ICD-9 coding on the claim form.

On the anesthesia record there are several important things that coders and billers verify before billing. First the record should identify the facility and the place of service. This is important, because each claim must identify the facility and whether services were performed in an outpatient, inpatient, ambulatory surgery, or office setting. Services should clearly detail the patient name, date of service, and the type of anesthesia administered. In addition, the anesthesia provider should record all procedures performed by the surgeon and the postoperative diagnosis so that correct coding can be ascertained. Anesthesia start and end time should be taken directly off the anesthesia record. Many times coders will need to look at the monitoring on the time line to verify the time reported or to support the time charged. It is best if monitoring occurs within 5 min of anesthesia start time and continues up until the time the patient leaves the room. Although this will not necessarily prove the medical necessity of the services, it does provide documentation of constant attendance with the patient. Other key services that may be pulled from the record are the delivery of ancillary lines or postoperative pain services.

From a billing standpoint, there is little to review on the postanesthesia care record. Currently the hospital conditions of participation and the ACS conditions for coverage have requirements regarding the elements of a postoperative anesthesia visit within a certain time frame. Anesthesia providers are required to be available to treat postoperative complication in the postanesthesia care unit but no specific documentation of availability is reviewed on an individual record.

Concurrency

Involved in anesthesia time is the Medicare definition of "concurrency." Concurrency is simply the reference to how many services an anesthesiologist is involved with at any one time. While originally a government term, most third-party payers have jumped on the bandwagon and actually now have some type of concurrency modifiers. These anesthesia-specific modifiers tell payers how anesthesia services are delivered in the operating room. Providers must pay close attention to their times because starting and ending on the same minute will cause the two cases to be concurrent. Concurrency is the reason why so many billing professionals harp on documentation of relief services. Anesthesia providers are to file under the provider who has the most time on the case, so tracking who is where and when plays a large component in anesthesia billing. The only exception in provider reporting is in the teaching rules, where Medicare has instructed to bill under the provider who starts the case.

The medical direction modifiers are as follows:

AA – anesthesia services performed personally by an anesthesiologist;

QY – medically directed by a physician: one CRNA;

QK – medically directed by a physician: two, three, or four CRNAs;

AD – supervision by a physician: more than four CRNAs;

QX – CRNA with medical direction by a physician;

QZ – nonmedically directed CRNA.

You cannot determine concurrency without looking at the elements of medical direction. Medical direction requirements were made clear in the Medicare Carriers Manual, MCM 15018.C. These requirements detail seven specific steps that an anesthesiologist must meet in order to file the claim as medically directed. These seven steps are:

1. perform a pre-anesthesia examination and evaluation;
2. prescribe the anesthesia plan;
3. take part personally in the most demanding procedures of the anesthesia service, including induction and emergence;
4. insure that any procedures in the anesthesia plan that he or she does not perform are performed by qualified anesthesia personnel;
5. monitor the course of the anesthesia administration at intervals;
6. be physically present and available for immediate diagnosis and treatment of emergencies;
7. provide the postanesthesia care indicated.

The government never makes a rule without creating a few exceptions, and the medical direction rules have six. While medically directing, a physician may:

1. address an emergency of short duration in the immediate area;
2. administer an epidural or caudal anesthetic to ease labor pain;
3. perform periodic, rather than continuous, monitoring of an obstetrical patient;
4. receive patients entering the operating suite for the next surgery;
5. check on or discharge patients from the recovery room;
6. coordinate scheduling matters.

The government believes that none of these exceptions substantially diminishes the scope of control exercised by a physician in directing the administration of anesthesia to surgical patients. Many carriers have added other items, such as placing invasive lines or postoperative pain blocks to these exceptions, but again you must check with your individual carrier to see if there are additional services allowed in your state.

Many people mistakenly use the words "medical direction" and "supervision" interchangeably. In anesthesia reimbursement, the two have very different meanings. Supervision specifically refers to an anesthesia provider who is involved in more than four concurrent procedures. Medical direction means that the anesthesia provider is involved with one, two, three, or four concurrent procedures.

If these seven steps are documented on the anesthesia record and the concurrency calculation is below four or less cases, the medical direction modifier QK or QY can be assigned to physician claims. Payers differ as to how they want claims submitted when the seven steps are not complete. Some require the case to be billed as a CRNA service alone (QZ modifier), whereas others allow the physician to claim supervision (AD modifier) for their work in the case. Every practice should check with their own state and local carriers before determining how to submit claims of incomplete medical direction.

In working with AAs, student registered nurse anesthetists (SRNAs), and residents, you must always document the steps of medical direction to qualify for payment. The teaching rules were amended for dates of service on or after January 1, 2010 to allow the AA modifier to be used when teaching two residents, which allows 100% reimbursement for each case. Although medical direction is allowed in cases involving residents of three or four concurrent cases, you will only be reimbursed for the physician portion (50% of the allowable) of the case. With SRNAs you are not allowed to medically direct more than two at any one time, and the QK modifiers would only allow the physician payment, as the SRNA and residents are paid through the graduate education program.

Important documentation factors for anesthesia billing

Appropriate anesthesia coding starts with the anesthesia provider documenting the procedure on the anesthesia record with a goal of matching the surgeon's postoperative procedure. Providers should think about location, site, position, approach, and technique used in providing enough information to code for anesthesia services. The next step in coding is to select the CPT procedure code (10021–99174) that most accurately describes the documented procedure. At this point the procedure code is cross-walked to the anesthesia code (00100–01999), which is provided by the ASA Crosswalk. Selection of the anesthesia code can be a bit tricky as the procedure code can link to multiple anesthesia codes, which are identified under "Alternate(s)." For example, CPT code 20680 (Removal implant; deep) links to 13 different anesthesia codes. This is why detailed documentation by the provider is crucial to accurate billing and reimbursement.

In the above example the provider needs to indicate the specific site where the implant was removed to select the correct alternate, which has been pointed out by italicized comments under the alternate codes. Base units for procedures on bones can vary depending on: (1) an open or closed procedure; (2) the site and location of the repair (i.e., humerus upper, shaft, or lower end); (3) a diagnostic or surgical arthroscopy; and/or (4) documentation of radical procedure. If the surgeon also performs an artery repair while repairing the fracture, this can increase the units by 1 unit or as much as 5 units, depending on the site of the fracture.

The documented site and position can also alter the anesthesia code and base units in the integumentary system. Procedures performed on the head, neck, and posterior trunk have a base unit value of 5, but 3 units are assigned for extremities, anterior trunk, and perineum. Position is helpful to support coding of the service as anterior versus posterior. It also helps support the RVG instruction that position other than supine or lithotomy is assigned 5 units regardless of a lesser base value.

Italicized comments are included in both ASA guides to help simplify assignment of alternative codes. Under procedure codes for mediastinoscopy, diagnostic thoracoscopy, and surgical thoracotomy procedures comments are included to "Consider single or double lung ventilation." Documentation by the anesthesia provider should include under the procedure to clearly document one lung ventilation for support of the additional 3-unit valuation. Incorrect reporting abbreviation can cause misunderstanding, which could lead to over- or underreporting of services (see Table 16.4). Only approved abbreviations should be used.

One example of an abbreviation that led to underreporting of the base unit is "CABG OP." Coronary artery bypass graft (CABG) codes have three alternatives: 00566 with pump oxygenator (25 units); 00567 with pump oxygenator (18 units); or 00562 with pump for reoperation for coronary bypass more than 1 month after original operation (20 units). The coder thought the code OP meant "on pump," but the provider intended the abbreviation as "off pump," which caused a loss of 7 units. If the coder had a copy of the anesthesia record, they could have checked the graph line to verify on/off pump – that is, if they had been trained in how to read an anesthesia record. As for the third alternative, to determine "1 month after original operation" the anesthesia providers would have to be a mind reader or ask the surgeon. This information can be easily overlooked by an anesthesia provider and disregarded by coding if not documented on the anesthesia record.

These examples are provided to help physicians understand the importance of documentation and understanding correct code selection. While these examples imply a loss in revenue by insufficient documentation, coders can easily overreport services from misunderstanding of abbreviation or new technology. At a minimum, providers should have a common working knowledge of anesthesia coding to understand the documentation needed to help facilitate correct coding, billing, and payment of services provided.

Ancillary services for anesthesiologists

In addition to the anesthetic, the providers place arterial, central venous, and pulmonary artery catheters. These services are not included in the basic unit value. Medicare and other carriers allow separate payment for invasive monitoring lines as long as they are not routinely inserted during anesthesia time. Per the Payment for Anesthesiology Services, Chapter 12, Section 50, F. Rev. 1859; Issued: 11–20–09; Effective Date: For services furnished on or after 01–01–10; Implementation Date: 01–04–10):

Payment may be made under the fee schedule for specific medical and surgical services furnished by the anesthesiologist as long as these services are reasonable and medically necessary or provided that other rebundling provisions (see subsection 30 and Chapter 23) do not preclude separate payment. These services may be furnished in conjunction with the anesthesia procedure to the patient or may be furnished as single services, e.g., during the day of or the day before the anesthesia service.

The anesthesia provider is responsible for documenting the insertion of the invasive monitoring lines in the patient's medical record. These are considered to be "surgical procedures," and a procedure note needs to include: (1) description of the nature; (2) extent and need of the procedure for the patient's condition; (3) medical assessment for the procedure; (4) method/technique utilized; (5) drugs and dosage; (6) time involved; (7) effort; and (8) the equipment necessary. Radiology guidance is sometimes needed to assist in line placements. Ultrasound guidance for vascular access can be reported in addition to a central venous catheter placement when guidance is utilized. The code descriptor indicates that the service requires the provider to indicate ultrasound evaluation of potential access sites, documentation of selected vessel patency, concurrent real-time ultrasound visualization of vascular needle

Table 16.4 Other common and not so common examples of documentation that caused a loss in base units based on the ASA *CROSSWALK* 2011

Procedure documented by anesthesia	Alternate choices of anesthesia coding	ASA codes	Base units
Cysto	Transurethral urethrocystoscopy	00910	3
	With manipulate and/or removal ureteral stone	00918	5
	Removal stone in upper one-third of ureter or kidney	00862	7
Abdominal wound closure	Integumentary system anterior trunk	00400	3
	Intraperitoneal procedure in lower abdomen	00840	6
	Intraperitoneal procedure in upper abdomen	00790	7
	Management of liver hemorrhage	00792	13
THR	Total hip arthroplasty	01214	8
	Total hip revision	01215	10
TAH	Intraperitoneal procedure in lower abdomen	00840	6
	(TAH, S&O, omentectomy, lymphadenectomy)	00846	8
Epigastric hernia	Hernia repairs upper abdomen	00750	4
	Strangulated epigastric hernia	00790	7
Placement interstitial radioelement prostate	Placement of needles, integumentary system perineum	00400	3
	Trans-rectal approach	00902	5
Anterior lumbar interbody fusion	Open procedures in lumbar region	00630	8
	ALIF with pins at L3, L4, L5	00670	13
	Use 00670 if performed with spinal instrumentation or on multiple vertebral levels		

entry with permanent recording and reporting. Use of a simple hand-held or other Doppler device that does not produce a hard copy is considered part of the examination of the vascular system and should not to be separately reported. Ultrasound utilized only to identify a vein, mark a skin entry point, or proceed with non-guided puncture should not be separately reported.

Transesophageal echocardiography (TEE) is also sometimes perceived as an extra ancillary service. Per the NCCI Policy, Version 16.0, Chapter 2 (4): "Transesophageal echocardiography for *monitoring purposes* is integral to anesthesia care." It would be inappropriate to bill for TEE services that are for monitoring purposes. There is one exception regarding the placement of a TEE. Pursuant to Medicare TEE National Coverage Policy Pub.100–4, Ch. 12, §30.4:

Diagnostic intra-operative TEE is indicated when the surgical procedure is expected to alter the anatomy or function of the cardiac or thoracic structures: 1. If the evaluation of cardiac function and/or thoracic structures is necessary for the safe conduct of anesthesia or surgery. 2. If the surgical technique will be affected by the intra-operative TEE findings, thus assisting in surgical management decision.

3. If thoracic structures and/or cardiac function were not adequately evaluated pre-operatively AND the information is necessary for the safe conduct of anesthesia and surgery.

It is the government's intent to require the surgical technique to be affected by the intraoperative TEE findings, thus assisting in surgical management decisions. The TEE is only billable during surgery when the surgeon requests the TEE for a specific diagnostic reason (determination of proper valve placement, assessment of the adequacy of valvuloplasty, placement of shunts or other devices, assessment of ventricular function, assessment of vascular integrity, or detection of intravascular air). Documentation should include a complete interpretation and report by the performing physician. The anesthesia provider may only be asked by the surgeon to place the probe and documentation would, in this instance, only include the placement.

Many individuals have questioned whether ancillary lines should be included in anesthesia time. Per *CPT Assistant*, Volume 17, Issue 5, May 2007 and as published in the ASA 2011 RVU "Reporting

Post-Operative Pain Procedures in Conjunction with Anesthesia":

- *If the service is conducted PRIOR to induction of the anesthesia for a surgical procedure being performed by another provider, the line is separately reportable, but should not be part of the anesthesia time.*
- *Sedation for placement of the line does not qualify as an event that starts anesthesia time.*
- *When lines are placed or performed AFTER anesthesia has been induced, the time spent performing these procedures does not need to be deducted from the anesthesia time.*

Providers should take reasonable care in documenting start and end times in placing invasive lines so that documentation can demonstrate that the services were done outside of anesthesia start time or done after the induction of anesthesia.

Acute pain management

Anesthesiologists are allowed to bill for postoperative pain services if the sole purpose of the service is management of postoperative pain. NCCI Chapter II (B)(3) states:

> Postoperative pain management services are generally provided by the surgeon who is reimbursed under a global payment policy related to the procedure and shall not be reported by the anesthesia practitioner unless separate, medically necessary services are required that cannot be rendered by the surgeon. Providers should clearly document medical necessity in the pre-anesthesia evaluation form to include or easily infer the services are provided for post-operative pain and at request of the surgeon. Modifier -59 is appended to the surgical CPT code to denote that the service was distinct and separate from the anesthesia service performed on the same day.

Postoperative pain services are to be billed under the provider who placed the block. Because these services normally fall under the surgeon's remit, it is important to document the request for the service from the surgeon. These services are considered surgical procedures and a procedure note needs to include: (1) description of the nature, extent, and need of the procedure for the patient's condition; (2) medical assessment for the procedure; (3) method/technique utilized; (4) drugs and dosage; (5) placement time; (6) effort; and (7) equipment necessary. Needle placement performed under ultrasound guidance can be reported in addition to the surgical procedure, if documentation supports imaging supervision and interpretation. Written documentation should include the fact that a hard copy of the image was taken. If fluoroscopic guidance is utilized it can also be separately reported and also must include written documentation. These blocks are never done within anesthesia time, as they are billed as separate and distinct surgical services.

Daily management of an epidural catheter has a special code that is not subject to E/M documentation guidelines. The CPT code 01996 represents follow-up care of an epidural catheter. There are no published requirements for documentation of 01996, other than there must be a catheter in place. Providers should consider supporting the service by documenting: (1) current regimen; (2) reported pain scale and pain relief; (3) current activity functions; (4) inspection of the catheter site; and (5) any side effects. Supporting documentation should include a medical plan such as continuing the epidural, removal, and/or transferring to oral analgesics. Other continuous catheter follow-up services should be billed with the subsequent hospital visit codes. Visit codes must meet documentation guidelines of E/M services.

The ICD-9-CM includes several acute pain diagnosis codes specific to postoperative pain. When postoperative pain services are provided, individual carrier guidelines for appropriate diagnosis reporting should be followed.

Although acute pain management is an important part of anesthesia services, documentation should be very clear that the block is not being used as part of a combine technique for the case. If used as a combined technique, no separate billing for the block is allowed and the time it takes to provide the regional technique for the case is then added to the case time (discontinuous anesthesia time) for billing.

Obstetric anesthesia

Obstetric services continue to be an issue in the billing arena. The ASA 2011 RVG states:

> Unlike operative anesthesia services, there is no single, widely accepted method of accounting for time for neuraxial labor analgesia. Professional charges and payment policies should reasonably reflect the costs of providing labor analgesia as well as the intensity and time involved in performing and monitoring any neuraxial labor analgesic. Four methods to help establish professional fees consistent with these principles are:
>
> A. Base units plus time units (insertion through delivery), subject to a **reasonable cap**.

B. *Base units plus one unit per hour for neuraxial analgesia management plus direct patient contact time (insertion, management of adverse events, delivery, and removal).*

C. *Incremental time-based fees (e.g., 0<2 hrs, 2–6 hrs, >6 hrs).*

D. *Single fee.*

The phrase "costs of providing labor analgesia" guides anesthesia practices to analyze their professional time, work, etc. for providing neuraxial labor analgesia. Labor services should be assessed to determine appropriate charges, especially since Medicaid and third-party carriers may differ in their requirements for reporting labor time and the appropriate methodology for payment. Without a specific labor time policy, a carrier may hold providers accountable to the anesthesia time definition to include constant attendance. Research of all local payer policies is a must to stay compliant in billing for obstetric anesthesia, specifically paying close attention to the definition of anesthesia time.

Physician Quality Reporting System

The Physician Quality Reporting System (PQRS) quality data code reporting, established by the CMS, is a statutory program that creates a financial incentive/penalty for eligible professionals who volunteer in this quality reporting program. Successful reporting of the identified quality measures may earn a bonus payment up until 2014, and after that date a reduction of the fee will be applied to the total allowed charges for covered services.

The 2006 Tax Relief and Health Care Act (TRHCA) (PL 109–432) required the establishment of a physician quality reporting system, including an incentive payment for eligible professionals who satisfactorily report data on quality measures for covered professional services furnished to Medicare beneficiaries during the second half of 2007 (the 2007 reporting period). The CMS named this program the Physician Quality Reporting Initiative (PQRI). The PQRI was further modified as a result of the Medicare, Medicaid, and SCHIP Extension Act of 2007 (MMSEA) (Pub. L. 110–275) and the Medicare Improvements for Patients and Providers Act of 2008 (MIPPA) (Pub. L. 110–275). In 2011, the program name was changed to the Physician Quality Reporting System.

For each program year, CMS implements physician quality reporting through an annual rulemaking process published in the Federal Register. Currently there are 190 measures that are possible for reporting. All reference information for the PQRS data collection program can be found by going to www.cms.hhs.gov/PQRS.

The ASA or surgical CPT code itself is the identifier to CMS that a provider is eligible for reporting the measure(s). Each measure has a set of CPT codes to report along with possible modifiers. The other key element to understand is that the bonus payment is for reporting, not in the performance of the measure. It is essential to understand the measures should be reported based on the ASA or surgical CPT code, not whether the measure has been performed.

Accurate reporting requires an understanding of PQRS modifiers. Modifier -1P indicates that the measure was not met owing to medical reasons; modifier -8P indicates that the measure was not met owing to reasons not otherwise specified.

Currently anesthesia has three measures that they can report on: (1) Measure 76, Maximal Sterile Barrier Technique for Catheter-Related Blood Stream Infections; (2) Measure 30, Timing of Prophylactic Antibiotic; and (3) Measure 193, Active Warming. These measures are allowed to be reported in what is termed as "clusters" in order for anesthesia providers to qualify for the bonus payment. The current three reporting options at the time of this writing are:

1) Report Measure 76, Maximal Sterile Barrier Technique for Catheter-Related Bloodstream Infections, alone.

2) Report on two measures: Measure 76, Maximal Sterile Barrier Technique for Catheter-Related Bloodstream Infections and Measure 30, Timing of Prophylactic Antibiotic.

3) Report on two measures: Measure 76, Maximal Sterile Barrier Technique for Catheter-Related Bloodstream Infections and Measure 193, Active Warming or at least one body temperature within 30 minutes before anesthesia end time or 15 minutes after anesthesia end.

Quality reporting is expected to continue to be a focus on reimbursement. Providers are encouraged to check the Medicare website for the most up-to-date information regarding PQRS.

Measurement of key billing benchmarks

The billing process is the heart of the revenue cycle and must be monitored consistently. Anesthesia groups should develop a business office scorecard to provide a foundation of measurements to insure processes and resources are aligned to achieve business goals. There are several business measures that should be calculated and measured in the billing cycle process. Below are suggestions of measurements that should be monitored.

Gross collection ratio is the amount paid to the practice divided by the total charges billed. This does not include any write-offs or adjustments. This ratio varies based on the practice and the payer mix. For example, a payer mix consisting of a larger percentage of Medicaid and Medicare may result in a lower gross collection ratio. Therefore this would not be a dependable metric to use for comparison to other practices. If this metric is used for comparison it is best to compare practices that are similar in nature; large shifts indicate that providers should immediately review the payer mix to see why the change is occurring.

Net collection ratio is the amount paid to the practice divided by the total charges after the adjustments due to contractual write-offs. Controllable adjustments (i.e., small balance write-offs, bad debt write-offs to outside collections) should not be included in these adjustments. This ratio basically measures what was collected versus what should be collected. For a high level of performance, this ratio is typically over 90%. A drop in this number would indicate a problem within the billing process.

Days in accounts receivable is the time elapsed between billing the charge and collecting the payment. This is an important metric to evaluate efficiency of a billing office/service. The number of days it takes to collect a bill varies by specialty and can be affected by timely follow-up with the payer and quick rectification of any issues that may arise. The lower the number of days in accounts receivable demonstrates the efficiency in the process. A good number of days in accounts receivable would be somewhere between 40 and 45 days.

Accounts receivable aging tracks past due accounts. The billing office/service should report this as a number and percent of accounts that are current, 30, 60, 90, 120+ days past due. It should have an effective analysis process to troubleshoot the reasons for accounts falling in past due status. A high-performing billing office/service should constantly improve upon its processes to reduce the aging of accounts. Ranges for accounts receivable breakdown in aging categories in general is current 50–55%;

30 days 12–15%; 60 days 8–12%; 90 days 4–7%; and 120+ days 15–18%.

The average charge per case is the total charges billed divided by the number of cases in the month. This metric should be reported and reviewed on a monthly basis to determine trends that impact the practice. A shift in this number would indicate volume problems within the operating room and should be addressed with the facility.

The average collection per case is the amount paid to the practice divided by the number of cases. Collection per case indicates actual money paid and the collection efforts of the practice. A decrease in this number would indicate problems within the billing process. Reviewing this metric monthly is important to determine collection trends that impact the practice.

The average collection per unit is the amount paid to the practice divided by the total number of units billed. This metric should be reported and compared on a monthly basis for the current year, and to the previous year's monthly average. Fluctuations in this metric may be an indication of a shift in payer mix and should be analyzed to determine the cause(s). The average charge per case, average collection per case, and number of cases should be used in conjunction to provide a clearer picture of trends within the practice.

Compliance

In today's medical environment one cannot discuss billing and coding without compliance. No matter what continues to unfold in health care, the government's activities indicate continued recoupment of monies that have been paid inappropriately. Every physician should realize that the government has a tremendous return on fraud and abuse dollars, and as keeper of the purse they will continue to scrutinize services. Physicians can be penalized monetarily, or in some cases where fraud is involved by jail time, a loss of medical licensure, or exclusion from the government programs. It is for this reason that all anesthesia groups should understand that it is critical to have an active compliance program.

The implementation of a compliance program can be a challenge, as many physicians are still unclear as to what makes an effective compliance program. The most effective programs will have integrated the compliance activities into the day-to-day operations of the group and will incorporate the seven federal sentencing guidelines.

The first of the sentencing guidelines requires written policies and procedures. The policies and procedures that have been written for the program need to be understood by all members of the group. How to complete the anesthesia record, definitions of anesthesia start and end time, and specific types of anesthesia delivered would all be examples of policies an anesthesia group might have. It is important that employees have guidance in understanding the basic concepts discussed in the plan. It is recommended that plan policies be tested and results kept in personnel files to assure that everyone knows the commitment of the group to the compliance program and the intention to bill only for services that are appropriately documented.

The second of the federal sentencing guidelines specifically asks that a compliance officer be designated for the group. The group must evaluate the performance of the compliance officer, and although the compliance officer does not necessarily have to be a physician, it does have to be someone who has the absolute authority to hire and fire personnel. The board should assess whether the compliance officer has sufficient knowledge and education to deal with the assigned responsibilities. It would be important for them to judge whether appropriate auditing and education is being carried out to fulfill the requirements of compliance. Compliance committee minutes and processes of handling any reported violations should be reviewed to insure all issues have been dealt with and recorded as to corrective action.

Education and training of all levels of employees must be done according to the third step in the sentencing guidelines. Courses and educational materials should reflect the important aspects of the group's compliance program. Ongoing training and demonstration of evaluation of knowledge should be recorded. Keeping accurate records of content, frequency, and attendees is very important in order to demonstrate educational efforts.

The fourth sentencing guideline stresses open communication, and it is considered an essential element in active compliance programs. You must have a way to receive feedback from employees on issues and concerns that they might have regarding activities within the group. It is not considered an effective plan if the program receives minimal or no feedback from employees. Simply recording that there have not been any violations reported would not be enough to qualify as open communication. A record of questions regarding policies, and any guidance given or research done by the compliance officer or committee members should be documented to show open lines of communication.

The fifth key component of the sentencing guidelines stresses ongoing monitoring and auditing. Auditing, both internal and external, is critical to a successful compliance program. The frequency and the extent of the audit function will vary depending on the size and issues identified by the group. Audits must not discriminate between providers and must address issues that are considered "hot spots" in the specialty. Things such as anesthesia time, postoperative pain, ancillary line placements and medical direction would all be appropriate topics for audits. Audits should insure that elements set forth in the compliance plan are being monitored and that auditing techniques are valid and conducted by objective reviewers. For example, we know that postoperative rounding for acute pain services use the E/M coding guidelines to bill for services. A compliance professional would want to audit these services based on the billing guidelines to see if they meet the criteria for billing. Medical direction elements would be another example of a focused audit that may be done evaluating the documentation of the seven required elements.

The sixth element of the federal sentencing guidelines requires suspected violations to be thoroughly investigated. In doing so groups must also insure that there is no retaliation to those who report violations. When a compliance officer learns of an issue, it is important to contact legal counsel to properly handle and circumvent any exposure to the group. Placing the audit under "attorney–client privilege" helps to maintain control of the investigation and documentation until a determination can be made regarding the errors. If evidence exists that misconduct has occurred, counsel will be needed to work through the process of self-disclosure.

Finally, the seventh factor that makes up the key ingredient to the federal sentencing guidelines is discipline. Disciplinary action must be taken against those employees who fail to adhere to the group's standards set forth in the compliance program. Discipline must be applied consistently among employees, regardless of the employee level in the corporation. Senior management must demonstrate a serious commitment to foster a climate that will require adherence to all federal and state regulations.

Summary

Correct coding and billing of services in today's medical environment is extremely important. Providers must insure that every service is documented appropriately and billed in compliance with a "who, what, and why" mentality regarding the services that were actually performed. All services require that a translation from the written record be made to CPT-4 procedural codes and ICD-9 diagnosis codes. In reviewing documentation, coders must review modifiers to see if there are components of the service that have additional reporting requirements regarding the service delivered. Each specialty will have special coding guidelines, which must be reviewed. Quality measures and the reporting of such measures are beginning to play a large part in physician coding. As reimbursement systems change, additional reporting will be required. Compliance programs are a necessity in every medical practice and must be incorporated into the day-to-day culture of the group. Always remember that the most important aspect of all coding is the provider documentation, which must accurately describe the services performed. Without accurate documentation, coding and appropriate reimbursement cannot be achieved.

Suggested reading

M. S. Diamond. *Mastering Coding: Tools, Techniques, and Practical Applications*. W.B. Saunders Company, 2001.

J. E. Steiner, ed. *Monitoring & Auditing Practices for Effective Compliance*, 2nd edn. Minneapolis: Health Care Compliance Association.

The Practice of Medical Billing and Coding, 2nd edn. ICDC Publishing Inc, 2006.

D. Walker Keegan, E. W. Woodcock, S. M. Larch. *The Physician Billing Process 12 Potholes to Avoid in the Road to Getting Paid*, 2nd edn. Englewood, CO: Medical Group Management Association, 2009.

Surgical coding

Bernadine Smith CPC, RCC, PCS

Understanding coding   183
Finding the correct code   184

Summary   185

Understanding coding

Understanding surgical coding along with documentation requirements, code edits, and associated rules and regulations is extremely valuable in the proper assignment of anesthesia codes. Once an appropriate surgical code is determined, the corresponding anesthesia code can readily be determined by using the American Society of Anesthesiologists (ASA) *CROSSWALK*.

Before assigning surgical codes, however, it is helpful to understand the general layout of surgery services in the code book. The surgery portion of the *Current Procedural Terminology* catalog (CPT) immediately follows anesthesia and comprises the largest section within the text. Surgery guidelines are described in the first few pages and provide guidance and other informational material helpful to providers when filing claims. The definition of a surgical package is included, and lists services that are inherently included in reimbursement for the surgery itself, thereby rendering them not separately reportable:

- local infiltration, metacarpal/metatarsal/digital block or topical anesthesia;
- subsequent to the decision for surgery, one related evaluation and management (E/M) encounter on the date immediately prior to or on the date of procedure (including history and physical);
- immediate postoperative care, including dictating all operative notes and talking with the family and other physicians;
- writing orders;

- evaluating the patient in the postanesthesia recovery area;
- typical postoperative follow-up care.

Needless to say, accurate code assignment is the primary goal. Complete, descriptive documentation is critical to properly code and capture billable surgical services. It has been said often that surgical coding is the most challenging of all.

Surgical services are mainly documented in a transcribed operative report, usually but not always independent of other documentation in the patient's medical record. In addition to personal information identifying the patient, the operative note should include the date of service, the pre- and postoperative diagnoses, the name(s) of attending surgeon(s), the name of the co-surgeon if applicable, the main body of the report, a signature line, and other pertinent information relative to compliance (i.e., date dictated, date transcribed, etc).

The body of the report must be clear and illustrative and, like a roadmap, should describe all body areas affected with details of the procedure(s), as well as pertinent observations.

The type of surgical technique should also be included. Reports describing "open" cases should indicate location, length, and type of incision, whereas laparoscopic cases should include a note to indicate establishment of pneumoperitoneum as well as the placement of trocars and laparoscope in the abdominal region. Such documentation is relative not only from a clinical perspective but also provides

Operating Room Leadership and Management, ed. Kaye A.D., Fox C.J. and Urman R.D. Published by Cambridge University Press. © Cambridge University Press 2012.

pertinent information for the coder relative to code choice.

Similarly, as excision of tissue and removal of body parts most often result in biopsy, documentation of excised tissue or specimens during surgery is also important documentation, providing quality clinical reporting and information useful in supporting subsequent claims for pathology billing. Similarly, for interventional services, documentation must include point of access, (i.e., vessel entered), arteries entered and traversed, arteries imaged, and documentation of any vascular anomaly or anomalies, which alters coding radically.

Describing the process of coding for surgery is not easily done. Ideally, coding is best accomplished in a quiet location – one with few distractions. It is suggested that the report be read over carefully and thoroughly in order to gain a complete understanding of the entire service. Depending on the complexity of the case, it may be necessary to reread the report one or more additional times to insure that the procedures are completely understood and that all services within the report are captured.

Coding from titles and headers alone is never recommended, as this usually results in incomplete and/or inaccurate coding; coding directly from a complete, concise operative report provides the best opportunity to capture services appropriately and also reduces the chance that money will be left on the table.

Finding the correct code

After reading the report, an experienced coder may know precisely where to go within CPT to find the specific procedure performed. The text is arranged in such a way as to assist in the code selection process. It is understood that there are 19 different subsections of surgical codes within CPT, ranging from the integumentary system to the auditory system, and everything in between.

Each section is arranged by body system first, then anatomically starting from the top of the body going downward. Procedures are often further broken down by type of procedure (i.e., excisions, repairs, manipulations, etc), making it somewhat easier to find a particular service once you have found the appropriate general area.

It is recommended that the guidelines for surgery be read before the assignment of codes. In general,

code selection may be made easier for some by referring to the index located at the back of the coding manual to get an overall idea of where to find a particular code. Search for the service in the index, then check the code descriptor to insure that the code matches precisely what was described by the surgeon. Keep in mind that CPT warns against selecting a code "that merely approximates the service." If no specific code exists, providers must use an unlisted procedure code to report services.

Sometimes it is necessary to further establish the appropriateness of a code by researching the use of it. There are various publications that describe surgical services in lay terms and are available to assist in appropriately choosing a code.

Multiple services performed on the same patient, the same day can also be problematic as often two or more services billed together are considered "bundled," resulting in claims denial. A standard practice should be employed to verify that the services are not bundled and indeed constitute separate, distinct, billable services. If two or more services are deemed as bundled, then some consideration is in order to determine whether or not they qualify for use of a modifier to "unbundle" the services. When documented appropriately, all services may be payable. For government claims, the national Correct Coding Initiative (CCI), instituted in 1996, serves to promote correct coding methodologies and "to control improper coding leading to inappropriate payment in Part B claims."

Coding for surgery is a complex and sometimes cumbersome assignment. Understanding how to proficiently navigate CPT is critical in accurately assigning codes for difficult cases. Situations are seldom unique and the proficient coder must know where to go to find information needed to properly code procedures.

Occasionally, for example, multiple services requiring use of the same code for the same patient on the same day are performed and must be billed. It is the coder's responsibility to determine the most appropriate way in which to bill such services. Do the services require application of modifier -50, -51, -59, or -76, or perhaps should the services be billed with a frequency of two or more? Also to be taken into consideration are payer requirements. These are typical scenarios encountered by the surgical coder on a daily basis.

Clearly, surgical coders must have a firm grasp of medical terminology and physiology, and an understanding of a multitude of medical abbreviations.

Good abbreviation manuals and medical dictionaries are great resources for the surgery coder, as well as other current, specialty-specific coding tools. Ongoing participation in continuing education is also critically necessary for the surgical coder in order to stay on top of coding challenges as they relate to changes in medical and surgical practice and ever-changing technology.

Summary

To run a financially sound operating room facility, it is important to get a thorough understanding of surgical coding along with documentation requirements, code edits, and associated rules and regulations. Coding for surgery is a complex and sometimes cumbersome assignment, and therefore it is critical to know how to navigate CPT to accurately assign codes for difficult cases. It is also important to be efficient and know where to find the information needed to properly code procedures.

Suggested reading

M. S. Diamond. *Mastering Coding: Tools, Techniques, and Practical Applications: A Worktext*. Philadelphia, PA: WB Saunders Company, 2001.

ICDC Publishing. *The Practice of Medical Billing and Coding*, 2nd edn. Upper Saddle River, NJ: Prentice Hall, 2006.

D. W. Keegan, E. W. Woodcock, S. M. Larch. *The Physician Billing Process: 12 Potholes to Avoid in the Road to Getting Paid*, 2nd edn. Englewood, CO: Medical Group Management Association, 2009.

J. E. Steiner Jr. *Monitoring & Auditing Practices for Effective Compliance*, 2nd edn. Minneapolis, MN: Health Care Compliance Association.

Chapter

18

Postanesthesia care unit management

Michael J. Yarborough MD
Henry Liu MD
Sabrina Bent MD, MS

Phases of recovery and discharge
from PACU   186

Design and staffing of the PACU   189
Financial considerations in the PACU   190

Comprehensive and integrated care of surgical patients involves many functional departments and specialized teams, including surgeons, anesthesiologists, and other anesthesia providers (certified registered nurse anesthetists [CRNAs], anesthesiologist assistants, and anesthesia residents), operating room (OR) nurses, and nurses in the surgical intensive care units (ICUs), regular wards, and postanesthesia care units (PACUs). Postanesthesia care units play an important role in the care of surgical patients; they affect not only the patient's continuing emergence from general anesthesia and the recovery of cognitive, sensory, and motor functions following anesthesia, but also the turnover rate of ORs and ambulatory surgery clinics or outpatient surgery, the patient's length of hospital stay, gate-keeping the discharge of ambulatory patients, and the overall efficiency of surgical services of a medical facility. Postanesthesia care units may ultimately affect the profitability of a hospital and overall patient satisfaction in a medical facility.

Phases of recovery and discharge from PACU

According to the American Society of Anesthesiologists (ASA) guidelines, all patients who have received general anesthesia, regional anesthesia, or monitored anesthesia care should receive appropriate postanesthesia management in a PACU, where intense monitoring almost equivalent to ICU care is offered [1], with the following potential exceptions: all open-heart-surgery

patients, who are transported to ICU directly from the OR after surgery; all other patients who have undergone major surgical procedures (prolonged intubation and mechanical ventilation, large quantity of volume resuscitation, delicate hemodynamic maneuvering) and potentially need a longer period of intensive care; and patients with significant vital organ dysfunction.

The concept of three phases of recovery from general anesthesia was initially developed for ambulatory surgery. Nowadays some of the concepts are gradually being adopted by hospital-based surgical procedures too. Traditionally hospital-based anesthesiologists tend to focus primarily on the initial recovery in PACU; however, the ambulatory anesthesia providers have to plan for, observe, and personally deal with patients' extended recovery and their readiness to be discharged from PACU and to return home [2]. This three-phase concept helps surgeons, nursing staff, and anesthesia service providers to better understand the importance of the surgical patient's step-by-step postoperative management but continual recovering process, to dedicate more time, resources, and efforts to the patient's recovery, and to better prepare patients for their discharge from the PACU. Realizing that patient recovery from anesthesia is a continual process, there will be some overlapping between the arbitrary phases.

Phase I, or early recovery, is the transition from the care mainly provided by anesthesia providers to that predominantly provided by PACU nurses. This phase spans from the discontinuation of anesthesia to the point at which the patient recovers from their

Operating Room Leadership and Management, ed. Kaye A.D., Fox C.J. and Urman R.D. Published by Cambridge University Press. © Cambridge University Press 2012.

Table 18.1 Aldrete score [3]

	2 points	1 point	0 points
Activity	Move four extremities	Move two extremities	Cannot move
Respiration	Able to breathe deeply and cough freely	Limited breathing, dyspnea	Apneic
Circulation	BP changes within 20% of baseline level	BP changes in 20% to 50% of baseline level	BP changes over 50% of baseline
Consciousness	Fully awake	Arousable on calling	Not responding
Color	Pink	Pale, dusky, blotchy, jaundiced	Cyanotic

mental ability, respiratory function, and protective airway reflexes. The patient undergoes a return of basic physiological functions within this period of time. Also during this phase of recovery, patients will demand a significant amount of attention from PACU nurses, and anesthesiologists potentially. Indeed, the intensity of care of this phase is almost equivalent to ICU care and requires almost all the same monitoring equipment as ASA standard care in the OR, except for gas spectrometry. The PACU Phase I monitoring includes at least electrocardiogram, noninvasive blood pressure, pulse oximetry, temperature, and urine output.

Patients in Phase I are likely to begin responding to verbal stimulations when alveolar anesthetic concentrations are decreased to about 0.5 minimum alveolar concentration (MAC) or less for the volatile anesthetic drug (MAC awake) if not impeded by other factors. The MAC is defined as the dose of an inhalational anesthetic in which 50% of patients will move in response to surgical stimulation. Increased ventilation results in a more rapid decline in alveolar anesthetic concentration, which hastens recovery, provided that the arterial carbon dioxide pressure is not so low that it may decrease cerebral blood flow and slow down the removal of anesthetic agent from the central nervous system. Recovery from neuromuscular blockade may be monitored by peripheral nerve stimulation and by clinical indices. Recovery from intravenous opioids and hypnotics may be more variable and difficult to quantify than recovery from inhalation and neuromuscular blocking agents.

The most common practice in most hospitals in determining whether to send a patient to the ICU or not is agreement between the surgery team and the anesthesia team. Often it may also depend on ICU bed availability. Commonly agreed criteria for admitting a patient to ICU include, but are not limited to, the following: (1) unstable hemodynamics, which require meticulous monitoring and intervention; (2) expecting prolonged intubation and mechanical ventilation; (3) long surgery, significant intraoperative blood loss, and a large quantity of fluid shifts; (4) multiple invasive monitoring and multiple inotrope/vasoactive medications.

Phase II, or intermediate recovery, is the phase of anesthesia recovery needed to get the surgical patient ready to be discharged from the medical facilities. Many different scoring systems have been used to evaluate the patient's recovery in this phase. The Aldrete score is a ten-point scale based on extremity movement, respiration, blood pressure, consciousness, and oxygen saturation (Table 18.1) [3]. Originally published in 1970, the Aldrete score has been widely used as a guideline for postanesthesia care for many years. However, the Aldrete score is far from an ideal guideline for postoperative patient recovery, especially for the ambulatory surgery patient, because it ignores the importance of pain and postoperative nausea and vomiting. The modified version of the Aldrete score (1995) is probably the most commonly used scoring system, with a score of 9 or higher required for discharge [4]. In the modified Aldrete score, a patient who is able to maintain oxygen saturation above 92% on room air scores 2 points, a patient needing oxygen inhalation to maintain oxygen saturation above 90% scores 1 point, and a patient with oxygen saturation less than 90% even with oxygen supplementation scores 0 points. The modified Aldrete score works well for the recovery from Phase I to Phase II. Other well-accepted scoring systems are the postanesthesia discharge scoring system (PADSS) and the White–Song score [5,6]. The PADSS serves as the scoring system getting the patient ready to be discharged home (Table 18.2). The White–Song score, which was published in 1999 (Table 18.3), was designed to qualify patients to bypass Phase I recovery and be discharged from the OR directly to the less-intensive Phase II recovery area. The PADSS uses five parameters

Table 18.2 The postanesthesia discharge scoring system (PADSS) for home readiness [5]

	2 points	1 point	0 points
Vital signs	BP & SpO$_2$ change <20%	BP & SpO$_2$ change 20–40%	BP and SpO$_2$ change >40%
Activity	Steady gait, no dizziness, meets preop level	Requires assistance	Unable to ambulate
Nausea and vomiting	Minimal, treated with p.o. medication	Moderate, treated with parental medication	Severe, continue despite treatment
Pain	Controlled with p.o. medication and acceptable to patient yes = 2	No = 1	
Surgical bleeding	Minimal, no dressing change	Moderate, up to two dressing changes required	Severe, three or more dressing changes

Table 18.3 The White–Song recovery score, 1999 [6]

	2 points	1 points	0 points
Mental status	Awake	Arousable	Unresponsive
Motor	Move all extremities	Some weakness	No movement
Blood pressure	Within 15% of baseline	15–130%	>30%
Respiration	Deep breathing	Tachypnea	Dyspnea
Pulse oximetry	>90% room air	Requires O$_2$	SpO$_2$ <90 with O$_2$
Pain	No pain	Moderate pain	Severe pain
PONV	No to mild nausea	Transient vomiting	Persistent vomiting

with a score of 0 to 10, whereas the White–Song score includes seven parameters with a total score of 0 to 14 and takes into account postoperative nausea and vomiting [7]. This scoring system and the PADSS seem to be more acceptable than many other scoring techniques published in the last decade.

However, there are many controversies regarding the currently used scoring systems and discharge criteria. Requiring patients to take oral fluid before discharge may not be necessary according to some recent observations. Eliminating drinking as a requirement before discharge can slightly shorten the Phase II recovery without convincing evidence of significant adverse effects, and there are studies supporting this practice [8,9]. If this practice can reach universal agreement, recovery room nurses should be educated to remove drinking requirement before discharging patients home. Another controversy is whether the ability to void is truly necessary before discharge. Several studies have demonstrated that even patients at high risk of urinary retention can be discharged before they have voided in the recovery room [10]. Eliminating

the requirement of voiding before discharge can significantly shorten recovery room stay without adding a negative impact to the clinical outcome.

Phase III, or late recovery, and psychological recovery extends from the discharge from hospital or ambulatory surgery center to full psychological, physical, and social recovery and return to work. This phase of recovery can have significant individual variations owing to various factors. Phase III recovery occurs outside the medical facility.

Fast track/PACU bypass is discharging a patient from the OR to Phase II recovery directly, bypassing Phase I recovery. According to the White–Song scoring system, the criteria for a patient to be a candidate for fast track or PACU bypass is a score of 12 or higher (Table 18.3) [6].

Generally, the following procedures qualify for fast track:

- most eye procedures;
- some cesarean sections;
- some cardiac catheterizations;
- most gastroenterological endoscopy;

Table 18.4 Clinical criteria for PACU discharge [11]

Stable vital signs for at least 1h
Alert and oriented to time, place, and person
No excessive pain, bleeding, or nausea
Ability to dress and walk with assistance
Discharged home with a vested adult who will remain with the patient overnight
Written and verbal instructions outlining diet, activity, medications, and follow-up appointments provided
A contact person and circumstances that warrant seeking the assistance of a health-care professional clearly outlined
Voiding before discharge not mandatory, unless specifically noted by physician (i.e., urological procedure, rectal surgery, history of urinary retention)
Tolerating oral fluids not mandatory, unless specified by physician (i.e., patient is diabetic, frail, and/or elderly; not able to tolerate an extended period of nil per os [NPO] status)

- most radiological special procedures with monitored anesthesia care;
- most patients with regional block as surgical anesthesia for their procedures.

The criteria for discharging patients from the PACU can be somewhat different depending on where the patients are discharged, patient age, and coexisting medical conditions. Table 18.4 gives the acceptable criteria for PACU discharge [11]. These criteria can be used, combined with the PADSS, to enhance patient safety during discharge from Phase II to Phase III recovery.

The criteria for discharging a patient from the PACU to the hospital ward can be slightly different. The patient does not need to be able to ambulate, void, or prove oral fluid intake. It is much safer to send a patient to the hospital ward than to discharge the patient home for recovery. Also, the criteria can be different for the pediatric patient population and the geriatric population. In Europe, the International Association for Ambulatory Surgery (IAAS) adopts the following guidelines [12].

Essential invariant criteria for patient discharge:

- stable vital signs;
- oriented to preoperative stage;
- minimal nausea and vomiting;
- controlled pain;
- without significant bleeding related to the procedure(s).

Variable criteria for discharging patient from PACU:

- micturition prior to discharge; essential following epidural or spinal anesthesia; may be deemed essential following certain surgical procedures;
- fixed length of stay in day unit following surgery; plays no part in the generality of surgical procedures; may be deemed necessary after certain procedures to minimize the risk of reactionary hemorrhage at home, e.g., tonsillectomy, thyroidectomy;
- individual for certain specific procedures.

Design and staffing of the PACU

There are as many variations of how to design a PACU structurally as there are architects to draw up the plans. However, there are certain guidelines that should be considered when the functionality of the PACU is taken into account. The first component to consider in the design of the PACU is what role it will play in the recovery of the postsurgical patient. Some PACUs are used strictly for Phase I and early Phase II recovery. Others function as the patient's room throughout their stay for the day, beginning as a preoperative assessment room, then becoming the Phase I recovery room, and progressing through Phase II and early Phase III until the patient is discharged, either home or to the floor. In addition, some hospitals have specialized PACUs, for general patients, pediatric patients, interventional radiology patients, etc.

When designing a PACU one common question pertains to the number of beds there should be per OR. The generally accepted ratio is 1.5–2:1. However, precise recommendations on the design of the PACU are lacking. In particular, the recommended ratio of PACU beds to ORs is not clearly defined [13]. Patient demographics and types of surgical cases affect those needs. Quick turnover surgery will provide a greater mass of patients to be admitted into the PACU over a shorter period of time, therefore resulting in a greater PACU bed requirement, whereas longer surgery will decrease the admission rate and thus decrease the PACU bed requirement. In addition, sicker patients will have the potential of requiring greater nursing care and a longer stay in the PACU than healthy patients, resulting in greater bed requirements. In contrast, simple surgeries should require less postoperative care routinely than complicated surgeries, which should decrease the PACU bed needs. In one study with unlimited resources available for the PACU patients, the required PACU bed to surgical room ratio came to less than 1:1 [13]. Of course, this was a simulated situation with unlimited resources, which is far from the situation in which most practitioners find themselves.

There are ways to try to minimize PACU time, and these should be considered whenever the opportunity avails itself, as a decrease PACU time results in a lower requirement for PACU beds. These include postoperative nausea and vomiting prevention, multimodal pain management, choice of anesthetic agent, etc. Delays in discharge from the PACU due to systems errors should be kept to a minimum. In addition, the ability to fast track should be considered if possible.

Most would agree that adequate nurse staffing is paramount to safe patient care. The American Society of PeriAnesthesia Nurses (ASPAN) Standards of Perianesthesia Nursing Practice, Resource 3, Patient Classification/Recommended Staffing Guidelines, offers staffing ratios that correlate to the level of care required in postanesthesia Phase I, Phase II, and extended observation settings [14]. In addition, ASPAN has established minimum staffing guidelines for these areas to provide a safe environment for patients during nonpeak hours, as well as a "position statement on on-call/work schedule" to address issues related to nursing fatigue and patient safety: ASPAN recommends that one nurse can care safely for up to two healthy, adult, conscious patients not requiring frequent cardiopulmonary intervention [15]. These recommended staffing ratios are based on the best available evidence: expert opinion and consensus. Although the nursing literature contained evidence on the relationship between nurse staffing ratios and nursing-sensitive outcomes, there was a paucity of scientific postanesthesia evidence that related to safe staffing ratios or nursing-sensitive indicators specific to the specialty practice [16].

It is extremely hard to calculate adequate PACU nursing staffing. Whereas other units in the hospital (floor, ICU, emergency department) have consistent

patient census, the PACU ideally starts and ends the day with a census of zero and along the way has a large variation in the census throughout the day. Therefore, some believe that the best way to generate proper staffing for each PACU is through computer modeling and aids that are based on historical data [17].

Other outside factors have been studied to see how they affect PACU staffing requirements. One of these is the sequencing of surgical cases, with the premise being that proper surgical sequencing should create a more predictable staffing requirement in the PACU. For small facilities with just a few ORs, the benefits of case sequencing are both seemingly obvious and impressive in practice. For large PACUs, however, whether case sequencing achieves benefits is unclear, particularly compared with the good performance of adjusting staffing and beds to match workload using statistical optimization [18].

Another factor that can affect PACU nursing requirements is delays in patient flow out of the PACU. Overwhelmingly, these delays appear to be system errors, with the most common being: orderly too busy; awaiting anesthesia assessment; PACU nurse too busy; receiving floor not ready; and patient awaiting radiographic interpretation.[19]. Putting in corrections for these systems errors at your institution should decrease the need for staffing and create a smoother flow of patients throughout the postsurgical period.

Financial considerations in the PACU

The PACU is a major component of OR process flow. Reimbursement for operative procedures continues to decline, while the costs of the operative process continue to increase. Efforts to improve margins and profitability in the OR depend on improvements in efficiencies in each component of OR process flow. Several strategies have been evaluated to decrease costs in the PACU. The effect of these strategies on fixed costs versus variable costs varies considerably: fixed costs are those that do not vary in relation to the surgical volume (e.g., capital equipment, physical plant, salaried personnel); variable costs include those costs that vary directly with the surgical volume (e.g., disposable equipment, pharmaceuticals, laboratory tests, and hourly personnel). The strategies for decreasing costs in the PACU include [20]:

1. changes in PACU nurse staffing, including both working hours and increasing productivity (i.e., increasing patient care hours without increasing work hours);

2. OR scheduling changes to decrease or modify the daily PACU peak number of patients admitted from the OR;

3. cost-reducing interventions, such as changes in medical practice patterns (e.g., to reduce PACU length of stay), affect only variable costs, whereas PACU nurse wages (i.e., hourly versus salaried), may be variable or fixed costs, respectively;

4. use of anesthetic drugs with favorable pharmacology, including those for pain and nausea and vomiting prevention;

5. improvements in Phase I PACU process flow, which depend on many factors, including inpatient bed availability, transport, and communication issues;

6. OR patients bypassing the Phase I PACU being directly admitted to phase II PACU;

7. fast-tracking patients to discharge directly from the PACU;

8. changing PACU discharge criteria or policies.

Although there are many studies and computer models intended to predict or suggest the effect of decreasing PACU costs, applicability and success of these strategies may be highly variable in different practice environments (i.e., ambulatory surgical centers, specialty surgery centers, tertiary care facilities, low-volume or high-volume facilities). The largest component of PACU costs is nursing staff wages. Nurse staffing is primarily dependent on the daily peak number of patients admitted to the PACU from the OR [21]. Therefore, the most effective strategies in decreasing PACU costs involve those that decrease the amount of nurse staffing (i.e., FTEs) either directly or indirectly.

The standards set by ASPAN, which state the number of patients that each nurse can simultaneously care for (i.e., one nurse per intubated patient or per two extubated patients) may prevent or decrease the ability to maximize nursing productivity in facilities with frequent high patient acuity levels [20,22]. Another factor affecting productivity is the increasing use of the PACU as an overflow location for ICU and patient wards. Ziser et al. prospectively studied patient overflow admission to the PACU over a 33-month period and found that lack of an available bed was the most common reason for PACU stay (85.5%) [23]. This results in variable acuity needs and can interrupt patient flow from the OR to the PACU, further contributing to inefficiencies in operative process flow and increased costs [24]. The ASPAN position statement on overflow patients in the PACU raises additional staffing concerns regarding maintenance of appropriate competencies for the patient population, maintenance of patient safety, coordination of OR scheduling, and appropriate staff utilization, further complicating this recurrent problem in some facilities [25]. Dexter et al. has suggested the use of computer optimization methods to determine staffing for Phase I PACU because of the complexity of staffing, especially when variability in patient acuity occurs [22].

PACU nursing staff wages generally fall into four categories [20]:

1. hourly employees with no minimum numbers of hours worked each week;

2. "full-time" salaried employees (no overtime pay);

3. "full-time" hourly (not salaried) employees with no minimum number of hours of work each day;

4. "full-time" hourly (not salaried) employees with frequent overtime.

Creative and flexible scheduling of nurses proportional to the predicted daily peak number of patients admitted to the PACU may allow some cost savings by reductions in staff hours during low admission periods [26]. However, the practice environment may not be conducive to the needed flexibility and creative scheduling that may be required for a given nursing staff wage category. Avoidance of frequent overtime and use of hourly employees with no minimum number of work hours may contribute to efficiencies. Additional strategies may include the use of a combination of more than one wage category in a particular PACU staffing model to add flexibility in scheduling. Improvements in surgical sequencing of cases, the sequence in which a surgeon performs his or her cases in an OR on one day, may also result in reduced PACU staffing needs [26]. However, surgeons may not be agreeable to loss of control over the order of their cases [20].

Waddle et al. studied medically appropriate PACU length of stay (LOS), defined as the time required to achieve a medically stable condition for safe PACU discharge compared to actual length of stay in 340 patients [27]. They found the actual LOS to be >30 min longer than the medically appropriate LOS in 20% of patients. The most frequent causes of excessive LOS were waiting for physician release or waiting for laboratory or study results (i.e., radiograph and ECG results). Other studies have implicated the PACU nurse being too busy, lack of transport, procedures performed in PACU, postoperative monitoring, pain management, bed availability, and nausea and vomiting as additional causes of increased LOS [13,19,20,28,29]. Improvements in the efficiencies in the largely administrative issues that result in increased LOS may lead to significant cost reductions. However, because of difficulty in scheduling full-time PACU nursing staff and wide variability in increased LOS it is difficult to fully assess the benefit of any single intervention aimed at decreasing LOS [20,21,30].

Several studies have suggested that strategies such as the use of short-acting drugs, multimodal antiemetics, and regional anesthesia may decrease LOS, allow fast-tracking of patient discharge directly from the PACU or bypassing of Phase I PACU to Phase II PACU, directly or indirectly decreasing PACU costs [24,30–32]. There is evolving evidence that regional anesthesia techniques can help to reduce costs in the ambulatory setting as a result of reduced postoperative complications, fewer unintended hospital admissions, and earlier home readiness of the patients [33]. However, the effectiveness of these strategies may vary significantly with the practice environment and PACU staffing needs. Often it is difficult to measure the true costs of implementation (i.e., drug, equipment, and staffing costs) when evaluating presumed cost savings [20,21,24,32–35].

Use of standard operating procedures and alternative definitions of discharge criteria may reduce surveillance time and improve fast tracking and bypassing of Phase I PACU, resulting in cost savings [19,20,33,36,37]. Many discharge criteria and policies (i.e., oral fluid intake, voiding, awaiting full return of motor function after regional block) may need to be altered based on outcome studies or planned location of discharge (i.e., inpatient versus home) [19,36].

In summary, the financial implications of the PACU, especially those involving cost savings, are complicated and mostly a function of nurse staffing, owing to its overwhelming proportion of cost in PACU operation. Many strategies to decrease costs may have potential benefit, especially if they result in improved OR-process-flow efficiencies. Future strategies to decrease PACU costs will probably require incorporation of the total OR process flow. It will be important that these strategies also incorporate maintenance of patient safety and good-quality outcomes.

References

1. American Society of Anesthesiologists. Postanesthesia Care Standards for 2009. www.asahq.org/For-Healthcare-Professionals/Standards-Guidelines-and-Statements.aspx (last accessed May 10, 2012).

2. J. Boncyk, J. Fitzpatrick. Discharge Criteria. In: S. R. Springman, ed. *Ambulatory Anesthesia: The Requisites in Anesthesiology*. Philadelphia: Mosby Elsevier, 2006; 109–17.

3. J. A. Aldrete, D. Kroulik. A post anesthetic recovery score. *Anesth Analg* 1970; **49**: 924–34.

4. J. A. Aldrete. The post anesthesia recovery score revisited [letter]. *J Clin Anesth* 1995; **7**: 89–91.

5. F. Chung, V. Chan, D. Ong. A post anaesthetic discharge scoring system for home readiness after ambulatory surgery. *J Clin Anesth* 1995; **7**: 500–6.

6. P. White, D. Song. New criteria for fast-tracking after outpatient anesthesia: a comparison with the Modified Aldrete's scoring system. *Anesth Analg* 1999; **88**: 1069–72.

7. M. S. Schreiner, S. C. Nicholson, T. Martin, *et al.* Should children drink before discharge from day surgery? *Anesthesiology* 1992; **76**: 528–33.

8. W. T. Fritz, L. George, N. Krull, J. Krug. Utilization of a home nursing protocol allows ambulatory surgery patients to be discharged prior to voiding [abstract]. *Anesth Analg* 1997; **84**: S6.

9. F. L. Jin, A. Norris, F. Chung, T. Ganeshram. Should adult patients drink fluids before discharge from ambulatory surgery? *Can J Anaesth* 1998; **87**: 306–11.

10. H. Ead. From Aldrete to PADSS: reviewing discharge criteria after ambulatory surgery. *J Perianesth Nurs* 2006; **21**: 259–67. Review. Erratum in: *J Perianesth Nurs* 2007; **22**: 154.

11. K. Korttila. Recovery from outpatient anesthesia: factors affecting outcome. *Anesthesia* 1995; **50**(Suppl): 22–8.

12. International Association for Ambulatory Surgery. Discharge Criteria Following Day Surgery. Available online at: www.iaas-med.com/index.php/recommendations/discharge-criteria

13. E. Marcon, S. Kharraja, N. Smolski, *et al.* Determining the number of beds in the postanesthesia care unit: a computer simulation flow approach. *Anesth Analg* 2003; **96**: 1415–23.

14. American Society of PeriAnesthesia Nurses. Practice Recommendation 1: Patient Classification/Recommended Staffing Guidelines. 2010–2012 Perianesthesia Nursing Standards and Practice Recommendations. www.aspan.org/ClinicalPractice/PatientClassification/tabid/4191/Default.aspx. (last accessed May 10, 2012).

15. F. Dexter, H. Rittenmeyer. Measuring productivity of the phase I postanesthesia care unit. *J Perianesth Nurs* 1997; **12**: 7–11.

16. M. E. Mamaril, E. Sullivan, T. L. Clifford, *et al.* Safe staffing for the post anesthesia care unit: weighing the evidence and identifying the gaps. *J Perianesth Nurs* 2007; **22**: 393–9.

17. F. Dexter, Why calculating PACU staffing is so hard and why/how operations research specialists can help. *J Perianesth Nurs* 2007; **22**: 357–9.

18. E. Marcon, F. Dexter, An observational study of surgeons' sequencing of cases and its impact on postanesthesia care unit and holding area staffing requirements at hospitals. *Anesth Analg* 2007; **105**: 119–26.

19. M. J. Tessler, L. Mitmaker, R. M Wahba, C. R. Covert. Patient Flow in the Post Anesthesia Care Unit: an observational study. *Can J Anesth* 1999; **46**(4): 348–51.

20. A. Macario, D. Glenn, F. Dexter. What can the postanesthesia care unit manager do to decrease costs in the postanesthesia care unit? *J Perianesth Nurs* 1999; **14**: 284–93.

21. F. Dexter, J. H. Tinker. Analysis of strategies to decrease postanesthesia care unit costs. *Anesthesiology* 1995; **82**: 92–101.

22. F. Dexter, R. E. Wachtel, R. H. Epstein. Impact of average patient acuity on staffing of the phase I PACU. *J Perianesth Nurs* 2006; **21**: 303–310.

23. A. Ziser, M. Alkobi, R. Markovits, B. Rozenberg. The postanaesthesia care unit as a temporary admission location due to intensive care and ward overflow. *Br J Anaesth* 2002; **88**: 577–79.

24. M. F. Watcha, P. F. White. Economics of anesthetic practice. *Anesthesiology* 1997; **86**: 1170–96.

25. American Society of PeriAnesthesia Nurses. A position statement for medical-surgical overflow patients in the PACU and ambulatory care unit. *J Perianesth Nurs* 2003; **18**: 301–2.

26. E. Marcon, F. Dexter. Impact of surgical sequencing on postanesthesia care unit staffing. *Health Care Manage Sci* 2006; **9**: 87–98.

27. J. P. Waddle, A. S. Evers, J. F. Piccirillo. Postanesthesia care unit length of stay: quantifying and assessing dependent factors. *Anesth Analg* 1998; **87**: 628–33.

28. P. Saastamoinen, M. Piispa, M. M. Niskanen. Use of postanesthesia care unit for purposes other than postanesthesia observation. *J Perianesth Nurs* 2007; **22**: 102–7.

29. K. Samad, M. Khan, Hameedullah, *et al.* Unplanned prolonged postanesthesia care unit length of stay and factors affecting it. *J Pak Med Assoc* 2006; **56**; 108–12.

30. F. Dexter, D. H. Penning, R. D. Traub. Statistical analysis by Monte-Carlo simulation of the impact of administrative and medical delays in discharge from the postanesthesia care unit on total patient care hours. *Anesth Analg* 2001; **92**: 1222–5.

31. B. A. Williams, M. L. Kentor, M. T. Vogt, *et al.* Economics of nerve block pain management after anterior cruciate ligament reconstruction. *Anesthesiology* 2004; **100**: 697–706.

32. W. S. Sandberg, T. Canty, S. M. Sokal, B. Daily, D. L. Berger. Financial and operational impact of a direct-from-PACU discharge pathway for laparoscopic cholecystectomy patients. *Surgery* 2006; **140**: 372–8.

33. M. Schuster, T. Standl. Cost drivers in anesthesia: manpower, technique and other factors. *Curr Opin Anesthesiol* 2006; **19**: 177–84.

34. D. Song, F. Chung, M. Ronayne, *et al.* Fast-tracking (bypassing the PACU) does not reduce nursing workload after ambulatory surgery. *Br J Anaesth* 2004; **93**: 768–74.

35. F. Dexter, A. Macario, P. J. Manberg, D. A. Lubarsky. Computer simulation to determine how rapid anesthetic recovery protocols to decrease the time for emergence or increase the phase I postanesthesia care unit bypass rate affect staffing of an ambulatory surgery center. *Anesth Analg* 1999; **88**: 1053–63.

36. F. Chung. Discharge criteria – a new trend. *Can J Anaesth* 1995; **42**: 1056–8.

37. R. I. Patel, S. T. Verghese, R. S. Hannallah, *et al.* Fast-tracking children after ambulatory surgery. *Anesth Analg* 2001; **92**: 918–22.

19

Pain practice management

Steven D. Waldman MD, JD

Introduction   194
Basic considerations   194

Summary   199

Introduction

Over the past several years there has been considerable interest in expanding the role of the pain-management specialist as an integral member of the health-care team. This interest has been stimulated in part by the increased availability of health-care professionals with a special interest and advanced training in pain medicine and in part by the unprecedented economic pressures of our rapidly evolving health-care system. These economic pressures have forced many pain-management specialists to explore new avenues of revenue generation as well as to examine new strategies to help improve the efficiency and cost-effectiveness of the care they provide.

The purpose of this chapter is to serve as a guide for the pain-management specialist who may be considering setting up a pain-treatment center or expanding the scope of services currently offered. Although many of the concepts presented in this chapter are basic, failure to take them into consideration may lead to high levels of professional frustration and dissatisfaction, damage to the professional image of the pain-management specialist, economic loss, and increased exposure to malpractice liability.

Basic considerations

Should pain-management services be offered?

There is no question that there is a huge demand for quality pain-management services. The Nuprin Pain Report, which to date is the only comprehensive evaluation of pain in the United States, reveals that there are four billion workdays lost due to pain in America alone [1]: 73% of the patients interviewed reported one or more headaches interfering with their ability to work; 50% of the people interviewed reported back pain that limited their ability to work; 46% reported abdominal pain that limited their ability to work. The Nuprin Pain Report further noted that 43% of Americans had seen a physician at least once in the year preceding the statistical analysis, and surprisingly 29% of those patients surveyed had sought the help of a physician for pain four or more times in that year. Of great interest to our specialty is the fact that of those patients who sought medical attention for more than an occasional pain: 58% saw their family physician; 18% sought help from a chiropractor; 12% sought help from their pharmacists; and 9% sought help from dentists or other health-care professionals. Only 3% sought the advice and help of a pain-management specialist. From these data, it is obvious that there are a huge number of patients that could potentially benefit from quality pain-management services, and equally obvious is the fact that our specialty continues to have a problem with recognition and identity.

Interfacing pain-management services with existing services

The first question that must be asked when considering the implementation or addition of new pain-management services is how the addition of this new service will interface with existing professional activities. One must take into account the impact of such new services on existing care. The addition or expansion of pain-

Operating Room Leadership and Management, ed. Kaye A.D., Fox C.J. and Urman R.D. Published by Cambridge University Press. © Cambridge University Press 2012.

management services requires a high level of commitment from *all* members of the health-care team. Even if additional professional members of staff are added to provide pain-management services, consideration must be given to such issues as call responsibilities, vacation coverage, etc.

As with all health-care endeavors, there must be sufficient expertise to provide an ongoing level of quality care. One would not implement an open-heart-surgery program or start a burn unit without adequate expertise and/or additional training. Pain management requires the same level of training, expertise, and commitment. In addition to the clinical expertise required to provide quality pain-management services, there must be the administrative expertise if the endeavor is to be economically viable. This is especially important when setting up a pain-treatment facility under the managed care paradigm [2].

Are there adequate personnel to provide quality care?

It is extremely important that when setting up a pain-treatment facility that the pain-management specialist recognize the high level of commitment in terms of the time and energy essential to provide quality pain-management services. For this reason, the pain-management specialist must insure that there are adequate personnel to provide high-quality coverage for any new services that are contemplated or to cover the expansion of existing services.

There is a common misconception that pain management can be done at the convenience of the pain-management specialist. This is simply not the case. This approach can only lead to high levels of dissatisfaction from both patients and referring physicians. Today's patient, or what has become affectionately known as today's "health care consumer," is unwilling to wait for extended periods of time in order to receive care. The proliferation and success of urgent care centers and walk-in clinics staffed by physician extenders attest to this fact. During implementation of a new pain-management facility or expansion of an existing one, a realistic appraisal of the time required to provide the proposed care must be undertaken to assure the provision of care in a timely manner. Just as there must be an adequate number of health-care professionals to provide high-quality pain-management services, there must also be a high level of motivation in order for the pain facility to ultimately succeed [3]. *All* members of the health-care team must be committed to quality and compassionate provision of pain-management

services. A lone pain-management specialist, no matter how motivated and caring, can do little to make up for the disinterest and lack of support of the remainder of the pain-management team. This statement applies not only to the clinical personnel but to the administrative personnel as well.

Is the support staff adequate?

When setting up a pain-treatment facility, care must be taken to be sure that the practice infrastructure is adequate to support a busy and growing pain-management service. If the pain-management specialist's existing billing office is unable to keep up with the volume of work generated from existing activities, the addition of billings from new or expanded pain-management service may throw the entire office into disarray and adversely affect cash flow. Additional help can be added to alleviate this situation, but this should be done in a prospective manner [4].

Services offered

Prior to setting up a new pain-treatment facility, the first decision that needs to be made is the decision as to which specific services (e.g., evaluation, neural blockade, behavioral interventions, drug management, and detoxification, etc.) should be offered. In order to delineate these services adequately, the pain-management specialist must take into account his or her existing expertise, experience, and preferences as well as those of other health-care professionals providing pain-management services within the group practice. The availability of support services such as physical therapy, occupational therapy, psychiatry, and radiology support services such as computerized tomography scanning, magnetic resonance imaging, ultrasound, and biplanar fluoroscopy must also be considered. Under the managed care paradigm, some services may not be reimbursed at levels adequate to justify their use from a purely economic viewpoint and may have to be subsidized from more profitable product lines.

It is very important to define clearly to the patient as well as the referring physician what a new pain-treatment facility can and cannot offer. Too often a pain-management specialist with limited experience and training tries to hold himself or herself out as a specialist in all areas of pain management. This is not only academically dishonest but often leads to high levels of patient and referring physician dissatisfaction [5]. It may also place the pain-management specialist and those with whom he or she practices in a potentially serious medicolegal situation. Services should not be advertised that are not available or cannot be provided with sufficient expertise to keep complications to a minimum. A clear policy regarding whether the specialist will prescribe controlled substances for chronic nonmalignant pain is mandatory to avoid upsetting patients and referring physicians.

Types of patients seen

The second decision that needs to be made is delineating the types of patients that the pain-management specialist feels are appropriate for the scope of pain-management services he or she has chosen to offer at the new pain-treatment facility. The pain-management specialist should determine whether he or she is comfortable treating cancer pain, headache and facial pain, chemical dependence problems, and acute and postoperative pain, etc. He or she must also determine whether they will accept patients who are involved in workers' compensation claims and patients who are involved in litigation. Thirdly, the pain-management specialist must decide whether he or she will accept self-referred patients or will require patients to be evaluated and then referred by another physician (see below). Finally, the pain-management specialist will also have to decide whether he or she will accept primary responsibility for patients who are admitted to the hospital. This decision has specific implications that must be carefully thought out from a quality of care viewpoint, because some pain-management specialists may be incapable or unwilling to deal with the many medical problems that may occur while the patient is hospitalized under their care. Political issues as to the appropriateness of pain-management specialists providing primary care may also have to be addressed [6,7].

Financial considerations

The following issues must be handled according to each pain-management specialist's existing financial situation, current policies, prior contractual agreements with the hospital and/or third-party carriers, and his or her own philosophical and ethical viewpoints on providing indigent care. To ignore these variables when starting a pain-treatment facility is to insure economic disaster.

In order for the pain-management service to remain on a strong economic footing in this period of ever-decreasing revenues, financial considerations must be carefully considered [8]. Some pain-management specialists have chosen to provide pain-management services on a cash-only basis. Although this may work in some affluent communities, by and large, in view of the high cost of many of the modalities offered, this represents an impractical approach for most pain-management specialists.

A decision must be made as to the desirability of accepting Medicare assignment as well as other third-party assignments of insurance benefits. Participation in managed care plans should also be carefully weighed [2]. Obviously local factors have to dictate the variables to be taken into account when making this decision. The pain-management specialist must also decide what provisions will be made for the indigent patient who has Medicaid or who is solely responsible for the payment of their health-care costs. The pain-management specialist is likely to be approached by attorneys who desire care to be rendered on a contingency basis. The economic impact of these decisions cannot be overstated.

Availability

It has been said that there are three "A's" of a successful practice of pain management: ability, amiability, and availability. From a patient-care viewpoint, ability is the most important issue. However, from a practice-management viewpoint, there is no question that availability is the most important. When starting a pain-treatment center, it is imperative that the clinical and administrative staff all agree on the appropriate levels of availability if the facility is to succeed. Most patients expect to see the same physician at each visit, and this fact has a specific impact on call schedule issues such as days off after call, vacation scheduling, afternoons off, etc. If *all* members of the pain-management care team are not motivated to facilitate the provision of quality pain-management services, it is impossible for a single member of the team to make the pain-management service successful. This statement also applies to the administrative staff. If the administrative staff refuse to factor in additional patients, or limit the hours of operation of the pain-treatment facility, adverse economic consequences will often result.

Additional issues that need to be determined when setting up a pain-treatment facility include the hours of operation for the pain-management center. The availability of evening hours has become more and more important and is increasingly expected by the health-care consumer in today's competitive market. Weekend and holiday coverage must also be clearly defined for both the patient and referring physician. Expectations of the pain-management specialist who is covering these periods should also be delineated to avoid friction between members of a group pain-management practice and to assure appropriate availability from *all* members of the pain-management care team. A clear protocol for how emergency referrals will be handled is mandatory in order to assure quality, compassionate care with a high level of satisfaction for both patient and referring physician.

How patient phone calls are handled will also impact on the ultimate success of the pain-management specialist. Calls from referring physicians, the pharmacy, and patients, as well as support services including laboratory, radiology, physical therapy, and occupational therapy are the rule rather than the exception. Again, it must be clearly defined as to how these calls will be handled by all members of the pain-management care team in order to provide consistent, quality care and avoid lost revenues through missed consults or unavailability. The use of answering machines and voice mail as a way to avoid dealing with patients and referring physicians is to be avoided and may require careful monitoring by the pain-treatment facility management team.

Coupled with the need for the prompt returning of phone calls is the timeliness in which outpatient appointments and inpatient consultations are handled. Although specific times may vary from community to community, seeing inpatient consults (other than emergencies) within 24 h of being called works well in most situations. Any consult requested on an emergency basis should be seen as soon as possible. Seeing all routine consults that are received before 16:00 h on that same day (this includes Saturdays, Sundays, and holidays) projects a very strong message that the pain patient will not suffer needlessly while waiting for the pain-management service to be implemented. The same reasoning applies to the availability of outpatient consultation. When setting up a pain-treatment facility, immediate appointments should be available on a same-day basis for patients with acute pain problems and pain emergencies. Such appointments should allow appropriate screening and triage for such patients without disrupting the flow of previously scheduled patients.

This approach also makes good sense from a time-management viewpoint. As the pain-treatment facility grows busier, if inpatient and outpatient consultations are put off, a large backlog of patients waiting to be seen may result. Given the competitive nature of pain-management services in most geographic areas, such delays will result in significant lost revenues and high levels of patient and referring physician dissatisfaction.

Support staff availability

Tandem to the issue of physician availability is the issue of support staff availability. How consultations and phone messages for the pain-management service are to be handled is of paramount importance to the ultimate success of the pain practitioner. In many hospital-based pain-treatment facilities, all scheduling activities have been made the responsibility of the hospital secretarial staff. Often this simply does not work, in terms of both efficiency and motivation, when applied to the pain-management service. The hospital employee may not be willing or able to provide prompt and courteous handling of phone calls from referring physicians as well as patients. Messages may get misplaced or lost. Generally the 07:00 to 15:30 h staffing patterns of the hospital does not meet the needs of the referring physician, who is often in his or her office until 17:00 or 17:30 h. For this reason it is desirable as well as cost-effective to hire a high-quality secretary whose prime responsibilities are the administrative aspects of the pain-management service. This will insure that the phone is answered courteously and promptly, that phone messages are handled appropriately, that patient records are readily available, and that there is an appropriate level of motivation to work in add-on and emergency patients.

The pain-management support staff must be available during regular clinic hours. The overuse of answering machines or voice mail is strongly discouraged, as most busy referring physicians are unwilling to make several phone calls trying to reach the pain-management physician to discuss or schedule a patient. Provisions for phone coverage during lunch and break periods by the pain-management support staff are mandatory.

Physician-referred versus self-referred patients

Pain-management specialists have traditionally felt that physician-referred patients are desirable. In fact, many practitioners will not accept self-referred patients. There are distinct advantages and disadvantages to this philosophical viewpoint, as outlined in Tables 19.1 and 19.2.

The physician-referred patient *may* be appropriately worked up and carry a correct diagnosis; however,

Table 19.1. Physician-referred patients

Advantages

1. The patient *may* be appropriately worked up.

2. The patient *may* be appropriately diagnosed.

3. The patient *may* be familiar with pain management services and the reason that they have been sent to the pain center.

4. The referral *may* be appropriate for the services and expertise of the pain center.

5. Patient acquisition is low cost relative to advertising for self-referred patients.

Disadvantages

1. The pain specialist has limited control over the appropriateness of the evaluation and treatment.

2. The patient may be inadequately worked up, which puts tremendous medicolegal responsibilities on the pain-management physician to complete the evaluation.

3. The patient may be sent to the pain-management specialist carrying the wrong diagnosis.

4. The patient may be an inappropriate referral to the pain clinic relative to the services being offered.

5. The pain-management physician may inherit a patient who has been inappropriately treated by a referring physician and assume significant medical liability if he or she continues this treatment.

Table 19.2. Self-referred patients

Advantages

1. The pain-management specialist may control the evaluation and treatment.

2. The pain-management specialist may choose consultants needed to help him or her make the diagnosis that are of a higher quality than those chosen by the referring physician.

3. The pain-management specialist has control over treatment and the use of prescription medication (especially controlled substances).

4. The pain-management physician may exercise a choice in diagnostic imaging facilities or for hospitals should admission for further evaluation be necessary.

Disadvantages

1. The pain-management specialist has sole responsibility for the evaluation and treatment.

2. The pain-management specialist assumes the role of primary care physician.

3. Once the patient is under the care of the pain-management specialist, transfer of the patient to a more appropriate specialist may be difficult should a problem arise.

4. Cost of patient acquisition is high relative to physician-referred patients if advertising is used.

the pain specialist has limited control over the appropriateness and quality of the evaluation and treatment of the physician-referred patient – the patient may be inadequately or inappropriately evaluated, which puts tremendous medicolegal responsibilities on the pain-management physician to complete the evaluation. These problems can be magnified under the managed care paradigm, as the managed care plan may want to save money by limiting diagnostic testing. Furthermore, the patient referral may not be appropriate for the services and expertise available at the pain-treatment facility chosen by the referring physician or managed care plan.

Advantages of the self-referred patient include the fact that the pain-management specialist maintains control over the evaluation and treatment and may choose consultants necessary to help him or her make the diagnosis who may be of a higher quality than those utilized by some referring physicians. The pain-management specialist has control over treatment and the use of prescription medication (especially controlled substances) when providing care for the self-referred patients. Furthermore, the pain-management specialist may exercise a choice in diagnostic imaging facilities or for hospitals, should admission for further evaluation be necessary. As an increasing number of patients under managed care have out-of-network or point-of-service benefits as part of their managed-care contract, such patients can choose the pain-management physician and/or pain-treatment facility in spite of the dictates of the managed care plan [9,10]. Such patients can represent a significant source of revenue for a pain-treatment facility, and care should be taken to identify patients with such benefits before assuming they cannot be seen at a pain-treatment facility.

Disadvantages of self-referred patients include the fact that the pain-management specialist and pain-treatment facility has sole responsibility for the evaluation and treatment, essentially assuming the role of primary care physician. Once the patient is under the care of the pain-management specialist and facility, transfer of the patient to a more appropriate specialist or facility may be difficult, should a problem arise.

The pain-management specialist and the pain-treatment facility must weigh these variables to determine the best course to follow. Should a pain-management specialist decide to accept self-referred patients, he or she must recognize that in essence one is assuming the role of primary care physician. Incumbent to this role is an increase in responsibility with its attendant nighttime phone calls, emergencies, talking with family members, etc. Regardless of the pain-management specialist's ultimate decision, it is my strong belief that the physician-referred patient requires the same level of vigilance and quality of evaluation that a self-referred patient does, especially under the managed-care paradigm.

Hospital-based versus freestanding facilities

As hospital administrators, government, managed-care plans, and third-party payers seek to exert greater control over hospital-based physicians, pain-management specialists have sought to limit their vulnerability to this situation, e.g. by opening of surgical centers, affiliating with rehabilitation centers, etc. [11]. An additional option is the development of a freestanding pain-treatment facility. By developing such a facility, the pain-management specialist may avoid the "label" associated with a given hospital. This can be good or bad, depending on the public perception of the specific hospital. It should be remembered that these perceptions can change over time, and what may be a desirable hospital to practice in at one point in time may represent a negative practice location at another.

An additional advantage of starting a freestanding pain-treatment facility is that the pain-management specialist may choose its geographic location. This is advantageous if the pain-management specialist's primary hospital practice is located in a less-desirable geographic area of the city [12].

In some localities, it is possible for the pain-management specialist to bill not only for his or her professional fees but also for the drugs, trays, radiology services, laboratory services, block room, and recovery room charges. Some third-party carriers in specific geographic locations in the United States, e.g. the east coast, allow the pain-management specialist to charge 150% of his or her professional fee to cover the cost of drugs, trays, and room charges. In other areas, local or state law as well as policies of the third-party carriers may require that the facility be licensed and accredited as an ambulatory surgery center in order for a facility fee to be paid. Medicare pays the pain-management physician a higher professional fee if he or she provides care in an office setting rather than an ambulatory surgical center or hospital-based pain-treatment facility. Changes in this policy may lead to a shift in where pain-management services are provided in the future.

In the freestanding pain-treatment facility, the pain-management specialist will have greater control of the space, staffing, hours of operation, capital expenditures, and utilization review/quality assurance activities. Obviously with this added control and flexibility, there comes an added measure of responsibility and risk [13].

The major disadvantage of the freestanding pain-treatment facility is cost. The pain-management specialist can anticipate a large capital expenditure to provide adequate space, equipment, and personnel to implement pain-management services at a freestanding location. In addition, the pain-management specialist assumes the added liability and cost of malpractice insurance of the facility as well as the liability for professional services offered. The pain-management specialist also inherits the liability for the actions of his or her staff. The advantages and disadvantages of the hospital-based pain-management practice versus the freestanding pain center are summarized in Table 19.3.

Summary

Starting a pain-treatment facility is a significant undertaking, in terms of both time and tangible expense. Although the risks are great, so can be the rewards if done properly. By addressing the above-mentioned issues as an integral part of the planning process, the

Table 19.3. Hospital-based pain center

Advantages

1. The rent is free.

2. The personnel are free.

3. The equipment is free.

4. There is high visibility to referring physicians.

5. There is a high level of convenience for inpatients.

6. There is excellent emergency support should problems arise.

7. There is high-tech equipment readily available.

8. Support services such as physical therapy, occupational therapy, etc. are available.

Disadvantages

1. There may be a lack of adequate designated space.

2. The pain-management specialist does not have control of staffing.

3. The hospital administration may be very unwilling to provide the capital expenditure necessary to provide appropriate diagnostic and therapeutic equipment.

4. If the hospital develops a negative perception in the community, this will be carried over to the pain-management services.

5. The pain-management specialist will be subject to hospital utilization review and quality assurance activities.

6. The pain management specialist is subject to medical staff rules, which may limit his or her ability to use operating room facilities, admit patients, etc.

7. The pain-management specialist receives no portion of the revenues from the facility, lab, radiology, and support service fees generated.

pain-management specialist will be better able to determine whether setting up a pain-treatment facility is the right decision.

References

1. J. Saper. A review of the Nuprin Pain Report. *Top Pain Manage* 1987; **2**: 2–4.

2. S. D. Waldman. Joining a managed care plan: a guide to the pain management specialist. *Am J Pain Manag.* 1992; **2**: 215–18.

3. S. D. Waldman. Motivating the pain center employee. *Am J Pain Manag.* 1993; **3**: 114–17.

4. S. D. Waldman. Hiring employees for the pain center. *Am J Pain Manag* 1992; **2**: 164–6.

5. S. D. Waldman. Total quality management for the pain center-an idea whose time has come. *Am J Pain Manag* 1993; **3**: 38–41.

6. S. D. Waldman. The antitrust implications of medical staff credentialling-Part I. *Am J Pain Manag* 1997; **7**: 22–7.

7. S. D. Waldman. The antitrust implications of medical staff credentialling-Part II. *Am J Pain Manag* 1997; **7**: 66–9.

8. S. D. Waldman. Reimbursement for chronic pain management service – the cloud's silver lining. *Reg Anesth* 1993; **18**: 227–8.

9. S. D. Waldman. Any willing provider laws-paradox or panacea Part I. *Am J Pain Manag* 1996; **6**: 54–61.

10. S. D. Waldman. Any willing provider laws-paradox or panacea Part II. *Am J Pain Manag* 1996; **6**: 93–6.

11. S. D. Waldman. N. A. Ford. Selling your medical practice-Part I. *Am J Pain Manag* 1998; **8**: 23–8.

12. S. D. Waldman. Selling your medical practice-Part II. *Am J Pain Manag* 1998; **8**: 53–60.

13. S. D. Waldman. The new OSHA regulations: implications for the pain management specialist. *Am J Pain Manag* 1993; **3**: 85–7.

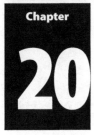

Chapter

20

Office-based surgery practice

Seth Christian MD
Charles J. Fox III MD

Introduction   201
Accreditation   201
Insurance coverage   202
Occupational hazards and risk management   203
Medical gases   204
Backup power and electrical wiring   204
Anesthesia and life-support equipment   204
Mobile anesthesia   204
Infection control   204
Controlled substances   205
Practice management   205
Billing methodology   206
Significant legislation   207
Clinical care   207
Postoperative care   208

Plastic surgery advisories and anesthetic training of dentists   208
Procedures performed in the office-based facility advisory   209
Physiologic stressors associated with surgery   209
Thromboprophylaxis   210
Postoperative recovery issues   211
Provider qualifications and facility standards   211
Patient selection advisory   211
Preoperative tests   212
The ASA physical classification   212
Pain management and prevention of postoperative nausea and vomiting advisory   212
Liposuction advisory   213
Office-based dental procedures   214

Introduction

Office-based surgery has increased in popularity over the last 10 years as a result of numerous factors. Managed care has embraced the cost containment that office-based facilities offer. Surgical procedures, thought only possible in traditional hospitals, have migrated to office-based facilities because of advancement in surgical techniques and equipment. These procedures are now safely performed in the nontraditional office-based environment. Patients and surgeons enjoy the ease of scheduling that office-based facilities provide, while cosmetic surgery patients relish the privacy that these facilities afford. Lastly, a lack of early state and federal regulations allowed rapid expansion of the office-based practice. This chapter will discuss pertinent issues necessary for today's office-based facility, detail practice advisories issued by the American Society for Plastic Surgeons (ASPS), and explain the unique training dentists undertake to insure office-based patient safety.

Accreditation

Accreditation may be obtained through the Joint Commission (JC), Accreditation for Ambulatory Health Care (AAAHC), or American Association

Operating Room Leadership and Management, ed. Kaye A.D., Fox C.J. and Urman R.D. Published by Cambridge University Press. © Cambridge University Press 2012.

Table 20.1 Suggested forms

Patient Demographics	Pregnancy Disclaimer	Notice of Privacy Practices
Medical Records Release	Preoperative Instructions	NPO Instructions
Preoperative Checklist	Surgery Consent	Anesthesia Record
PACU Record	Postoperative Instructions	Intraoperative Record
Health History Questionnaire	Bloodborne Pathogen Testing Release	Patient Satisfaction Survey
Photo Release	Acknowledgement of Preoperative Instructions	Universal Protocol Verification
PACU Orders		

for Accreditation of Ambulatory Surgery Facilities (AAAASF). Accrediting agencies address the facility layout, patient records, personnel records, peer review, quality assurance, operating room (OR) personnel, equipment, operations and management, and environmental safety. Although the AAAASF is the only accrediting body that requires mandatory reporting of adverse events, all three organizations are working to create standardized definitions of adverse events.

The facility should have a medical director or governing body that establishes policy and is responsible for the activities of the facility and staff, for insuring that facilities and personnel are adequate and that all applicable local, state, and federal laws, codes, and regulations are observed. All health-care practitioners and nurses should hold a valid license or certificate to perform their assigned duties. The supervising operating practitioner or other licensed physician should be specifically trained in the office-based surgery being performed as well as sedation, anesthesia, and rescue techniques appropriate to the type of sedation being provided. It is recommended that anesthesiologists and surgeons practicing in an office-based setting maintain current advanced cardiac life support with hands-on airway training.

All patient records must be kept on file and available for review. Preoperative and postoperative evaluations must be documented in the patient record. All medical information must be maintained in a fashion that is compliant with the Health Insurance Portability and Accountability Act (HIPAA). The list of forms that may be required is shown in Table 20.1.

Office-based anesthesia practices should have a written quality improvement plan in place to continually assess, document, and improve outcome. The quality improvement plan should utilize peer reviews, benchmarking, and risk-management strategies. The quality improvement plan should also include review of morbidity and "adverse" or "sentinel" events (Table 20.2). The review of quality indicators should also include measures of patient satisfaction.

Insurance coverage

Insurance providers do not discriminate against office-based practitioners, but because office-based practices are an emerging concept, insurers may lack many of the traditional tools utilized to establish rates and plans. Insurers may lack an established peer-review structure to examine the quality of the exclusively office-based practitioner and a facility accreditation system to assess risk related to adequacy of the equipment, supplies, and protocols and procedures. Underwriting calculations are complicated, because providers often work in an office-based setting only part time, at multiple sites, or across state lines.

Individual practitioners should be familiar with all practice guidelines. Insurance providers will cite standards and guidelines and require adherence to these as a condition of coverage. For example, pulse oximetry, electrocardiogram, end tidal CO_2, and blood pressure measurement are considered standard monitors, and noncompliance with these standards may void coverage and payment. Requirements for obtaining professional liability insurance are listed in Table 20.3.

Practitioners should also understand the concept of vicarious liability, which is the legal liability that

Table 20.2 Adverse and sentinel events suggested for review

Death	Cardiac arrest	Respiratory arrest
Unplanned reintubation	Central nervous system deficit within 2 days of anesthesia	Peripheral nervous system deficit within 2 days of anesthesia
Myocardial infarction within 2 days of anesthesia	Pulmonary edema within 1 day of anesthesia	Aspiration pneumonia
Anaphylaxis or adverse drug reaction	Postdural puncture headache within 4 days of neuraxial anesthesia	Dental injury
Eye injury	Surgical infection	Excessive blood loss
Unplanned admission to a hospital or acute care facility	Drug error	Wrong surgical or regional block site
Wrong procedure or patient		

Table 20.3 Professional liability insurance agents requirements

Clinic ownership and practitioner list	Assurance that all patients will be discharged in the care of a responsible adult
Policy and procedure manual for routine and emergency situations	Assurance of adherence to all applicable ASA standards and guidelines
Policy and procedure manual for record review	Presence of a defibrillator if general anesthesia, regional anesthesia, or parenteral sedation/analgesia is to be administered
Policy and procedure manual for outcome analysis	On-site inspection by the company's consultant anesthesiologist
Types of anesthesia to be administered	Compliance with all applicable federal and state statutes
Description of equipment and monitoring capabilities	Any voluntary accreditation obtained
Evidence that all patients give informed consent to the surgeon and anesthesiologist	Procedures for resuscitation and arrangements for transport to an emergency facility in a timely manner
Evidence of adherence to a formal credentialing policy	

may exist for the actions of others involved in the same incident. Individual practitioners should personally examine all liability insurance policies for limitations or restrictions on the type of surgery to be performed and inquire of the state medical board about any limitations placed on the operating surgeon's license. Individual practitioners should also compare coverage limits with those of the other practitioners. A wide disparity in coverage could invite disproportionate accusations of liability (i.e., the "deep-pocket" phenomenon). It is vital that practitioners in an office be absolutely certain of the license status, training qualifications for the procedures performed, and professional liability insurance of the operating surgeon and all assisting personnel.

Occupational hazards and risk management

Office-based facilities are typically constructed differently. The OR environment has a high degree of occupational hazard risk, and unfortunately most of the safeguards and redundancies designed to protect patients and providers do not exist in the office-based setting. Office-based practices should be compliant with the National Fire Protection Association (NFPA) 99 Health Care Facilities document, which details the requirements for health-care facilities.

Because most office buildings are built with the assumption of an ambulatory population, office-based practices must have a plan for evacuating patients who may be under the effects of anesthesia during an emergency. An office-based practice's policy and procedures manual must include a plan for transporting a ventilated patient on a stretcher, either because of a medical necessity or because the building must be evacuated. Elevators in a medical or commercial building may not have adequate capacity to transport a ventilated patient on a stretcher.

Medical gases

The logistics of using volatile anesthetics and/or nitrous oxide introduce an additional level of complexity for many office-based practices, most of which do not have the level 1 medical piped gas systems found in classic hospitals, so if the anesthesiologist plans on using volatile anesthetics for general anesthesia, a system must be developed to access and then eliminate these gases. Many office-based practices use portable tanks – if such tanks are used, storage must conform to NFPA guidelines and an adequate volume of gas must be on hand to meet the day's needs. The Compressed Gas Association (CGA) and the Department of Transportation (DOT) provide the information and regulations that address the transportation of compressed or liquefied gases. The NFPA standards for eliminating medical gases are not required in the office setting unless the accrediting organization requires it. Most office-based facilities do not have the capability to actively vacuum and pipe gases or passively direct gases into the facility ventilation exhaust system, so an office-based practice may run an exhaust hose to an outside window, but must insure that the gases do not reenter or enter another living space. Many office-based practices opt for total intravenous techniques to eliminate the need for medical gas waste systems.

Backup power and electrical wiring

The backup power in most medical or commercial office buildings is only required to allow a safe and orderly exit from the building, but appropriate backup power should be in place for life-support equipment. A minimum of two independent sources of power is required. When general anesthesia and electrical life-support systems are used, a type I essential electrical system (EES) is typically required. The Joint Commission recommends that the generator should be tested 12 times a year for at least 30 min under a dynamic load of at least 30% of the nameplate rating on the generator. In the absence of line-isolation monitors, the use of ground fault circuit interrupters (GFCI) should be used to limit the shock hazard.

Anesthesia and life-support equipment

All anesthesia and life-support equipment should be fully factory supported and include current factory technical support, parts availability, and continued factory service training. A biomedical technician or equivalent should annually inspect all of the equipment. The manufacturer's specifications and requirements are kept in an organized file. All equipment should be on a preventative maintenance schedule. A biomedical technician or equivalent should perform all equipment repairs and changes. Anesthesia machines should not be obsolete.

Mobile anesthesia

Mobile anesthesia may be defined as a practice in which the anesthesiologist transports all anesthesia equipment from office site to office site. A site visit should be conducted before the start of mobile anesthesia services. Mobile anesthesia practices are considering accrediting themselves as a separate entity, as a means of enhancing the credibility and value of the anesthesia practice. Mobile anesthesia providers cannot bill a facility fee or share a facility fee, but may recoup the costs of durable and disposable equipment/supplies provided by the practitioner. Many anesthesia machines are not meant for frequent transport, and many calibrations may be invalidated by spillage of gases. The Food and Drug Administration (FDA) has approval for anesthesia machines that are suitable for "mobile" anesthesia use.

Infection control

Practices should adhere to the Centers for Disease Control and Prevention (CDC) Standard Precautions for Infection Control, which summarizes methods for body substance isolation (BSI) and universal precautions to prevent transmission of a variety of organisms. The office-based practice should have policy and procedure for sterilization of surgical equipment, cleaning and disinfecting procedure rooms, and managing patients with multidrug-resistant organisms (MDROs).

Table 20.4 Infection control suggested policy and procedure

Sterilization of surgical equipment and supplies	Managing patients with multidrug-resistant organisms
Cleaning and disinfecting procedure rooms	Occupational health and bloodborne pathogens standard
Protective clothing appropriate to the procedure	Safe injection practices and appropriate aseptic techniques

Table 20.5 List of DEA forms

DEA Form 222	Schedule I & II drug order form
DEA Form 223	The DEA Controlled Substances Certificate of Registration issued to the practitioner or entity.
DEA Form 224	Application for registration. Renewed every three years on form 224a. The address on the form is important. DEA registrations are issued for principle place of business or professional practice where controlled substances are distributed or dispensed.
DEA Form 106	Report of Theft or Loss of Controlled Substances Form
DEA Form 41	Request to Dispose of Stocked Controlled Substances Form.

Table 20.4 shows a suggested infection policy and procedure. Lastly, employees should be compliant with all Occupational Safety and Health Administration standards.

Controlled substances

Policy and procedures are required to comply with laws and regulations pertaining to controlled drug supply, storage, and administration. The Federal Drug Enforcement Administration (DEA) requires separate registration certificates for manufacturing, distributing, and dispensing and administering controlled medications, and a separate state-controlled drug registration may also be required. Office-based practices probably do not need a registration certificate for manufacturing, but some practices may choose to function as a distributor.

Controlled substances may be supplied by the office-location or by the anesthesiologist. If the office supplies the controlled substances, the site will have a DEA 223 registration number and will order controlled substances with their DEA 222 order form. If the anesthesiologist provides the medication at different locations under the practitioner's DEA license, a separate DEA registration for each site is not needed. Narcotics must be stored in a double-locked box. Any person or place acting as a "dispenser" of controlled drugs must take an inventory on the date of DEA registration and every 2 years thereafter.

A daily drug-use inventory must be maintained that accounts for the use and wastage of all controlled medications on each patient for each date. The recording method and any backup media should be specified, and records are subject to DEA inspection. Loss or theft of a DEA Controlled Drug Order Form 222 must be reported immediately. Expired drugs can be disposed of by filing a form 41 with the DEA. Important DEA forms are shown in Table 20.5.

Practice management

Outcomes-based accountability practitioners will often get asked to help in facility operations, such as scheduling, equipment and supply ordering, medical directorships, and accreditation. It is usually advantageous to be involved in facility operations, but it should be viewed as more a consultative role and contractual arrangements can be made with facilities for anesthesiologists to serve in that capacity. Such services must be provided at fair market value by the practitioner, and must not be construed as a "bonus" service, which may be viewed as a kickback, to facilities.

Patients who choose to have surgery in the office-based setting will expect excellent clinical care, availability, flexibility, and reliability – all for a reasonable price. Because of limitations in scope, this chapter assumes excellent patient care and reliability, and focuses on improving availability and reducing prices. Availability is largely associated with the size of the anesthesia group. Large anesthesia groups can provide more availability, but many surgeons prefer having a consistent core group of anesthesiologists. Utilization benchmarking data are available from The Ambulatory Surgery Center Association, and percent utilization should be agreed upon and included in negotiation. Price differentiation is much more complex, but the management of nonbillable downtime has a major impact on the price transferred to the patient.

A variety of unique payment plans may be created for office-based procedures. Patients may make direct cash payments to the provider for purely elective cases or may make hybrid insurance/cash payments for combined procedures that are both medically necessary and elective (ventral herniorraphy and abdominoplasty). Medicare pays only for covered services that are medically necessary, and often pays less than one's standard fee for covered services. Because it is illegal to bill Medicare patients directly to cover the difference, it is very important to get an accurate picture of the payer mix during the initial negotiation phase.

Although commercial third-party payers have higher reimbursement rates, there are additional complexities to understand. Office-based providers must decide whether or not to become a participating provider in a particular insurance plan. Provider participation with CMS or any insurance company is strictly voluntary, although some hospitals or facilities may require an anesthesiologist to participate. Surgeons and/or the facility would prefer an upfront agreement that all anesthesia providers must be a participating provider with all contracted insurance plans of the facility.

Anesthesiologists must consider many factors before accepting such an upfront agreement. In the office-based setting, insurers do not have to pay the traditional facility fee, and otherwise poor insurance plans are often able to lure surgeons with an additional nonprofessional fee that is paid to surgeons who perform procedures in the office-based setting. Every effort should be made to insert language such as "agree to negotiate in good faith with all insurance companies" into the contract, in order to protect from being bound to participate in undesirable insurance plans.

If the anesthesiologist is not a participating provider, often the insurance company will send the payment directly to the patient, who then pays the anesthesiologist his/her fee. This can result in delays at best and total nonpayment at worst. Patients are often charged an "out-of-network" fee when the anesthesiologist is a nonparticipating provider, and this frequently causes lots of complaints from patients and surgeons.

When considering becoming a participating provider, first compare the rates of the third-party payer with the rates the anesthesia providers charge. Analyze the payer mix. Compare the rates paid by the third-party payer for participating providers with the rates paid for nonparticipating providers. Determine if the patient is billed an "out-of-network" fee for nonparticipating providers.

Billing methodology

Billing for services should be clear to all participating parties during negotiations to provide services. Anesthesia providers may perform their own billing, engage a billing service, or have the facility/owner(s) collect anesthesia fees and pay the anesthesia provider in a prearranged fashion. If anesthesia providers choose not to perform their own billing, it is important to understand that the anesthesiologist is responsible for all claims submitted in his or her name.

Individual anesthesiologists or practices must set their own fees for services, because coordination of charges among groups can be viewed as illegal price-fixing. A methodology must be established for charging for services. Anesthesiologists typically bill by base time with modifier units, by case, or by the hour.

Billing by base time with modifier units is an accepted methodology and generally used when billing third-party payers and insurance companies. However, when billing the patient or facility directly, practices may chose to bill by hour, by case, or by an all inclusive "package fee" to provide additional convenience to the patient. Providers must negotiate his/her global and professional fees in advance when billing the patient by hour, case, or package fee. Providers should be familiar with his/her state legislation regarding billing HMO patients. Providers should be prepared to accommodate insurance companies that require pre-authorization for both surgery and anesthesia.

Significant legislation

A federal law known as Stark II prohibits certain physician self-referrals for "designated health services" and prohibits physicians from making referrals for such designated health services to an entity in which the physicians or their immediate family members have financial interest, either by way of ownership or compensation, unless an exception applies.

The federal anti-kickback law prohibits offering, paying, soliciting, or receiving any "remuneration" to induce referrals of items or services that are reimbursable by federal health-care programs. Because it is a criminal statute, it requires proof of intent, unlike Stark II. Situations involving the provision of drugs and supplies may raise concerns for potential anti-kickback law violations, and individual providers should seek legal counsel if questions arise regarding anti-kickback laws. Because of the current lack of oversight in the office-based setting, individual providers may find themselves in questionable ethical situations. Direct employment relationships may jeopardize the autonomy of office-based practices if economics influence medical judgment.

Clinical care

The levels of surgery have been loosely defined earlier in this chapter, but many times the health-care practitioners themselves establish written policies governing the specific surgical procedures that may be performed in the office. Longer procedures should be scheduled early in the day, because they may require longer recovery periods. Any procedures involving significant blood loss, major intra-abdominal, intrathoracic, or intracranial cavities, postoperative pain, or postoperative nausea and vomiting are not appropriate for the office-based setting. Ideally, the procedure should last no longer than 6 h, to allow for adequate recovery and discharge.

There are two classifications that are common to office-based surgery facilities. One classification deals with the anesthetic being administered, and the other classification describes the complexity of surgical procedure and level of anesthesia required for the given office-based procedure. Class A anesthesia includes topical and local infiltration blocks with oral or intramuscular preoperative sedation; Class B anesthesia includes oral, parenteral, or intravenous sedation; and Class C anesthesia includes regional and general anesthesia.

Office-based surgery is similarly classified as level I, II, or III depending on the complexity. Level I surgery includes minor surgical procedures performed under topical, local, or infiltration blocks with preoperative oral anxiolytic medications. Level II surgery includes minor or major procedures performed with oral, parenteral, or intravenous sedation or under analgesic or dissociative drugs. Level III surgery includes major surgical procedures that require deep sedation/analgesia, general anesthesia, or major conduction blocks and support of vital bodily functions.

Each office should establish patient selection guidelines based on the patient's medical status, stability of medical status, psychological status, social support system, post-procedure monitoring, and risk of deep vein thrombosis/pulmonary embolism (DVT/PE) (Table 20.6). Generally, ASA physical status 1 and 2 patients can proceed by protocol, but ASA 3 and 4 must have a direct consultation and the conditions must be medically optimized (Table 20.7). The history and physical should be within 30 days of the procedure and reassessed by the surgeon on the day of surgery. Appropriate fasting protocol and specific perioperative medication instructions should be clearly explained.

Sedation is recognized on a continuum from anxiolysis, moderate sedation/analgesia (conscious sedation), deep sedation/analgesia (MAC), to general anesthesia. Patients under conscious sedation respond purposefully to verbal commands or light tactile stimulation and require no airway support. Patients under deep sedation respond purposefully to painful stimulation and may require assistance in maintaining a patent airway. Patients under general anesthesia cannot be aroused and may require respiratory and cardiovascular support.

The anesthesiologist should focus on providing an anesthetic that will give the patient a rapid recovery to normal function, with minimal postoperative pain, nausea, and other side effects. The intraoperative record must document anesthetic agents, medications, and supplemental oxygen used, vital signs, oxygen saturation, electrocardiogram (ECG) interpretation, end-tidal carbon dioxide, inspired oxygen, and temperature measurements when required. Pain should

Table 20.6 Risk factors for PE

Age > 40	Venous insufficiency	Factor V Leiden mutation
History of PE or DVT	Elevated factor VIIIc	Protein C deficiency
Protein S deficiency	Hypercoagulable states	Lupus anticoagulant
Polycythemia	Oral contraceptives	Postmenopausal HRT
History of >3 pregnancies	Previous miscarriage	Current pregnancy
Chronic heart failure	Malignancy	Obesity
Trauma	Bedbound	Radiation therapy to pelvis
Infectious disease	Abdominoplasty	Recent long-distance travel
Use of general anesthesia		

Adapted from: Iverson RE, and the ASPS Task Force on Patient Safety in Office-based Surgery Facilities. Patient Safety in office-based surgery facilities. Procedures in the office-based surgery setting. *Plast Reconstr Surg* 2002; **110**: 1337–42.

Table 20.7 Medical conditions requiring additional consideration

Difficult airway	Morbid obesity	Obstructive sleep apnea
Hx anesthetic complications	Malignant hyperthermia	Anaphylactic drug allergy
Latex allergy	Inadequate NPO status	Alcohol abuse
Substance abuse	Inadequate social support	

be managed proactively. Multiple modalities should be used to manage pain, including nonsteroidal anti-inflammatory drugs (NSAIDs), opioids, local anesthetics, acetaminophen, gabapentin or pregabalin, and regional or neuraxial anesthesia.

Postoperative care

The Standards for Post-operative Care and Guidelines for Ambulatory Anesthesia and Surgery on the ASA website apply to all anesthesia services, but in the office-based setting providers must recognize that differences in the facility structure and/or support services may present unique challenges to successful postanesthesia care. In many office-based practices, patients recover in the surgical room or procedure room without transport to a postanesthesia care unit. Oxygenation, ventilation, circulation, and temperature should be monitored on all patients, including a quantitative method of assessing oxygenation (pulse oximetry). The anesthesiologist should be immediately available until the patient has been discharged from anesthesia care and deemed medically appropriate for discharge. If the patient remains in the facility after discharge from anesthesia, personnel trained in

basic life support/advanced cardiac life support should be present until the person leaves.

Postoperative discharge instructions should include the procedure performed, information about potential complications, telephone numbers and names of medical providers, instructions for any medications, instructions for pain management, date, time, and location of the follow-up or return visit, and pre-determined places to go for treatment in the event of an emergency. Office-based practices do not have to have a designated area for recovery and the modified Aldrete score and fast-tracking criteria are often combined (Table 20.8).

A patient that meets all of these criteria can be discharged from anesthesia care. Each category is worth 2 points, and a cumulative score of 12 is required for discharge. Each category has intermediate criteria worth 1 point, but this was not described as it is beyond the scope of the chapter.

Plastic surgery advisories and anesthetic training of dentists

Many hospitals have become extremely complex organizations as patient surgical options have expanded and

Table 20.8 Combined modified Aldrete score and fast-tracking criteria

Moves all extremities voluntarily

Breathes deeply and coughs freely

Blood pressure within 20 mm of pre-anesthetic level

Fully awake

Pulse oximetry of >92% on room air

Postoperative pain: none or mild discomfort (VAS <3)

Postoperative emetic symptoms: none or mild nausea with no active vomiting

Adapted from: White PF, Song D. New criteria for fast-tracking after outpatient anesthesia: a comparison with the modified Aldrete's scoring system. *Anesth Analg* 1999; **88**: 1069.

evolved. Some have limited block times for "new" surgeons or possess service lines that necessitate emergent OR time. This can result in issues with efficiency and convenience for patients and surgeons trying to access the hospital OR. Also, hospital costs have escalated, and, with many procedures left uncovered by conventional insurance carriers, patients have gravitated to the more cost-competitive option that office-based surgery offers. Additional potential advantages of office-based surgery include greater privacy for the patient and consistent specialty-specific nursing care. Because of this, today's patient undergoing dental or plastic surgery commonly has his or her procedure performed in an office-based facility.

The advancement of surgical equipment, technique, and knowledge has permitted increasingly complex surgical procedures to be successfully completed in an office-based surgery facility. This "new" frontier for medical care had limited regulations and few guidelines for the office-based surgeon. As the "surgical envelope" was pushed, several highly publicized bad outcomes were reported that necessitated an immediate need for regulation and guideline development. The guidelines developed by the American Dental Association and the ASPS are not considered standards of medical care, but rather, a strategy for patient care based on a review of current literature.

The ASPS quickly met and assembled a task force to address the issues present in the office-based practice. The task force determined that patient safety should serve as the cornerstone for crafting their actions. Over several years, the task force developed four office-based surgery advisories. The first practice advisory addresses procedures performed in the office-based facility, whereas others deal with patient selection, pain management, and liposuction. An overview of the advisories is discussed below. This is a distilled version of their recommendations and is meant to give the reader knowledge of each advisory, but not serve as a replacement for the whole thing.

Procedures performed in the office-based facility advisory

In the ASPS practice advisory for procedures for the office-based surgical suite, the ASPS task force delineates common issues, relative to most plastic surgery procedures, thought to affect patient safety. The degree of concern for each factor varied depending on the specific procedure performed. The issues found most pertinent to plastic surgery patients' safety were physiologic stressors associated with surgery, provider qualifications, surgical facility standards, thromboprophylaxis measures, and postoperative recovery issues.

Physiologic stressors associated with surgery

All surgical procedures produce physiologic stress for the patient. The degree of stress seems more linked to the severity of the physiologic derangement rather than the procedure. The task force was unable to exclude certain plastic surgery procedures from being done in the office-based setting owing to lack of data but felt that the surgeon should base the degree of surgical involvement on the facility resources. They acknowledged that hypothermia, blood loss, duration of surgery, and liposuction, in combination with other procedures, were factors that should be considered when selecting the appropriate facility.

Hypothermia and blood loss are two common intraoperative issues faced by surgeons. The body's protective thermoregulatory measures to conserve heat loss are blocked by regional or general anesthesia. Combined with colder temperatures, common to most ORs, these factors increase the patient's risk of developing hypothermia. Because of this, the surgical facility should have forced air warming blankets and intravenous fluid warmers. The operating room should have the equipment and ability to monitor and regulate room temperature. Surgery, without the use of hypothermia prevention measures, should be of short duration (1–2 h) and not involve more than 20% of the patient's body surface area.

When a general or regional anesthetic is planned, the patient should be actively prewarmed and core temperature should be measured throughout the procedure. Additionally, one should cover as much body surface area as possible with blankets or drapes to minimize radiant or convective heat loss during the procedure. If large volumes of irrigating or infiltrating fluids are used, they should be warmed. Postoperative shivering should be aggressively treated with forced air warming or resistive heating blankets and pharmacologic intervention if needed.

Surgical blood loss occurs to varying degrees, depending on the type and duration of each procedure. For the average-sized adult, anticipated blood loss of 500 cc or more may necessitate blood and blood component replacement. So when scheduling the procedure the surgeon should select a facility with this capability.

Liposuction is routinely performed safely in office-based surgical procedures. However, when liposuction is combined with multiple procedures during a single operative experience, the potential for complications may increase. Because of this, some states have developed policies clearly delineating procedural limits. The ASPS feels that liposuction can be done safely in the office-based facility as long as the volume of aspirant (supernatant fat and fluid) is 5000 cc or less and that large-volume liposuction combined with other procedures, especially abdominoplasty, should be avoided in the office-based facility.

The anticipated duration of surgery is an extremely important factor that may affect patient outcome. Most plastic surgery procedures performed last more than 1 h. Often, multiple procedures are performed during the same operative period. The ASPS task force advises that longer procedures should be performed early in the morning to maximize recovery time for the patient before discharge. Also, they suggest that office-based surgical procedures should be completed in under 6 h. Lastly, although duration of surgery can affect outcome, other factors such as patient selection, intraoperative management, and postoperative management play a role in the outcome of surgical procedures of longer duration in the office-based surgery.

Thromboprophylaxis

Most patients presenting for office-based surgery have a small chance of developing a DVT/PE, but the significance of such an event led the task force to develop guidelines for the office-based surgeon. These guidelines should help physicians when evaluating the patient preoperatively. Numerous studies have identified risk factors thought to predispose patients to developing DVT/PE (see Table 20.6). A careful preoperative history and physical examination should be done, which may uncover subtle clues of past DVT/PE or identify risk factors associated with their development.

A history of dyspnea, syncope, or pleurisy may indicate past PE, whereas a history of calf pain or leg swelling may indicate past DVT. A detailed list of medications past and present, paying close attention to patients taking oral contraceptives or on hormone replacement therapy, should be ascertained preoperatively. A detailed family history may uncover valuable clues concerning past thrombotic events or hypercoagulable states that may require further investigation before proceeding with surgery. Physical examination of the lower extremity should pay attention to leg swelling, edema, or calf pain in the absence of trauma. Lower extremity skin discoloration or ulceration may warrant further analysis.

The information gathered from the history and physical examination will allow the surgeon to classify the patient as low, moderate, high, or very high risk for developing DVT or PE. Based on the risk classification, the task force developed thromboprophylaxis for each. Low-risk patients are usually under 40 years of age and have no risk factors. For these patients, thromboprophylaxis includes positioning the lower extremity in a comfortable position with knees slightly flexed and avoiding constriction or external compression of the lower extremity. Optional therapy for these patients includes the use of graduated compression stockings at home.

Patients categorized as moderate risk are 40 years of age or older undergoing procedures longer than 30 min. Patients taking oral contraceptives or on hormone replacement therapy are also found to be at moderate risk. Prophylaxis for this group includes the use of lower extremity pneumatic compression devices for the calf and ankle, which should start before the induction of general anesthesia and continue until the patient is awake and active postoperatively, along with those recommendations used for lower-risk patients. These patients should also qualify for pre- and postoperative chemoprophylaxis with low-molecular weight heparin continued until fully ambulatory.

High-risk patients include those over 40 years of age with one risk factor who are undergoing surgical procedures lasting longer than 30 min. Thromboprophylaxis for these patients should include those advised for low- and moderate-risk patients as well as a preoperative hematology consultation and preoperative and postoperative antithrombotic drug therapy. Chemoprophylaxis for this group may be warranted for up to 10 days postoperatively.

Very-high-risk patients include those over 40 years of age with more than one risk factor who are undergoing procedures lasting longer than 30 min. These patients should have the same thromboprophylaxis as the high-risk group. Additionally, they may require longer prophylaxis with agents such as warfarin. This may necessitate anticoagulation monitoring using the blood test for international normalized ratio (INR).

Postoperative recovery issues

The most common issues for office-based surgery patients resulting in hospital admission are dizziness, nausea and/or vomiting, pain, and postoperative bleeding. Pain control for these patients should take into account body mass and type of procedure performed. One study found breast augmentation and liposuction to be the two procedures associated with the most pain postoperatively. Although not mentioned in the task force report, numerous studies indicate that prevention of postoperative nausea and vomiting starts with various pharmacologic therapies preoperatively. Patients presenting for surgery have intravascular volume depletion from fasting. This, coupled with intraoperative blood loss, requires adequate preoperative, intraoperative, and postoperative fluid replacement to lessen the occurrence of postoperative hospital admission.

Provider qualifications and facility standards

The ASPS lists numerous qualifications and standards that the surgeon and organization must achieve before opening an office-based facility. The ASPS states that the surgeons performing the operation should have hospital privileges for that procedure and either board certification or qualifications leading to board certification by a surgical specialty board recognized by the American Board of Medical Specialties. Other qualifications for the surgeon are listed in the accreditation section of this chapter, as are the office-based surgery facility standards. Additionally, the facility should be certified to participate in the Medicare program in accordance with Title XVIII.

Patient selection advisory

Preoperative history and physical examination

Appropriate patient selection starts on the preoperative visit. A thorough preoperative history and physical examination allows the medical staff to select the appropriate time and facility for the patient's procedure. Also, it should identify risk factors and establish baseline preoperative values that will be used by the staff when caring for the patient intra- and postoperatively.

A vital part of patient selection is the ability to identify comorbidities preoperatively, which may affect the procedure planned or increase the incidence of intra- or postoperative complications for the patient. The preoperative history and physical examination should include age and body mass index (BMI) determination and careful questioning and examination of the cardiac and pulmonary systems. Additionally, a history of diabetes mellitus or risk factors for thromboembolism should be ascertained preoperatively. It is not uncommon for significant comorbidities to be discovered in the preoperative period that warrant further investigation by medical specialists.

Patients over the age of sixty, those considered severely obese (with a BMI >35), or those suspected of having obstructive sleep apnea (OSA) are at increased risk for intra- and postoperative complications. Because of this, some of these patients should not have their surgery performed outside the hospital setting. Those patients over the age of sixty are at increased risk for cardiac events, other complications, and unanticipated admissions. They can have their procedure at an office-based setting, but this determination depends on a multitude of factors, such as type of procedure planned, anticipated length of surgery, and availability of equipment for intra- and postoperative monitoring. However, it is strongly advised by the ASPS task force

Table 20.9 ASA physical status classification system

ASA Physical Status 1 – a normal healthy patient

ASA Physical Status 2 – a patient with mild systemic disease

ASA Physical Status 3 – a patient with severe systemic disease

ASA Physical Status 4 – a patient with severe systemic disease that is a constant threat to life

that patients with a BMI >35 have their procedure performed in a hospital.

Patients with OSA can be extremely challenging intra- and postoperatively, and because of this, certain factors should be weighed preoperatively. The factors include, but are not limited to, severity of their sleep apnea, presence of other comorbidities, type of surgery, type of anesthesia, need for postoperative narcotics, and resources of the office-based facility. These patients may need an extended postoperative recovery time, sophisticated respiratory care, or extensive postoperative pain management. Obviously, these needs are met most easily in a hospital. For those patients without a diagnosis of OSA, careful questioning of them and family members should take place preoperatively. A history of loud and frequent snoring, airway obstruction during sleep, daytime somnolence, or falling asleep in a nonstimulating environment should raise suspicion for OSA. These patients warrant further investigation before proceeding with surgery.

Preoperative tests

After a preoperative history and physical examination and consideration for the procedure planned, preoperative testing may be warranted. Common preoperative tests include a complete blood count (CBC), basic metabolic profile, and an ECG. The ECG is needed for anyone over 45 years of age or patients of any age with known cardiac disease. Baseline labs are needed for evaluation of patients diagnosed with diabetes mellitus, anemia, and hypertension. Patients taking certain medications, such as diuretics, should have preoperative lab evaluation. Lastly, the procedure being performed may dictate lab evaluation to establish baseline values.

The ASA physical classification

Once the preoperative physical examination, history, and test results are completed, the patient should be

assigned an ASA code. Table 20.9 lists the ASA physical classification system. Patients classified as ASA physical status 1 or 2 are the best candidates for office-based surgery. Patients classified as ASA physical status 3 can have their procedure performed in the office-based facility if the surgery can be performed using local anesthesia with or without sedation. Patients classified as ASA physical status 4 can have their procedure in an office-based surgery facility if the surgery can be performed using local anesthesia only.

Pain management and prevention of postoperative nausea and vomiting advisory

Two frequent reasons for postoperative hospital admission, after office-based surgery, are failure to control postoperative pain or nausea and vomiting. Therefore, prevention of these two factors is vitally important to physicians treating patients in the office-based facility. This advisory offers suggestions that should lessen the incidence of these issues.

Prevention and treatment of these disorders starts preoperatively. A thorough preoperative history will uncover factors such as: a history of motion sickness, previous postsurgical nausea and vomiting, or allergies and/or reactions to certain analgesics. Patients with a prior history of motion sickness or postoperative nausea and vomiting require a multimodal pharmacologic plan for prevention. Also, an adequate explanation of pain management and postoperative pain management expectations allows the patient to understand the process better, which decreases postoperative anxiety. Lastly, patients are frequently fearful of becoming addicted to postoperative narcotics. Because of this, they should be counseled on the appropriate need and use of postoperative narcotics.

Successful intraoperative management starts with efficient and atraumatic surgical technique. The use of local anesthetic either locally infiltrated by the surgeon or as a regional technique by the anesthesiologist can reduce postoperative pain. Avoidance of fentanyl and nitrous oxide decreases the incidence of postoperative nausea and vomiting, especially in patients with a history of motion sickness or nausea and vomiting. The use of NSAIDs reduces the need for narcotics and helps avoid their side effects.

Postoperative pain and nausea and vomiting are treated quickest with intravenous medications. When NSAIDs are combined with narcotics, they reduce unexpected postoperative pain admission and expedite discharge. Home management of pain and postoperative nausea and vomiting must be discussed with the patient and a capable adult before discharge.

Liposuction advisory

Liposuction is a procedure commonly performed by plastic surgeons. However, the ASPS task force acknowledges that little scientific information exists concerning patient safety issues for individuals undergoing liposuction. The purpose of this advisory is to provide an overview of techniques, practices, and management strategies thought to improve and insure patient safety.

Techniques

Multiple liposuction techniques were discussed in this advisory. No single technique was considered best or applicable for all patients undergoing liposuction. However, some general recommendations were made by the task force. Factors such as the patient's coexisting diseases, BMI, anticipated volume aspirated, and number of sites used for aspiration must be considered by the surgeon when crafting a surgical plan.

The "dry" technique, which involves inserting the catheter into the subcutaneous fat and applying suction, creates considerable edema, bruising, and blood loss. Owing to the amount of blood loss that occurs with this technique, the task force recommends this technique only for surgeries with an anticipated aspirate volume of 100 cc or less. Furthermore, the dry technique should never be used with ultrasound-assisted liposuction, which alone can cause collateral tissue damage and blood loss.

As noted above concerning the liposuction technique, there is, also, no liposuction cannula that best fits every patient regardless of liposuction technique. The cannula should be matched to a multitude of factors, which include but are not limited to: liposuction technique; site of planned liposuction; anticipated volume of aspirate; number of sites; and health of the patient involved. Liposuction technique varies, as do the cannulas used with each technique. Surgeon preference, based on experience, may influence selection.

Infiltrate solutions

Various substances are injected into the subcutaneous fat. Local anesthetics are used to produce preemptive and postoperative pain relief, whereas epinephrine is added to produce vasoconstriction, which promotes hemostasis and reduces systemic absorption of local anesthetics. Although various local anesthetics (lidocaine, bupivacaine, and prilocaine) have been used, none have proven more beneficial than lidocaine. When a solution containing epinephrine is used, lidocaine may be utilized in doses up to 35 mg/kg (ideal body weight). This dose is not advisable for patients with low protein levels or patients whose medical conditions render them incapable of handling the metabolites of lidocaine. In these patients, the dose of lidocaine should be reduced. Lidocaine is not needed if general or regional anesthesia is employed.

Epinephrine can be used safely in liposuction solutions. The infiltrate solutions vary in dosage from 1:100 000 to 1:1 000 000 based on the liposuction technique, volume of infiltrate, and type of alkalinized fluid utilized in the infiltrate. Epinephrine doses should not exceed 0.07 mg/kg. In patients with pheochromocytoma, hyperthyroidism, severe hypertension, cardiac disease, peripheral vascular disease, or cardiac arrhythmias its use should be avoided.

Management

Anticipated liposuction aspirate volume is a point of consideration before selecting a facility for the procedure. When an aspirate volume greater than 5000 cc is anticipated, the patient should have their procedure performed in either an acute care hospital or in an accredited or licensed facility. Their urine output and vital sign should be monitored overnight in an appropriate facility by competent and knowledgeable staff familiar with postoperative liposuction care. In certain patient populations, it may be prudent to have procedures done serially and not as multiple procedures on the same day.

Fluid management is dependent upon multiple factors. An accurate charting of the patient's preoperative fluid deficit, along with intake and output should follow the patient through their perioperative experience. In large aspirate cases preoperative and postoperative hemoglobins are drawn to follow blood loss. However, it may take 24 h for the patient's hemoglobin to equilibrate postoperatively. For patients with less than 5000 cc of aspirate, the task force recommends maintenance fluid replacement plus subcutaneous infiltrate volume. For those having greater than 5000 cc of aspirate, they should receive 0.25 cc of intravenous fluid for each milliliter of aspirate plus maintenance and subcutaneous infiltrate volume

Office-based dental procedures

Office-based procedures have been the mainstay of dentists for many years. Because of this, the practice of dentistry has had involvement with the administration of sedation and general anesthesia. In the 1840s, nitrous oxide was first used by the Hartford dentist Horace Wells. His student, William Morton, revolutionized surgery by unveiling the anesthetic capabilities of ether. Today dentistry continues to build on this rich foundation. The American Dental Association has multiple venues where dentists can train to become knowledgeable and adept at the delivery of sedation and/or general anesthesia.

Dentistry realized the need for specialization training in anesthesiology many years ago. A large number of the patients presenting for procedures were either pediatric or physically and/or mentally challenged. These patients traditionally had trouble accessing the standard hospital OR. Today dental anesthesiologists provide anesthetic services for a multitude of patients undergoing dental procedures. They undergo 2 years of postdoctoral anesthesiology training at one of eight recognized training programs in North America. During their training, the majority of their training time is spent in hospital OR anesthesiology rotations. Additionally, they spend the remainder of their time in ambulatory centers caring for medical and dental patients undergoing various procedures. They have an ongoing dialogue with the ASA and share their views concerning delivery of anesthesia and sedation in the office-based facility.

Suggested reading

American Academy of Pediatric Dentistry. Guideline on behavior guidance for the pediatric dental patient. *Pediatr Dent* 2008; **30**(suppl): 125–33.

American Academy of Pediatrics, American Academy of Pediatric Dentistry. Guideline for monitoring and management of pediatric patients during and after sedation for diagnostic and therapeutic procedures. *Pediatr Dent* 2008; **30**(suppl): 143–59.

American Dental Association. Policy statement: The use of conscious sedation, deep sedation, and general anesthesia in dentistry. 2005. Available at: www.ada.org/prof/resources/positions/statements/useof.asp (last accessed October 30, 2011).

American Dental Association. Guidelines for the use of conscious sedation, deep sedation, and general anesthesia for dentists. 2005. Available at: www.ada.org/prof/resources/positions/statements/anesthesia_guidelines.pdf (last accessed November 3, 2011).

American Society of Anesthesiologists. Guidelines for ambulatory anesthesia and surgery. 2003. Available at: www.asahq.org/publicationsAndServices/standards/04.pdf (last accessed November 3, 2011).

American Society of Anesthesiologists. Guidelines for office-based anesthesia. 2004. Available at: www.asahq.org/publicationsAndServices/standards/12.pdf (last accessed October 25, 2011).

American Society of Anesthesiologists. *Office-Based Anesthesia: Considerations for Anesthesiologists in Setting Up and Maintaining a Safe Office Anesthesia Environment,* 2nd edn. 2008.

American Society of Anesthesiologists. ASA physical status classification system. Available at: www.asahq.org/clinical/physicalstatus.htm (last accessed May 10, 2012).

P. C. Haeck, J. A. Swanson, R. E. Iverson, *et al.* Evidence-based patient safety advisory: patient selection and procedures in ambulatory surgery. *Plast Reconstr Surg* 2009; **124**(4 Suppl): 6S-27S.

R. E. Iverson, ASPS Task Force on Patient Safety in Office based Surgery Facilities. Patient safety in office-based surgery facilities: I. Procedures in the office-based surgery setting. *Plast Reconst. Surg* 2002; **110**: 1337.

R. E. Iverson, D. J. Lynch, ASPS Task Force on Patient Safety in Office-based Surgery Facilities. patient safety in office-based surgery facilities: II. Patient selection. *Plast Reconst. Surg.* 2002; **110**: 1785.

R. E. Iverson, D. J. Lynch, the ASPS Committee on Patient Safety. Practice Advisory on Liposuction. *Plast Reconstr Surg* 2004; **113**: 1478–90.

R. E. Iverson, D. J. Lynch, ASPS Committee on Patient Safety. Practice advisory on pain management and prevention of postoperative nausea and vomiting. *Plast Reconstr Surg* 2006; **118**: 1060–9.

D. Nick, L. Thompson, D. Anderson, L Trapp. The use of general anesthesia to facilitate dental treatment. *Gen Dent* 2003; **51**: 464–8.

S. Wilson. Pharmacologic behavior management for pediatric dental treatment. *Pediatr Clinic North Am* 2000; **47**: 1159–73.

Chapter

21

The future of perioperative medicine

Michael R. Hicks MD, MBA, MS, FACHE
Laurie Saletnik RN, DNP

Introduction 216
The perioperative system 217
Current system 217
System theory research 217
Blurring of specialty lines 218

Technology 219
Telemedicine 219
Implications of payment reform 220
Summary 220

Introduction

Historically, the surgical patient has received care as if moving down a conveyor belt, much like a manufactured product in a quasi made-to-order industrial factory. Initial referrals by primary care providers to surgeons, decisions for referrals for imaging, labs, medical screening and preparation, scheduling and facility registration, the procedure itself, and post-operative pain management and rehabilitation are all essentially treated as separate stations along the surgical assembly line. This segmentation, while meeting the needs of the staff of each station, produces an overall experience that is inadequate for its intended purpose, wasteful of resources, and confusing to patients and their family members. Modern management science that has addressed these issues in other industries has been slow to be embraced by the health-care system. Fortunately, increasing numbers of clinicians and administrators are adding management expertise and experience to their clinical abilities. Clinicians are in an ideal position to best understand the clinical and financial needs of direct care provision and must have a voice in the decision-making process. A collaborative team with an extensive skill set is essential for the changes necessary as health-care evolves. This chapter explores integrative options for the future for improving or redesigning the surgical patient experience.

As in nearly all aspects of US health care, the perioperative system's structure has been driven by the volume-based fee-for-service payment system. Since payment has been directed at what one actually does to the patient instead of on the total process itself, it is not surprising that little attention has been given to the system as a whole. In addition, the culture of US medicine has been for a physician to care for a patient's needs. While those of us working in the area of perioperative medicine are somewhat familiar with a team-based approach inside the operating room (OR), once outside this environment the degree and extent of collaboration begins to decline markedly. Unfortunately, the trend for increasing levels of subspecialization across both medicine and nursing has made it rare for a patient's care to be coordinated across all areas. This is certainly true for the perioperative experience.

Similarly, the current reimbursement system – and its attendant system of incentives, intended or not – is responsible for the lack of anesthesiologist involvement in the care of the surgical patient at points temporally distant from the actual surgical procedure and the OR. As a result, perioperative management of patients outside the actual anesthetic itself has been largely provided by physicians and nurses who are compensated in ways that anesthesiologists are not (for example, physician evaluation and management codes as opposed to American Society of Anesthesiologists (ASA) base units plus time) or who have differing skill sets, training, and intellectual interests from those of anesthesiologists.

Limited access to patient information before the day of surgery has also presented a challenge and created a greater reliance on integrated electronic records to insure adequate, patient-specific planning and preparation has taken place.

The perioperative system

A discussion of the future of perioperative medicine requires the exploration of many subtexts for completeness. Clinicians tend to focus on the delivery and quality of clinical care that they provide while devoting minimal attention to basic throughput measures such as frequency of unnecessary testing, case cancellation rates, and OR start and turnover times, as well as basic customer satisfaction. Although vitally important, however, these topics are only part of an overall system of perioperative care. A focus on our own individual aspects of the process will not result in the changes that are required – rather, a collaborative team working together on each step of patient care delivery is essential. A more holistic approach to the analysis and management of the perioperative delivery system is needed if we are to truly meet the expectations of consumers and payers for increased quality, safety, efficiency, and effectiveness. Understanding clinical delivery as a system and thinking strategically, beyond the individual successes, will lead to more sustained programmatic success. Most importantly, from a patient satisfaction perspective our current model, with its heavily siloed approach does not place patients where they rightfully belong, at the center of the delivery system. Moving toward patient-centered care will refocus our efforts and assure that we are individualizing our care by incorporating each patient's values, preferences, and decisions.

At its basic level the care of the surgical patient consists of a collection of processes and interconnected components (subsystems) that act with and upon a patient desiring a surgical solution to a health issue (the input) to produce a satisfied patient, who is ideally returned back to the postsurgical environment in the best possible health status at the most economical cost (the output).

Largely because of the reimbursement system and its inherent incentives, both explicit as well as implicit, perioperative clinicians and managers have focused upon optimizing their own particular subsystems (e.g.,

preoperative testing, admitting, preoperative holding, the OR, postanesthesia care unit [PACU], etc.) and have given minimal thought to how these subsystems interact with each other, particularly from the perspective of the patient. The resulting effect of this, called suboptimization in systems theory [1], is that the system is designed to maximize the efficiency for those providing care in the various silos and not for improving the patient experience or enhancing the system's performance or value.

Current system

In the case of planning for surgery, activities are scheduled for the convenience of the surgeon, other consultants, the preoperative clinic (if one exists), and finally time availability in an OR – again, usually around the schedule of the surgeon. In this model each provider segment can and frequently does optimize workflow for its own self-benefit. Issues such as office and clinic hours, staff compensation including overtime, and equipment availability all require consideration. While resource constraints are real issues in all systems [2], this approach unfortunately makes little sense for patients in terms of ease of use or clarity of purpose. Likewise, insurers and employers paying for the services often subsidize inefficiencies at a system level that result from this desire to achieve optimization at the subsystem level. When viewed as a whole, this approach to managing the perioperative system is generally inefficient and results in decreased satisfaction, wasted efforts, decreased quality, increased risk, ineffective use of resources, and increased cost at the macro level. As resources continue to shrink, appropriate and efficient utilization become more critical.

System theory research

Fortunately, more perioperative medicine clinicians are gaining knowledge and experience in operations management and system theory. Familiarity with the work of Shewhart and Deming in quality improvement and statistical process control is allowing many health-care organizations to improve their processes in substantial and significant ways [3,4]. Tools such as Lean, Six Sigma, Continuous Quality Improvement, Toyota Production System, and Statistical Process Control that have driven advances in other industries are now proving their value in the health-care environment. Examples of this in health care are now increasingly common and the evidence is more than suggestive that sound clinical care is the result of a well-managed perioperative process [5].

Blurring of specialty lines

A primary issue as the field of perioperative medicine evolves is the question of how care is actually provided, by whom, and with what level of coordination. Historically, surgeons have been responsible for directing the preoperative and postoperative care, either directly or through consultation, and anesthesiologists and certified registered nurse anesthetists (CRNAs) have controlled the process from the time immediately prior to the surgical procedure through the PACU experience or admission to a critical care unit. Even here, however, there has been great disparity as to the role of the anesthesia providers' involvement after leaving the OR, despite long-standing suggestions that anesthesiologists will play a bigger role in perioperative care [6].

However, other than the anesthetic care itself, the bulk of patient care is actually delivered by nurses that have assumed specialized roles throughout the system. According to the Institute of Medicine report on the Future of Nursing, as health-care reform brings more people into the health-care system, it needs to bring to bear all of the high-quality practitioners available [7]. Nurses are the largest component of the health-care workforce. They spend the most time with patients, making them an essential partner in transforming the way that Americans receive health care. Nurses will require new competencies to deliver high-quality care such as leadership, health policy, system improvement, research and evidenced-based practice, teamwork, and collaboration. Nurses, as well as staff in other disciplines, should be given the opportunity to further develop their leadership skills and competencies. It is important to focus on making sure nurses have multiple pathways to advanced degrees that are affordable and accessible. Having enough nurses with the right kind of skills will contribute to the overall safety and quality of a transformed health-care system. Currently business and management training for nurses and others are acquired on the job. A more educated workforce would be better equipped to meet the demands of an evolving health-care system. Focus should expand beyond those in system leadership positions and include many additional clinicians who are managing programs and service lines on a daily basis.

As clinical care progresses, clinicians themselves must adapt by changing their skill sets to meet the demands. Clinical leaders will need to expand their skill sets in order to help manage the operations and set the future strategic agenda. At the same time, assuring that the workload is delegated to the appropriate level of health-care worker will be required to assure that the demands can be met. *Training must be transformed to include the multidisciplinary team and to incorporate simulation experiences.*

Preoperatively, there has been reluctance for anesthesiologists to engage in the care of the patient. As previously mentioned, one of the key drivers of this reticence is the way anesthesia providers are currently compensated. In addition, fears of malpractice litigation as well as concerns about the adequacy of anesthesia training vis-à-vis the handling of chronic medical conditions have also contributed to the lack of anesthesiologist involvement in patient preparation.

Not surprisingly, other medical and nursing specialties have begun to fill the void that anesthesia providers have ignored. Emergency medicine physicians, gastroenterologists, and registered nurses now perform sedation analgesia, which was previously the domain of anesthesia professionals. Even more striking is the degree of similarity between the care offered in intensive care units by critical care nurses working under the direction of intensivists and the care delivered in the OR by anesthesiologists and CRNAs. In many respects the care provided, and the physical effect on the patient, is indistinguishable from that offered in the OR except for the training of the provider and the location in which it is offered.

Aside from the actual administration of anesthetic and sedation agents, primary care providers, especially hospital medicine specialists, now play a major role in the care of perioperative patients. The Society of Hospital Medicine, for example, now offers educational programming to address the role played by hospitalists in caring for surgical patients. In addition, primary care physicians have developed novel approaches to the care of the surgical patient [8]. Several well-known health-care systems, such as the Cleveland Clinic with its Internal Medicine Preoperative Assessment Consultation and Treatment Center (IMPACT Center), have formal preoperative clinics that are managed and staffed by hospitalists. Likewise, hospitalists now increasingly "co-manage" surgical patients along with the surgeons. This type of collaborative approach allows surgeons to focus on surgical issues while hospitalists and, to a lesser extent anesthesiologists, manage medical issues, the patient's transition through the hospital experience, postoperative pain control, and the nonsurgical discharge planning and follow-up [9,10].

Management of the OR will continue to require clear structure, strong leadership, and interdisciplinary communication and collaboration. This often means negotiating between competing agendas of clinicians and the institution. The growing list of quality and regulatory expectations demands constant oversight and engagement of the key stakeholders. Provision of accurate data, received in a timely manner, will allow for appropriate data analysis so that evaluating progress and changing course when necessary can be done in real time.

Technology

The future evolution of perioperative medicine depends on developing and enhancing collaborative care. For this to reach its maximum potential, collaborative care requires an integrated health information management system capable of deliverable pertinent, accurate, and actionable information so that appropriate clinical and process decisions can be made. Decision-support systems, both clinical and managerial, allow decision makers to collect and analyze data in real time and make meaningful interventions to enhance care, safety, and throughput. An important component of this will be the ability to monitor outcomes on a clinical level, thus allowing the appropriate use of the immediate feedback needed in a robust continuous quality improvement process. In addition, health information management systems must promote adherence to evidence-based treatment protocols by providing relevant information for clinical decision making and the ability to track deviances from the protocols as well as clinical outcomes.

Nurses should be engaged to work with developers and manufacturers in design, development, purchase, implementation, and evaluation of medical and health devices and health IT products. Sharing clinical expertise and outlining current challenges during the design phase of development assures a more relevant product that meets the needs of patients and health-care providers. The health-care evolution and constantly changing technology will require nurses and others to commit to lifelong learning. As the complexity of the technology increases, other specialized roles may be added to support the environment and the multidisciplinary team.

Telemedicine

Perioperative medicine, much like medical and nursing practice as a whole, is replete with treatment practices of questionable value that are based on personal anecdote and not on formal controlled clinical studies. Widespread adoption of electronic health records as part of wholesale adoption of health information technology initiatives will illuminate some of the variability in perioperative practices as well as remove some of the mystique that accompanies the surgical patient's passage through the OR.

Most importantly, advances in telemedicine capabilities that are already being utilized in areas such as enhanced intensive care units and field medicine in the military and combined with telemetric sensor capabilities currently under development will probably transform the way anesthesia services are delivered. When viewed in the context of projecting knowledge and experience over a distance, telemedicine will radically change the entire specialty of anesthesiology by allowing fewer anesthesiologists to provide more care to more patients over larger geographic areas.

Indeed, only the physical or technical component of anesthesia administration requires the actual presence of a caregiver with the patient. The cognitive or intellectual component, with the appropriate technology, can be provided from practically anywhere in the world. There are several potentially striking aspects of the ability to place-shift expertise across the continuum. First, it could lead to the use of nontraditional caregivers to physically provide the care heretofore requiring the presence of an anesthesiologist or CRNA. This could serve to mitigate the feared shortage of anesthesiologists that has long been predicted [11].

Second, patient care that currently requires transfer to facilities offering more specialized or sophisticated care may be unnecessary as long as someone on site has the capability to perform relatively routine functions such as vascular access placement and airway control. For example, most emergency medicine physicians have the requisite skill set to establish a controlled airway and place invasive monitoring lines. The expertise of a critical care physician such as an anesthesiologist at some distant site could provide the necessary fund of knowledge and experience to direct the patient care and remove the need for transfer.

Third, advances in surgical technology, when combined with the continuing advances in pharmacology and monitoring, will accelerate the existing outmigration of procedures to physician offices. This will redefine the nature of surgery and perioperative medicine not only in terms of location but also in terms of the skill set needed to provide safe care. This migration will continue to challenge the historical reticence for anesthesia providers to leave the safety of the traditional OR and may result in other types of providers assuming the responsibility for providing this care.

Finally, much of the routine care of the postoperative patient, using existing telemetric capabilities, can be shifted out of the acute care hospital setting to environments that are more patient and family friendly as well as potentially less problematic from a risk perspective. Many aspects of the preoperative experience can be performed over a distance with the widespread availability of broadband Internet [12]. This may lead to a higher acceptance rate among patients and surgeons of the value of preoperative anesthesia consultation by the elimination of an additional clinic or office visit.

Implications of payment reform

Finally, many policy makers predict the decline of fee-for-service medicine, if not its elimination completely. Coupled with the dissociation of consumers from the actual payment for health care and the moral hazard issues of higher proportions of Americans having health coverage under the Affordable Care Act, it is unlikely that the current health-care financial system will remain financially viable. Furthermore, the current system of reimbursement encourages higher resource consumption. The effect of health-care reform and increased insurance coverage on the utilization rate of surgical procedures remains to be seen. However, changes in payment methodologies are already under way. The most likely mechanisms to date are payments for episodes of care or other payment bundling programs, in which a total payment is issued for a procedure and all related care. This payment must be adequate to cover all costs and be inclusive of all services.

This type of reimbursement system will demand a perioperative medicine program that is streamlined, efficient, cost-effective, and quantifiable. Classic business concepts such as strategic and financial planning as well as return on investment analysis will be required skills. Currently, expertise in these areas is still largely lacking in health-care management [13]. However, this deficiency offers opportunities for current leaders in perioperative medicine to provide creative and constructive solutions for the future. Organizational

commitment, both in terms of time and financial support, to the development and refinement of these skills will assure sustainable progress toward the future of the health-care environment.

Summary

As health care becomes more patient centered with greater emphasis on, and reimbursement for, an episode of care rather than individual services, a new skill set as well as updated tools to enhance decision making will be required. This transformation does not stop at the OR doors, but rather encompasses the perioperative environment. Appropriate decisions regarding resource acquisition and allocations, including individual members of the health-care team, will become even more critical to assure quality health care is delivered. This will require engagement and development of not only the multidisciplinary leadership team, but inclusive of front-line clinicians. A more holistic approach to the analysis and management of the perioperative delivery system with broader collaboration, extending beyond the immediate care setting, is what will be required of future leaders. Investment in these health-care team members will assure a successful transformation to meet the requirements for the future of health care.

References

1. B. Ronen, J. S. Pliskin, S. Pass. *Focused Operations Management for Health Services Organizations*. Jossey-Bass, 2006.

2. E. Goldratt, J. Cox. *The Goal: A Process of Ongoing Improvement*. Gower Pub Co, 1996.

3. W. A. Shewhart. Economic Control of Quality of Manufactured Product. American Society for Quality Control, 1980.

4. W. E. Deming. *Out of the Crisis*. The MIT Press, 2000.

5. J. Toussaint. *On the Mend: Revolutionizing Healthcare to Save Lives and Transform the Industry*. Lean Enterprise Institute, Inc., 2010.

6. P. Rock. The future of anesthesiology is perioperative medicine. *Anesthesiol Clin North America*. 2000; **18**: 495–513.

7. IOM (Institute of Medicine). *The Future of Nursing: Leading Change, Advancing Health*. Washington, DC: The National Academies Press, 2011.

8. D. G. Silverman, S. H. Rosenbaum. Integrated assessment and consultation for the preoperative patient. *Anesthesiol Clin* 2009; **27**: 617–31.

9. M. Magallanes. The perioperative medicine service: an innovative practice at Kaiser Bellflower Medical Center. *The Permanente Journal*. 2002; **6**: 13–16.

10. K. Hinami, C. T. Whelan, R. T. Konetzka, D. O. Meltzer. Provider expectations and experiences of comanagement. *J Hosp Med* 2011; **6**: 401–4.

11. L. Daugherty, R. Fonseca, K. B. Kumar, P. C. Michaud. *An Analysis of the Labor Markets for Anesthesiology*. Santa monica, California: RAND Corporation, 2010.

12. J. A. Galvez, M. A. Rehman. Telemedicine in anesthesia: an update. *Curr Opin Anaesthesiol* 2011; **24**: 459–62.

13. P. H. Song, J. Robbins, A. N. Garman, A. S. McAlearney. High-performance work systems in health care, Part 3: The role of the business case. *Health Care Manage Rev* 2012; **37**: 110–21.

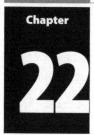

Chapter

22

Nursing
Organizational structure, staffing, resource management, metrics, and infection control

Melissa Guidry RN, MPH, CNOR
Lesley Bourlet RN, MSN, CNOR

Organizational structure and design   222
Perioperative staffing model   222
Resource management   223
Operating room finance – operational budget and capital budget   225

Efficiency metrics   226
Sterilization   230
Infection control   232
Summary   234

Organizational structure and design

Hospitals can be very different – building structure, patient care delivered, organizational structure, control, and ownership. Based on these differences, the operating room (OR) team must understand their roles and responsibilities within the department.

To provide structure within the department, policies and procedures must be developed to support a safe environment for the care of each individual patient and provide guidelines for nursing practice. The Association of periOperative Registered Nurses (AORN) publishes the Perioperative Standards and Recommended Practices to be used as a guide for ORs and the Joint Commission also publishes standards. These standard statements and recommended practices describe the registered nurses' responsibilities within the perioperative setting. They serve as a base for maximizing patient outcomes and represent an optimal level of practice. However, specific policies and procedures must be written for each recommended practice and available for use within the practice settings. Developing policies requires collaboration with the appropriate clinical disciplines or administrative groups and must include current scientific knowledge and consideration of ethical and legal concerns and

utilize findings from quality improvement and assessment activities. Figure 22.1 gives an overview of the table of contents to consider what policies and procedures are needed for an individual facility. Another publication providing resource materials for OR management and development of policies and procedures comes from the Association for Professionals in Infection Control and Epidemiology (APIC), which develops standards of practice to promote patient safety. Before developing departmental structure, one must refer to one's own facility manuals to eliminate duplication and streamline information.

Perioperative staffing model

The AORN is considered the go-to resource for information and guidance. Perioperative staffing guidelines have been developed to accommodate safe patient care and promote a safe work environment. The first point of order is to develop operating rules and regulations. These rules must define the number of allocated rooms to be staffed and the hours required to provide the service. The writing of these rules and regulations must be done in collaboration with the anesthesia department. The AORN has written recommendations for staffing. These can be used as a guide for determining the number of full-time equivalents (FTEs). Several pieces

Operating Room Leadership and Management, ed. Kaye A.D., Fox C.J. and Urman R.D. Published by Cambridge University Press. © Cambridge University Press 2012.

Introduction
AORN Vision, Mission, and Values
Section I: Standards of Perioperative Nursing
  practice
Section II: Recommended Practices for
  Perioperative Nursing

  Recommended Practices for....
    Aseptic Practice
      Attire, Surgical
      Hand Hygiene
      Maintaining a Sterile Field
      Traffic Patterns
    Equipment and Product Safety
      Electrosurgery
      Gowns and Drapes – Selection
        and use
      Laser Safety in practice Settings
      Minimally Invasive Surgery
      Pneumatic Tourniquet
      Product Selection
      Surgical Tissue Banking
    Patient and Worker Safety
      Environment of Care
      Environmental Cleaning
      Reducing Radiological Exposure
      Retained Surgical Items – Prevention
        of Specimen Care and Handling
      Transmissible Infections, Prevention of
        Patient Care
      Documentation of Perioperative Nursing
        Care
      Hypothermia, Prevention of
      Local Anesthesia, managing the Patient
        Receiving
      Moderate Sedation/Analgesia, Managing
        the Patient Receiving
      Positioning the Patient
      Preoperative Patient Skin Antisepsis
      Transfer of Patient Care Information

Sterilization and Disinfection
  Anesthesia Equipment – Cleaning, Handling,
    and Processing
  Disinfection, High-Level
  Flexible Endoscopes – Cleaning and Processing
  Instruments and Powered Equipment –
    Cleaning and Care of
  Packaging Systems – Selection and Use
  Sterilization

Section III: Guidelines and Guidance Statements
Do-Not-Use Abbreviations
Environmental Responsbility
Health Care Industry Representative – Role of the
Implanted Electronic Device – Care of the
  Perioperative Patient With an
Latex Guidelines
Malignant Hyperthermia Guidelines
Patient Safety Culture – Creating a
Perioperative Staffing
Postoperative Patient Care in the Ambulatory
  Surgery Setting
Preoperative Patient Care in the Ambulatory
  Surgery Setting
Safe Medication Practices
Safe On-Call Practices
Safe Patient Handling and Movement
Sharps Injury Prevention
Single-use Devices – Reuse of
Venous Stasis – Prevention of
Section IV: Additional Resources
Appendix A: Listing of AORN Position Statements
Appendix B: Policy and Procedure Template for Use
  with Recommended Practices
Appendix C: AACD Procedural Times Glossary
Appendix D: Standards for RN First Assistant
  Education Programs
Appendix E: Quality and Performance Improvement
  Standards
Index

Figure 22.1 Perioperative standards and recommended practices for inpatient and ambulatory settings – table of contents. Perioperative Standards and Recommended Practices: Published by AORN.

of information will be needed before completing this calculation, including number of rooms, benefit time, and indirect caregivers. A guide with example is shown in Figures 22.2 and 22.3. This can be used to develop FTE needs for any size of OR.

Resource management

To perform surgery in a safe, efficient, and economical manner, all necessary instruments, supplies, and equipment must be reliably brought together at the correct

AORN, Inc.

Revised July 1997

Formulas:

Step 1. # of Rooms multiplied by # of Hours per Day multiplied by # Days per Week = Total Hours to be Staffed per Week

Step 2. Total Hours to be Staffed per Week multiplied by # of People per Room = Total Working Hours per Week

Step 3. Total Working Hours per Week divided by 40 Hours = Basic FTE

Step 4. Calculate Benefit Relief

Step 5. Basic FTE multiplied by Benefit Hours/FTE/Year divided by 2080 Hours = Relief FTE

Step 6: Basic FTE added to Relief FTE = Total Minimum Direct Care Staff

NOTE 1: To determine the number of personnel per room:

1. If half of the procedures done in your OR require a third person, you will need to use a figure of 2.5 persons per room in computing your staffing needs.
2. If more or less than half of the procedures done in your OR require a third person, or if a percentage of procedures require a fourth person, the number of personnel per room will need to be adjusted accordingly.
3. In the following example, a figure of 2.5 persons per room is used.

NOTE 2: If your institution's FTE is greater or less than 2080 hours per year, this must be adjusted in the formula.

Direct Care Staff

* Personnel who are involved with "hands on" care of the surgical client. In the operating room this includes registered nurses, licensed practical nurses, and surgical technicians.
* The staffing policy for the operating room should state the minimum number of nursing personnel which will be provided for different types of surgical procedures. Complexity of the procedure may necessitate more than the minimum number of nursing personnel identified.

Indirect Care Staff

* Personnel who support the activities of the operating room. In the operating room this includes the director, the supervisor, the nurse manager, the charge nurse, the staff development instructor, secretaries, unit manager, aides, orderlies, and environmental service personnel if on your budget.
* Supervisory and educational personnel will vary according to work load.
* Indirect care staff will vary according to functions, but a rule of thumb is one indirect care giver to two direct care givers.

Benefit Hours

* Benefit hours are those hours such as vacation time, holiday time, available sick time (whether paid or unpaid), and any other time that personnel policies determine an employee might take off.
* In the operating room, benefit hours also include breaks and lunches unless the operating room ceases work production during those times.
* When relieving for lunch, it is necessary to add about 15 minutes to the allotted time at either end to allow for nurse-to-nurse reporting as to what has transpired during the procedure in progress. It may take less than seven minutes for one circulating nurse to report to her relief, but the relief of the scrubbed person must include the time needed to scrub, gown, and glove, so 15 minutes is average.
* When computing Benefit Relief for breaks and lunches, the amount of minutes is multiplied by 260 days (52 weeks multiplied by 5 days per week = 260 days).

Figure 22.2 Guidelines for computing OR staffing requirements. Perioperative Standards and Recommended Practices: Published by AORN.

time and place and must be available for case after case. Historically, the OR provides supplies and equipment specific to the operation and physician. With an ever-increasing emphasis on reducing the cost of providing health care, many ORs are working with surgeons to standardize instrument sets and supplies to help reduce the costs of procedures. Other factors known to influence the viability of the OR are the scheduling system, preference cards, inventory management, and budget development. The effective manager will utilize their knowledge of strategic planning to maximize resources and revenue for the department.

Preference cards

An ideal situation is to have scheduling, materials management, and perioperative computers linked to

```
13 rooms, Monday–Friday, 7a–3p,  13 × 8 × 5 = 520
6 rooms, Monday–Friday, 3p–7p,   6 × 4 × 5 = 120
1 room, Monday–Friday, 7p–11p   1 × 4 × 5 = 20
1 room, Monday–Friday, 11p–7a   1 × 8 × 4 = 40
Total hours per week                        = 700
```

Basic FTEs = 700 × 2.25 = 1575/40 = 39.38 basic FTEs

Note: 2.25 = 25% cases require additional personnel

Basic benefit/employee – varies by facility

```
Average vacation hours        = 184
Holiday hours                 = 56
Available sick hours          = 96
15 min break × 260 days/60    = 65
30 min lunch × 260 days/60    = 130
Total                         = 531
```

Relief FTEs = 39.38 × 531/2080 = 10.05 relief FTEs

Direct care givers = 39.38 + 10.05 = 49.43

Calculate indirect care givers – includes Director, Manager, Clinical Supervisor, Charge Nurse, OR Assistants, RN Holding, Video Tech, Scheduler, Secretary, etc. = 21.0 FTE

49.43 + 21.0 = 70.43 Total FTEs

Figure 22.3 An example of computing OR staffing requirements based on 13 rooms

a network that interfaces with the hospital's information system. This interface will provide support and the necessary backup for the information stored. The basis for building this system is the preference cards, which identify nursing plan, supplies, instrumentation, and equipment routinely needed for any type of procedure. The cards also list physician-specific information that can be used to capitalize on efficiencies during the procedure. The OR nurses and surgical technologists use the surgeon's preference card in their selection and preparation for their assigned case. It is imperative that they consult the preference cards to avoid forgetting an item vital to the operation.

Inventory

The OR has the highest inventory cost and may have as many as 30 000 items in stock, probably closely followed by the catheterization lab. Supply inventory is likely to be the second largest budget allocation after personnel. Inventory management is a massive responsibility and requires the efforts of an educated and knowledgeable

team to adhere to the organizational goals, to practice fiscal responsibility, and to meet the needs of the health-care team and the patients. Probably the greatest challenge for the OR management team is to run an efficient and low-cost OR without an absence of critical items at the time of surgery. However, these can be conflicting goals because low cost means reduced inventory, and never running out is most easily achieved with a large inventory. One mechanism for minimizing the size of the inventory is to standardize as much as possible. This means that the facility does not carry several different types of a particular item from different suppliers just to satisfy the personal preferences of various surgical staff. The advantages of standardization are that it will aid in pursuing additional discounts for the facility and that it decreases the amount of time spent on training nurses and technicians. Standardizations also aid the scheduling office by reducing the complexity of scheduling personnel who are knowledgeable of the equipment.

Operating room finance – operational budget and capital budget

Operational budget

The operational budget can be developed using two main methods: zero-based budgeting or a budgeting based on previous years. Zero-based budgeting is where a budget is built from scratch: you develop staffing, volume, supplies, equipment, implants, and any other item associated with the operations of the department, excluding capital expenditures. Many facilities build a budget based on the previous 6 or 9 months and annualize and project it throughout the following year. It is important to review the projections for any deviations and adjust prior to approval. Changing a budget already approved can be difficult, not easily controlled, and would need ongoing justification.

Capital budget

Operating rooms require a tremendous amount of expensive equipment. Individual facilities determine what is considered a capital purchase based on the cost of an item. Items costing greater than $500 can be considered capital. Capital equipment can be obtained through direct purchase or through capital and/or operating leases. A capital lease is an installment purchase, usually with a loan from the company. The facility must pay taxes and insurance costs, and generally has an option to purchase the equipment at the termination of the lease. With an operating lease, the equipment is obtained for a designated period of time, a monthly fee is paid, and the facility maintains and services the equipment. An operating lease is a viable option to be used when technology is changing or when evaluating new diagnostic or therapeutic technology. The facility's finance department can assist the OR management team when determining whether to purchase versus lease equipment. An example of cost differences in purchase versus leasing is shown in Table 22.1.

When developing a capital budget, consideration must be given to a plan for new technology based on the facility's strategic plan and also end-of-life replacement, which may be over a 5-year period. Each facility has an established decision-making process for capital equipment. A recommended process is completing a capital equipment request form. This request form should include priority (whether it is urgent, needed, or desired) and whether the request is for replacement of an item, an upgrade to existing equipment, or a new technology. The request should also state the reason for the request, how often the equipment will be used, and the impact on services. Other information listed on the request may include whether multiple departments can utilize the requested equipment and any training or other special requirements. Based on the type of equipment, operating costs (such as maintenance and disposables) will need to be included. If the request is for new technology, a pro forma may need to be completed based on the finance department's policies. The next step would be to prioritize the requests and submit to the OR Committee for review and decision prior to submitting to the senior leadership. Other valuable processes to use would be to meet with department chairs, discuss their individual departmental needs, prioritize the requests and have a capital oversee committee make the purchasing decision.

Developing an equipment replacement plan for the department is a vital step in a strategic planning process. The recommendation should be to establish a physical inventory of all equipment within the department. Clinical engineering services (BioMed) at each facility can assist with this list.

Efficiency metrics

First case starts

Operating room time is very expensive, and is one of the biggest revenue generators in the hospital. Improving

efficiency can be beneficial to all. To improve the first case starts in a surgery department, there are several other factors to consider and several steps that must be in place in order for that patient to roll into the OR suite on time.

The first step in the process is the scheduling of the procedure. This process may seem very simple, when in actuality it is very complex. The scheduler must be able to put the procedure in the appropriate room at the time that is being requested and also document any special requests that are being made for that particular procedure. The scheduler must also insure that the time that is being allotted for that procedure is appropriate, so that if there is a case to follow an accurate time can be given. Most schedulers use computers to book cases, which can be very helpful in predicting case time. Each surgeon's procedure will have cleanup and setup time built into it, which will provide an accurate average procedure time. The scheduler can also schedule the preop visit, which is also an important factor in starting the first case on time.

The preop visit consists of the patient being preadmitted to the hospital with consent to treat and bill being done at that time by the admitting department. The surgeon also sends preop orders for each individual patient to identify specific laboratory and other tests that are necessary. The preop visit can be done 5 to 30 days before the procedure to insure that all tests are done in an appropriate time frame. The preop nurse will do a head-to-toe assessment and take the patient's history. Anesthesia will do a comprehensive history and physical as well as consent the patient and order any additional labs or tests that would be necessary to put the patient to sleep safely. The preop visit can take anywhere from 2 to 8 h depending on what type of tests are ordered and any complications that may occur related to insurance. At this point there are several different departments that have been involved in the process of starting this procedure on time and we are still days away from the start time; any deviation at any point can cause a delay, which can be costly in a multitude of ways.

On the day of surgery, the patient is usually asked to arrive 1.5 to 2 h before the procedure start time. This allows the patient to be assessed for any history or physical changes that may have occurred since the preop visit, an IV to be started, and one last check to make sure all documents are on the chart and available to all. The surgeon will need to update any history and physical (H&P) that has been done prior to

Table 22.1 Comparison of purchasing versus leasing of equipment

A. Projected cost of purchasing item

Year	Principal	Interest @ 3.25%	Maintenance	Depreciation (useful life = 8 yrs)	Revenue	Allowable costs	Net cash flow	Cost of capital	Present value
1	40 000	5200	600	25 000	50 000	30 800	4200	0.95	3990
2	40 000	3900	600	25 000	50 000	29 500	5500	0.95	5225
3	40 000	2600	600	25 000	50 000	28 200	6800	0.95	6460
4	40 000	1300	600	25 000	50 000	26 900	8100	0.95	7695
5	40 000	0	600	25 000	50 000	25 600	9400	0.95	8930
Total	200 000	13 000	3000	125 000	250 000	141 000	34 000		32 300

B. Projected cost of leasing item

Year	Lease payment	Maintenance	Depreciation	Revenue	Allowable costs	Net cash flow	Present value
1	42 000	0	0	50 000	42 000	8000	8000
2	42 000			50 000	42 000	8000	8000
3	42 000			50 000	42 000	8000	8000
4	42 000			50 000	42 000	8000	8000
5	42 000			50 000	42 000	8000	8000
Total	210 000	0	0	250 000	210 000	40 000	40 000
	30 000	Buy-out option					10 000

the patient being admitted; this is because the patient has not been in his or her care and he or she must assess the patient for any history or physical changes that may have occurred. The consents are also verified with the patient for accuracy. The patient will have repeated checks for consent, H&P, lab work, additional tests that may have been ordered, and correct identification by every member of the perioperative team. At this point we have still not rolled the patient into the room; the OR team has to prepare for the actual procedure.

Ideally, the OR team will arrive 45 min to an hour prior to the time on the schedule. The team, in most cases, would have prepared and evaluated supplies and equipment the day before and then completed preparation on the morning of the procedure. The team will have organized and arranged the equipment and furniture, created and maintained a sterile field, and checked all appropriate implants and specialty items, if any, that were ordered for this patient. Anesthesia, the OR circulator, and surgical scrub will agree on readiness and when the surgeon is present they will then roll the patient into the OR suite.

The patient has finally made it into the OR. There are many factors that can prevent the patient from getting into the room on time, and most of these are out of the control of the OR staff. The following are factors that will affect rolling into the room on time:

1. the case has been scheduled at an incorrect time;
2. the H&P has not been dictated or transcribed;
3. the consent has not been completed, either for surgery or anesthesia;
4. the diagnostic test results are not on the chart;
5. the patient has not shown up or scheduled a preop appointment;
6. anesthesia has not prepared the patient;
7. abnormal results have not been reported that can potentially cancel the case;
8. equipment is unavailable or has failed;
9. the surgeon is late;
10. the OR team is late;
11. the equipment has not been prepared or supplies are not available.

There are many checks and balances along the way to insure that everything is in place so that the first case can start on time. Starting the first case on time will set the pace for the rest of the day and allow for a better chance to end the day on time, also making everyone happy: the surgeon finishes on time, the OR team goes

home on time, and the families are pleased because the plan of care is proceeding as expected. The first cases that do not start on time will lead to many being dissatisfied. Let us not leave out the fact that working less efficiently and leaving an OR suite vacant costs a great deal of money. In 1998 the Clinical Advisory Board reported that an outpatient procedure cost was $5.23 per minute. Today that cost has just about tripled and reimbursement has decreased at about the same rate as the increase, so it would be in the best interest of all to improve efficiency within the OR suite.

Turnaround time

Turnaround time can be a huge satisfier as well as a revenue enhancer if done efficiently. The same factors that can prevent the first cases from starting on time can also affect turnaround time. The term "turnaround time" can have different meanings depending on who you are. For the circulator and scrub in the OR it usually means the time it takes for one patient to roll out and another patient to roll in to the suite. The surgeon has a different perspective: to him or her it means the time between closing one patient and making an incision on the next patient. The anesthesia team views turnaround time as the time that one patient is rolled into the recovery area until the next patient receives his or her anesthetic induction. Turnaround time can be very complex, and a very busy time for all involved. A number of functions need to be completed during turnover time [1]:

- the room needs to be cleaned;
- the OR table needs to be set up with sterile equipment;
- the anesthesia equipment needs to be cleaned and restocked;
- the patient needs to be taken to the postanesthesia care unit (PACU)/intensive care unit (ICU), their vital signs need to be checked, and they need to be signed off to PACU nurse;
- medications need to be reconciled and new ones checked out;
- the next patient needs to be greeted (by the anesthesiologist and OR nurse);
- the preoperative assessment, including surgical and anesthesiology consent, surgical reassessment, review of plans, and site verification need to be done;
- intravenous lines/block need to be placed;
- the anesthesia equipment needs to be checked out.

From the list above, it should be apparent that turn-around time is dependent on many different factors. To improve or optimize OR availability by improving turnaround time we must develop a multidisciplinary team with clearly defined roles that will occur simultaneously. The team must first define the time on the schedule or at the start and the goal for room turnover. The team must next each define their process and agree upon methods to improve efficiencies. The team must develop an overlapping or parallel work flow in order to be successful with improving the overall turnaround time. The team must then put their processes in place and document their outcomes. The team should also set goals and all agree to be committed to the workflow process to improve turnaround time.

Block utilization

Block utilization allows surgeons or services to have secure time in the OR on certain days of the week. Block utilization must be consistently monitored for use. The surgery schedule and its accuracy can affect the entire organization, not just the OR; anesthesia services to other locations, the availability of hospital beds (either surgical or ICU), the productivity of the surgeons and anesthesiologists, and the marketability of available OR time can all be affected.

The OR schedule must be able to balance the needs of the surgeons, nursing, administration, and anesthesia, who all have a different interest in the efficiency and availability of the OR schedule. The surgery schedule can become out of balance by any of the following factors:

1. late surgeons;
2. high rate of add-on procedures;
3. extended preop;
4. gaps in the schedule;
5. increased demand to schedule first cases;
6. increased demand for two rooms with staggered starts and one surgeon;
7. lack of anesthesia coverage.

Nursing and anesthesia must work in unison to make block utilization of the schedule effective. There are also several components related to scheduling that must be in place. The first thing that must be incorporated into a schedule that utilizes blocks is some variable time to accommodate add-on cases that are emergent or urgent. The computer system should be able to estimate the time for a procedure accurately. This must also be monitored manually, because many factors that

can affect the time cannot be consistently captured by a computer. There must be policies and procedures in place for assessing blocks and reassigning block time. The policies and procedures must be supported by a strong surgery committee with a supportive chairman in order for the block utilization to be successful.

The policy regarding block utilization should contain certain elements that are clearly defined, as follows:

1. the actual block time in relation to the hours of the day;
2. the process for booking in a block;
3. how blocks are assigned and who assigns them;
4. utilization targets for maintaining blocks;
5. the mechanism for data collection and reporting of block utilization;
6. the process for release of a block;
7. the process for requesting a block.

It is important that all elements be understood by all using the OR scheduling system. There should also be a procedure for bumping a case on the OR schedule to accommodate emergency or urgent cases that cannot wait for the first available time slot.

In order for block utilization to be effective, it must constantly be monitored and maintained. The system is not flawless, but if utilized consistently and fairly it can be very helpful in managing utilization of the OR.

Open scheduling versus block scheduling

Traditionally, OR schedules were filled on a "first-come, first-served" basis that assumed any case could be performed in any room and that all anesthesiologists and nurses could handle the different surgeries equally well. Increasingly complex cases with specialized equipment and teams have led to a more organized system of assigning rooms to specific surgeons or services and guaranteeing them specific time slots. This allows specialized equipment to remain in designated ORs (e.g., cardiopulmonary bypass circuits, laparoscopic equipment/displays) and for specific teams to work in these areas consistently. Block scheduling smoothes the variability in OR case volume by giving greater predictability to surgeons when booking their cases. It also creates more accountability when evaluating case volume expectations and targets for the hospital, surgeons, nurses, and anesthesiologists. In general, blocks appear to work more efficiently when they are assigned to specific services rather than particular surgeons. Additionally, full-day blocks are preferable to partial-day blocks, because they eliminate the possibility of delayed starts for a second service as a result of preceding cases running longer than expected. Block booking may not work well in ORs with high numbers of emergent cases that disrupt the schedule; in such situations, open scheduling for one or more rooms may lead to higher OR utilization and patient satisfaction.

A key part of block scheduling is having specific rules in place that govern how OR time is allocated. *Release time* is defined as the number of hours before the scheduled time of surgery when a block of time must be either booked or released for use by others. Release times for specific services should reflect the nature of their cases. For example, cardiac surgery typically has very short release times because of the urgent nature of many of their cases, whereas plastic surgery has longer release times as their cases are almost exclusively elective [1].

Sterilization

There are numerous sterilization mechanisms used in the OR – steam, sterrad, steris, and limited availability of ethylene oxide. Steam sterilization can be flashed, gravity displaced, or pre-vacuumed. There is an expectation of any health-care facility to use a deliberate, thoughtful sterilization process that is clear and evidence-based. Any process used must be documented and monitored for completion of appropriate parameters.

Flash (just-in-time) sterilization is when the sterilization cycle has no dry time or a 1-min dry time, so the items are considered wet at the conclusion of the cycle and should be used immediately. No current benchmark exists for flash sterilization. This form of sterilization should not be done as a matter of convenience. It is the responsibility of the facility's leadership to insure adequate resources are provided for an effective sterilization process. Factors to remember when using this method of sterilization are decontamination of items, choice of correct parameters, documentation of cycle, and transfer of items to the sterile field. Managers must monitor how well flash sterilization documentation is being maintained. The AORN-recommended practices for sterilization state that flash sterilization documentation should include: item being processed; patient receiving item; cycle parameters used (e.g., temperature, duration of cycle, and the date and time the cycle is run); operator information; and reason for flash sterilization. Figure 22.4 shows an example of documenting a sterilization cycle when using a flash (JIT) sterilization method. This log can be used to trend what is being flashed and why. Utilization of these data can assist in developing a flash reduction strategy, supplying a rationale for requests of additional instrumentation, a change in scheduling, or other strategies to reduce flash sterilization. Figure 22.5 gives a list of examples of sterilization cycles to be used as a guideline for processing instruments and equipment. Always refer to the manufacturer's guidelines when deciding on sterilization parameters.

Time, temperature, and moisture are three identified factors in steam sterilization. *Time* is the exposure time required to reach a 6 log reduction. For example, in a 4-min cycle at 132 °C, a 6 log reduction is achieved at 2 min. All microorganisms should have been killed at this point. There are situations that require an extended cycle because of the complexity of the device, lumen size, configuration of a set, or resistance of an organism such as a prion. The manufacturer's recommendations must be reviewed and followed when determining sterilization time. *Temperature* directly correlates to length of exposure. The lower the temperature, the longer the time required for sterilization to occur. The steam must be saturated in order to kill the microorganisms, even if the time and temperature are appropriate. If a failed biological indicator occurs, increasing the exposure time is not the proper corrective action, because it does not insure the presence of saturated steam. Saturation is achieved by organization of instruments within containers and placement of sets within the autoclave. At the end of the sterilization cycle, the sterilizer printout must be checked to determine if the proper time and temperature were achieved and whether the exposure time was sufficient. The operator must know what the normal values should be and understand their meaning. *Moisture* reduces the time necessary to denature or coagulate proteins, which causes microorganisms to be killed in steam. One impediment to adequate moisture is trapped air. Air and steam do not mix well, and air can prevent steam contact with a device. In sterilizers, air is removed from the chamber by gravity, vacuum, or pulse pressure. Positioning of devices in a gravity displacement sterilizer or cycle is critical. Concave devices must be inverted to prevent air entrapment. In a vacuum cycle, concave items are inverted to prevent pooling of condensate.

Sample
OPERATING ROOM
FLASH STERILIZATION RECORD

PLEASE NOTE THE FOLLOWING INFORMATION:
>Each load must be recorded on this sheet. The first load is *always* a Bowie Dick test.
>Prior to placing an item on the sterile field, sterility must be confirmed by the surgical team.
>All loads containing implantable items require a biological test.

Cells 1–10 (form blocks, each containing):

STERILIZER / DATE / STERI-GAGE / ACCEPT/REJECT / PATIENT LABEL

CYCLE: __3 MIN __5MIN __10 MIN __20 MIN __22 MIN __25 MIN __30 MIN __35MIN __BOWIE DICK TEST

ITEM: / REASON: / BIOLOGICAL: Y/N RESULT: POS/NEG INITIALS: / INCUBATOR SLOT # TIME PLACED IN INCUBATOR

Figure 22.4 An example of documenting a sterilization cycle.

Residual air in a vacuum cycle must be tested. A Bowie–Dick test can be used to test air removal in a cycle where air is removed by vacuum. Class 5 and 6 indicators are available as testing mechanisms to insure the autoclave has met the parameters set. Class 5 integrating indicators are designed to react to all critical variables (time, temperature, and the presence of steam) and have stated values that correlate to a biological indicator (BI) at three different time/temperature relationships. Class 5 integrating indicators must have three stated values at 121 °C, 135 °C, and at one temperature in between that correlates to a BI. Additionally, that stated value at 121 °C must not be less than 16.5 min. This guarantees the time/temperature response for a Class 5 integrating indicator will respond like the BI when exposed to ideal, saturated steam. Therefore, if the exposure temperature was not achieved where the class 5 chemical integrator is located and the BI result was positive (a sterilization failure), the Class 5 chemical integrator will respond like the BI performance and also indicate that a failure had occurred. Class 6 uses a chemical ink formulated to change abruptly when the indictor reaches the stated values for the sterilization cycle.

The stated values correspond to the critical variables the sterilizer manufacturer has defined for the sterilization process. They are designed and validated for specific sterilization cycles (see Figure 22.5 for a list of various sterilization cycles). However, it is important always to check the manufacturer's recommendations before cleaning and sterilizing any item. Autoclave testing should be performed at the same time each day. A suggestion is to have the testing performed during the night shift immediately before the start of the day

Type of autoclave	Instruments/Equipment	Temperature C/F	Time in mins
Gravity-displacement	Wrapped	121/250	30
Gravity-displacement	Wrapped	132/270	15
Gravity-displacement	Wrapped	135/275	10
Gravity-displacement flash	Unwrapped non-porous	132/270	3
Gravity-displacement flash	Unwrapped non-porous	135/275	3
Pre-vacuum flash	Wrapped	132/270	4
Pre-vacuum flash	Wrapped	135/275	3
Pre-vacuum flash	Unwrapped non-porous	132/270	3
Pre-vacuum flash	Unwrapped non-porous	135/275	3

NOTE: Always check manufacturer's recommendations prior to cleaning and sterilization

Figure 22.5 Sterilization cycles

shift. Principles of steam sterilization, including basic functioning and proper operation of equipment, must be completed yearly to validate staff knowledge. Safety and consistency in the departmental process are key to providing quality patient care and facilitating positive outcomes.

Infection control

Throughout the years there have been processes developed to make surgery an aseptic event: wearing gloves to protect the patient and gowns and masks to prevent microbial soilage, and using sterilizers to insure that any item coming into contact with the patient is sterile. According to the literature, by 1910 these processes were standard practice within university hospitals.

Asepsis is designed to assist in eliminating all microorganisms. Aseptic technique is a practice that restricts microorganisms in the environment and on equipment and supplies to prevent contamination of the surgical wound. The goal of every surgical team should be to prevent surgical infections, optimize wound healing, and reduce the length of recovery from surgery. These principles are the basis for infection control in the surgical arena.

Controlling infections within the perioperative area must focus on prevention. According to *Alexander's Care of the Surgical Patient* [2], infection control practices involve both personal and administrative measures. Personal measures include fitness for work and application of aseptic principles. Administrative measures include provision of adequate physical facilities, appropriate surgical supplies, and operational controls.

Universal, standard, and enhanced precautions have been developed to assist in enhancing patient care and reducing exposure to infectious processes. Universal precautions dating to 1985 applied blood and body fluid precautions universally to all persons regardless of their known infection status. Universal precautions recommended personal protective equipment, including gowns and gloves. In 1987, the Centers for Disease Control and Prevention (CDC) proposed body substance isolation (BSI) of all moist and potentially infectious body substances, such as blood, feces, urine, saliva, drainage, and other body fluids. Because of the confusion with trying to separate universal and body substance isolation, standard precautions were developed by the CDC. This action would provide one process that would combine both universal precautions and BSI. The intention of this action was to reduce transmission risk for bloodborne pathogens and all pathogens from moist body substances. Standard precautions should be applied to all patients regardless of their diagnosis or presumed infection status and include hand hygiene, gloves, masks, eye protection, face shields, gowns, sharps, patient-care equipment, linens, environmental control, and patient placement. Additional precautions, called enhanced precautions, have been developed for patients with known or suspected infection with highly transmissible pathogens. These enhanced precautions include airborne infection isolation precautions, droplet precautions, and contact precautions. For patients identified with any of these types of infections, standard precautions still apply.

Engineering practices to control infection generally start with the construction and design of the OR.

Items to consider when designing the department are: storage of sterile supplies and equipment; separation of sterile and contaminated items; wall and floor covering; selection of doors; location of scrub sinks; heating, ventilation, and air conditioning. Work practices to control infection are sterilization processes, which have already been discussed, and environmental cleaning of the ORs. Aseptic practices to control infection start with minimizing or eliminating the patient's exposure to external organisms when performing surgical procedures. Principles of asepsis must be followed – AORN recommended practices outline principles and include the rationale for each statement. Using sterile surgical prep, drapes, and instruments, wearing appropriate surgical attire, practicing good handwashing techniques, following surgical hand-scrub procedures, and managing traffic patterns within the operative suite will provide good processes for reducing or preventing infection.

The Centers for Medicaid & Medicare Services (CMS) has published guidelines for reducing surgical site infections through the Surgical Care Improvement Project (SCIP). The areas of review are cardiac, vascular, orthopedic (hip and knee replacements), colon, general surgery, urologic, gynecologic, and neurosurgery procedures. Recommendations are listed below.

- Appropriate antibiotic selection: different antibiotics work on different body parts (for example, ciprofloxacin is usually used to treat urologic or lung issues; using ciprofloxacin for cardiac surgery would not be indicated). Antibiotic selection must be safe, cost-effective, and cover probable intraoperative contaminants. Vancomycin is not recommended routinely owing to the risk of antibiotic resistance. It is appropriate in certain situations, which must be documented before surgery.
- Prophylactic antibiotic must be given within 1 h prior to incision: multiple studies indicate that antibiotics administered within 1 h prior to incision greatly decrease the risk of infection postoperatively.
- Prophylactic antibiotics must be discontinued within 24 h of surgery end time unless documented appropriate reason for continuation: the patient must be provided with low risk and high benefits of antibiotic administration – excessive doses of antibiotics provide no additional benefit to the patient, and can put them

at risk for infection with *Clostridium difficile* or a multidrug-resistant organism.
- Pharmacological venous thromboembolism (VTE) prophylaxis (lovenox, heparin) must be given within 24 h of surgery end time: VTE (or deep vein thrombosis [DVT]) is the most common postoperative complication, yet prohylaxis is often overlooked. All surgical patients should have some form of VTE prophylaxis within 24 h of their surgery (most effective). Pharmacologic prophylaxis is recommended for all colon and hip surgeries in addition to mechanical. This is also considered a "never event" (a hospital-acquired condition). For patients who develop a DVT post-hip or -knee surgery, Medicare/Medicaid will not reimburse the facility.
- Beta-blocker perioperatively: if the patient is on a beta-blocker at home, they must receive it before surgery – even if the patient is nil per os (NPO). Patients on a beta-blocker at home who are not beta-blocked prior to surgery have a significantly higher mortality rate.
- Urinary catheter should be removed on postoperative day 1 or 2: if this does not happen there must be a documented reason why this could not be completed. Patients often have a urinary catheter longer than necessary. Every day a catheter is in place, the patient is at risk of a urinary tract infection – another "never event." Patients should be evaluated every shift for the necessity of the catheter.
- Cardiac patient's blood glucose at 06:00 h on postoperative days 1 and 2 should be less than 200: hyperglycemia is associated with an increased risk of morbidity and mortality postoperatively. The risk of infection is also greatly increased when glycemic control is not maintained, as well as renal failure, and general intensive care stays.
- Preoperative hair removal: no razors should be used when preparing patients. Shaving patients leaves microscopic nicks in the skin, which have proven to increase the risk of infection. Patients should have no hair removal or be "clipped" with electric clippers prior to surgery.
- Perioperative temperature management: normothermia must be maintained or patients can be at risk for poor wound healing, adverse cardiac events, coagulopathy, and other negative outcomes. Temperature should be monitored and

documented. A patient's temperature should be at 36 °C within 15 min after surgery ends.

Summary

This chapter is an overview, but not an exhaustive list, of topics for managing the OR. The AORN, APIC, American Society of Anesthesiologists, OR manager, CDC, and the Joint Commission are all valuable resources to utilize for guidance. The OR is a complex area that involves many people, with a common goal of always doing what is best for the patient and keeping the patient at the center of all decisions. The best knowledge comes from actually working in the OR and experiencing the complexity of the systems. Critical thinking and problem-solving skills are the keys to success.

References

1. R. Urman, S. Eappen. Operating room management: Core principles. In: C. A. Vacanti, P. K. Sikka, R. D. Urman, M. Dershwitz, B. S. Segal. *Essential Clinical Anesthesia*, 1st edn, Cambridge University Press, 2011.

2. J. C. Rothrock. *Alexander's Care of the Patient in Surgery*, 14th edn. St. Louis, MO: Mosby, 2010.

Chapter

23

The Joint Commission, CMS, and other standards

Shermeen B. Vakharia MD
Zeev Kain MD, MBA, MA (Hons)

The Joint Commission   235
The Centers for Medicare &
Medicaid   235

The CMS and JC standards in the OR   236
Emergency and disaster response   241
Summary   243

Operating rooms are subject to several standards set by governmental and private not-for-profit agencies. Accreditation by these agencies is a way through which a health-care organization is recognized as offering quality health care that meets established standards. This chapter provides a brief history of Centers for Medicare & Medicaid Services and the Joint Commission and the influence of their standards on the perioperative arena.

The Joint Commission

Almost a century ago, in 1919, minimum standards for hospitals were developed by the American College of Surgeons (ACS). These standards were a result of Dr. Earnest A. Codman's vision for standardization based on "end result" of treatment. Over the next 30 years, the standard of care in the hospitals improved, and more than 3200 US hospitals approved and embraced these standards. In 1951, ACS collaborated with the American College of Physicians, the American Medical Association (AMA), the American Hospital Association (AHA), and the Canadian Medical Association to form the Joint Commission on Accreditation of Hospitals (JCAH). In 1952, ACS formally transferred their Hospital Standardization Program to JCAH and the accreditation process began in 1953. As the scope of JCAH expanded, it was renamed in 1987 as the Joint Commission for Accreditation of Health Care Organizations (JCAHO), which was then shortened to the Joint Commission (JC) in 2007.

In 1965, the Congress passed the Social Security Amendments with a provision that hospitals accredited by JCAH were "deemed" to be in compliance with most of the Medicare Conditions of Participation for Hospitals. This gave the commission authority and power to determine whether a health-care organization would be eligible to receive Medicare reimbursement. Over the years, the JC standards have improved and expanded to hold hospitals to optimal standards rather than minimal standards. The Comprehensive Accreditation Manual for Hospitals (CAMH) has all of the JC standards, of which there are more than 250 standards that pertain to patient safety and quality of care. These standards are divided into chapters for each accreditation program, for example the Hospital Accreditation program has 17 chapters. The JC assesses both processes and outcomes during their inspection, the philosophy being that good processes lead to favorable outcomes and not all outcomes are easily measurable. Surveys by the JC are random and unannounced and held at least once every 3 years.

The Centers for Medicare & Medicaid

In 1965, President Lyndon Johnson signed the Social Security Act, and Medicare and Medicaid were enacted as Title XVIII and Title XIX of this act. As a result, health coverage was extended to almost all Americans aged 65 or older, low-income children deprived of parental support, the elderly, the blind, and individuals with disabilities. In 1966 when Medicare was implemented more than 19 million individuals enrolled. In 1977, the government established the Health Care Financing Administration (HCFA), which was responsible for

Operating Room Leadership and Management, ed. Kaye A.D., Fox C.J. and Urman R.D. Published by Cambridge University Press. © Cambridge University Press 2012.

the coordination of Medicare and Medicaid. In 2001, HCFA was renamed Centers for Medicare & Medicaid (CMS) to reflect increased emphasis on responsiveness to beneficiaries and providers, and on improving the quality of care that the beneficiaries received.

The CMS establishes conditions of participation (CoP) for all facilities that participate in the Medicare and Medicaid programs. The CoPs are first published in the federal register and then the standards with interpretive guidelines and survey procedures are published in the State Operations Manual (SOM) for certification of hospitals.

All facilities participating in the Medicare and Medicaid programs are required to undergo an initial CMS inspection, followed by surveys on a regular basis to insure compliance with federal health and safety standards. The CMS contracts with state agencies to conduct these inspections. If any deficiencies are found during the initial certification or recertification process, the facility has to bear the full cost of a revisit survey to ascertain that corrective action has been implemented. Initially, the JC was given authority by Congress to determine whether hospitals met the requirements for Medicare reimbursement. In 2008, this automatic authority was eliminated. Since July 2010, the JC's accreditation program is required to meet all CMS standards.

With a few exceptions, the majority of the CMS and JC standards apply directly or indirectly to the operating room (OR). The OR managers have to familiarize themselves with these standards and establish policies and procedures to ingrain these standards into the daily practice and culture of the OR environment. Discussion of all applicable standards is beyond the scope of this chapter. Instead, the chapter gives a broad overview of some of the standards as they apply to the OR suite. The reader is encouraged to look up the SOM and the CAMH for details and also be aware that the standards and interpretive guidelines are subject to periodic change and updates.

The CMS and JC standards in the OR

Patient rights

The CMS and JC have several standards that protect and promote patients' rights. Many of these standards apply throughout the perioperative period, including the right to privacy, confidentiality of medical records, the right to participate in decisions about their care,

treatment, and services, and the right to receive safe care (CMS §482.13, JC RI.01.01.01, EC.01.01.01-EP3,EP4, IM.02.01.01, EP 1–5). Informed consent process is a right that the patients or their representatives may need to exercise after receiving adequate information and disclosures about anticipated benefits, risks and alternative therapies. Federal and state laws or regulations set minimum requirements for informed consent (CMS §482.24(c)(2)(v)). Hospitals are required to have policies and procedures that also protect the patient's right to request or refuse a procedure or treatment.

Per CMS and JC standards, medical staff are responsible for determining which procedures or treatments require informed consent. Owing to the procedural nature of the OR, the physicians and staff taking care of operative patients should be aware of the policies that apply when documenting various forms of informed consent – particularly consent for surgery and anesthesia, consent for transfusion of blood or blood products, consent for producing images or recordings of the procedure for purposes other than patient care, and consent for participation in perioperative research and clinical trials. Inspections of the perioperative area by the JC and CMS include determining the proper execution of informed consent.

Although not directly applicable to the OR, restraints are used on rare occasions in the postanesthesia care unit (PACU). Both CMS and JC require that hospitals have policies regarding the use of restraints, including documenting the rationale for use, using least restrictive interventions, age-specific monitoring, early discontinuation, and staff training and reporting requirements (CMS §482.13(e), JC PC.03.05). The PACU staff must be appropriately trained and be aware of the policies and procedures that apply to the use of restraints.

Surgical services

Scope and standards for surgical services

The CMS recommends the ACS definition of surgery and requires that hospitals have appropriate organization, equipment, and qualified personnel to insure the health and safety of the patient (CMS CoP §482.51, JC LD.03.06.01-EP3, IC.01.01.01-EP3). The accreditation survey generally includes observation of practices in the inpatient and outpatient OR suites for adherence to acceptable standards of practice. Acceptable standards of practice include recommendations by nationally recognized professional organizations (ACS, AMA, the American Society of Anesthesiologists [ASA], the Association of Operating Room Nurses, etc.), federal agencies, and state regulations. The needs of the population should guide the types of surgical services provided directly or through referral and agreements (CMS §482.51(b) JC LD.04.03.01). Policies governing surgical care, including postoperative care (CMS §482.51(b)(4), JC PC.01.03.07), should be designed to achieve the highest standard of clinical practice. The CMS interpretive guidelines for standard §482.51(b) in SOM provides a comprehensive list of policies governing surgical care that OR staff could be asked about during survey.

Provider qualifications and scope of practice

Per CMS, the OR supervisor has to be either a registered nurse, doctor of medicine, or doctor of osteopathy. Both the JC and CMS require that the hospital determines the appropriate qualifications for OR supervisors and is able to provide surveyors with a position description with required qualifications (CMS §482.51(a)(1), JC HR.01.02.01). The CMS regulations require that all scrub and circulatory duties performed by technologists or licensed practical nurses must be supervised by a qualified registered nurse (CMS §482.51(a)(2), §482.51(a)(3), JC PC.03.01.01-EP5).

The process of privileging and credentialing all practitioners, including surgeons, is a function of organized medical staff and is subject to surveyor review. The JC requires that information from ongoing professional practice evaluation (OPPE) be factored into the decision to maintain privileges (MS.08.01.03). A current roster of each practitioner's privileges must be maintained in the OR suite, and at the request of the surveyors the OR staff must be able to demonstrate how to check a practitioner's privileges (CMS §482.51(a)(4), JC MS.03.01.01, MS.06.01.07, MS.06.01.09).

Patient assessment and documentation requirements

This section pertains to CMS standard §482.51(b) (1) and the JC standards also reflect CMS requirements for patient assessment and timely documentation (PC.01.02.03-EP4 and EP5, RC.01.03.01-EP4). According to these standards, before surgery or administration of anesthesia a medical history and physical exam must be completed and documented no more than 30 days before or 24 h after admission (or registration). If the medical history and physical exam is completed and documented within 30 days of admission,

an updated physical exam must be completed and documented within 24 h of admission. These standards apply to all cases even if surgery occurs within 24 h of admission, the only exception being emergency surgery. Survey procedures include a review of the patient's medical records to confirm compliance with these standards. The standards were prevalent when this chapter was written, and the reader is advised to look for the most recent updates.

The JC requires that the operative report be written or dictated before the patient leaves the operative suite for the next level of care, unless accompanied by the practitioner to the next area of care, where it can be completed. It is common practice for surgeons to write a brief operative summary immediately after the surgery, in which case a detailed report can be completed and authenticated in a time frame specified by the hospital (CMS §482.51(b)(6), RC.02.01.03-EP 5 and EP 6). The surgeons should be aware of the minimum requirements of an operative report. Generally a review of approximately six surgical reports is performed during CMS surveys to verify it includes specified information and is signed and dated by the surgeon.

Informed consent for surgery

CMS and the JC specify minimal requirements for informed consent policy (CMS §482.51(b)(2), JC RI.01.03.01). A properly executed surgical consent is required to be in the patient's medical record before surgery. The only exception to this regulation is emergency surgery to save a patient's life or limb. Appropriate documentation in the patient's medical record by the surgeon is considered acceptable under most circumstances; however, different approaches may be used, depending on the local regulations and hospital policy.

As most surgeries are performed under anesthesia, CMS recommends that the hospitals extend their surgical consent policy to include anesthesia. The CMS and JC recommend that hospitals have policies for handling do-not-resuscitate (DNR) patients in the perioperative period. As survival and functional outcome of resuscitation in the OR differs greatly from resuscitation on the hospital wards, automatic upholding or discontinuation of DNR is no longer practiced. The ASA's Ethical Guidelines for the Anesthesia Care of Patients with Do-Not-Resuscitate Orders or other Directives That Limit Treatment were published in 1991 and recommend that in keeping with the patient's autonomy and self-determination of course of treatment, a discussion should transpire before surgery and DNR orders be revised to allow intubation and resuscitation that would constitute a part of administering anesthesia (the ACS and Association of periOperative Registered Nurses [AORN] guidelines formulated later also reflect ASA standards).

Anesthesia services

Scope and standard of anesthesia services

Standards on anesthesia services are perhaps among the most complex and controvertible, and the interpretive guidelines have undergone several updates. The scope of anesthesia services was expanded in the December 2009 update of CoP, into two categories: (1) anesthesia, including general, regional, and monitored anesthesia care; and (2) analgesia and sedation, with increased emphasis being on the ability to rescue if the level of sedation becomes deeper than intended. The CMS requires that anesthesia services throughout the hospital, including all off-site locations, be organized into a single service under the direction of a doctor of medicine or doctor of osteopathy (CMS §482.52). Services provided should be consistent with the needs of the hospital. Anesthesia services policies must designed to insure the delivery of care is consistent with recognized standards (for example, the ASA standards) and address important issues pertaining to staff responsibilities, documentation and reporting requirements, protocol for supportive life functions, patient safety, and consent issues.

Qualifications and scope of practice

The hospital's policies and procedures must define the circumstances when a non-anesthesiologist doctor of medicine or doctor of osteopathy can administer or supervise anesthesia services (for example, procedural sedation as determined by the state scope of practice law). Medical staff bylaws must specify criteria obtaining and maintaining privileges. The type and complexity of procedures for each individual practitioner who may administer anesthesia must be specified in his/her privileges (CMS §482. 22(c)(6), JC MS.03.01.01-EP 2). Staff with sedation privileges should have credentials for rescuing patients from various levels of sedation (JC MS.06.01.01-EP1). The CMS requires supervision of anesthesiologist assistants and certified registered nurse anesthetists while providing anesthesia services, by an anesthesiologist who is available to furnish assistance and direction (or supervision in case of a CRNA) throughout the performance of the procedure (CMS §482.52 (a), JC PC.03.01.01). Such CRNA supervision by an anesthesiologist is not obligatory in states that have opted out of the CRNA supervision requirement (see www.cms.hhs.gov/CFCsAndCoPs/02_Spotlight.asp for a list of opt-out states).

Patient assessment and documentation requirements

Anesthesia standards for preoperative evaluation and postoperative check have undergone several revisions. This section refers to the February 2011 update, which aligns preoperative assessment and documentation with standards for surgical services. According to these standards, before administration of anesthesia, a pre-anesthesia evaluation must be completed and documented no more than 30 days prior to the procedure requiring anesthesia; however, certain elements of the history, risk assessment, physical exam, and discussion of risks and benefits have to be completed within a 48-h time frame before administering anesthesia (CMS §482.52(b)(1), JC PC.03.01.03-EP8 and EP 18). Per CMS standards, pre-anesthesia evaluation can only be performed by a practitioners qualified to administer anesthesia.

Postoperative evaluation should be performed by a practitioner qualified to administer anesthesia, and completed within 48 h of the patient being moved to the designated recovery area. The postoperative evaluation is performed after the patient has sufficiently recovered from anesthesia (CMS §482.52(b), JC PC.03.01.07-EP1, EP2, EP7, EP8). The 48-h time frame for postoperative evaluation also applies to outpatients unless state law and hospital policy specify more stringent standards. The CMS, JC, and ASA specify minimal requirements for pre-anesthesia evaluation, intraoperative anesthesia documentation and postanesthesia evaluation. Accreditation surveys generally include review of anesthesia records to verify that current documentation standards are met. Owing to frequent updates to anesthesia standards, the reader is advised to check for latest updates.

The JC National Patient Safety Goals patient safety standards

The National Patient Safety Goal (NPSG) program was developed by the Patient Safety Advisory Group of the JC in 2002. The goal was to help accredited hospitals address the most challenging patient safety issues. The

NPSG (2011) standards that apply to the perioperative environment are summarized below. Where CMS or TJC has corresponding or related standards, a reference is to the standard is provided. NPSG standards are revised annually and new goals may be added.

Identify patients correctly

NPSG.01.01.01: *Use at least two patient identifiers when providing care, treatment, and services.* This also applies to labeling of blood samples and specimens.

NPSG.01.03.01: *Eliminate transfusion errors related to patient misidentification.* This NPSG requires verification by two people (qualified per hospital policy and state law) that the blood component matches to the order and patient, with one verifier being the transfusionist.

Improve communication

NPSG.02.03.01: *Report critical results of tests and diagnostic procedures on a timely basis.* This is important during the perioperative period, when the patient's condition can change rapidly and handoffs also occur during the episode of care.

Safe use of medication

NPSG.03.04.01: *Label all medications, medication containers, and other solutions on and off the sterile field in perioperative and other procedural settings.* Recommendations for labeling include medication name, strength, quantity, diluent and volume (if not apparent from the container), expiration date when not used within 24 h expiration time or when expiration occurs in less than 24 h. A two-person verification is required when the person is preparing the medication if not prepared by the person administering it. This safety goal also requires that medications be reviewed by entering and exiting staff.

NPSG.03.05.01: *Reduce the likelihood of patient harm associated with the use of anticoagulant therapy.* Perioperatively, this standard requires use of approved protocols for the initiation, maintenance, and monitoring of anticoagulant therapy and the use of an infusion pump when heparin is administered continuously.

NPSG.03.06.01: *Maintain and communicate accurate patient medication information.* Transferring accurate medication information is critical in the perioperative period, when several handoffs can occur during the episode of care.

Other medication safety standards in the OR are discussed later in this chapter.

Prevent infection

NPSG.07.01.01: *Comply with either the current Centers for Disease Control and Prevention (CDC) hand hygiene guidelines or the current World Health Organization (WHO) hand hygiene guidelines.* The standard requires implementation of a hospital-wide hand hygiene program based on CDC or WHO guidelines with goals for improving compliance (JC IC.01.04.01-EP5, IC.03.01.01-EP3).

NPSG.07.03.01: *Implement evidence-based practices to prevent health care-associated infections due to multidrug-resistant organisms in acute care hospitals.* The standard requires implementation of policies and practices that apply to the whole organization as well as to the perioperative environment, aimed at reducing the risk of transmitting multidrug-resistant organisms.

NPSG.07.04.01: *Implement evidence-based practices to prevent central line-associated bloodstream infections.* Per this standard, the policies and practices aimed at reducing the risk of central line-associated bloodstream infections must be implemented and complied with. These policies and practices must be aligned with state and national regulatory requirements and professional organization guidelines. Some provisions in this NPSG are the use of standardized supply cart or kit that contains all necessary components for the insertion of central lines, use of standardized protocol for hand hygiene, aseptic skin preparation and sterile barrier precautions, use of a standardized protocol to disinfect catheter hubs and injection ports before accessing them, and avoiding femoral vein for central line insertion unless other sites are unavailable.

NPSG.07.05.01: *Implement evidence-based practices for preventing surgical site infections.* Elements of performance include implementation of educational, preventive, and surveillance strategies. This goal encompasses ORYX core measures (such as the Surgical Care Improvement Project [SCIP]) and is generally a part of the hospital-wide performance improvement program.

The CMS condition of participation §482.42 on infection control requires that health-care-associated infection prevention be a part of the hospital-wide infection control program. Hospitals that employ alcohol-based skin preparations in anesthetizing locations are required to have appropriate policies and procedures to reduce the associated risk of fire. Failure to implement appropriate measures to reduce the risk of fires associated with the use of alcohol-based skin preparations in anesthetizing locations is considered a condition-level noncompliance.

Prevent mistakes in surgery

UP.01.01.01: *Conduct a pre-procedure verification process.* This standard requires implementation of a pre-procedure protocol to verify the correct procedure, for the correct patient, at the correct site, with patient involvement if possible. Use of a standardized list to verify at a minimum relevant documentation (for example, history and physical, signed procedure consent form, nursing assessment, and pre-anesthesia assessment), diagnostic and radiology test results, and any special requirements, matched to the patient.

UP.01.02.01: *Mark the procedure site.* This standard requires marking of procedure site, side, and level if applicable, before the procedure is performed, and with patient involvement if possible. Marking should preferably be done by a licensed practitioner who is ultimately accountable for the procedure and will be present when the procedure is performed. If hospital policy allows, a designated qualified practitioner may perform site marking to meet this standard. The mark should be visible after skin preparation and draping. Exceptions for site marking include mucosal surfaces, perineum, teeth, premature infants, and patient refusal.

UP.01.03.01: *A time-out is performed before the procedure.* This requires performing a standardized time-out immediately before the procedure, initiated by a designated member of the team. The members of the procedural team should agree on at least three elements: correct patient, correct site, procedure to be done. The completion of the time-out should be documented.

Medication safety

Medication safety presents a unique challenge in the OR environment. Medication errors are among the most common errors in anesthesia because of the unique situation in which a person orders, dispenses, and administers a drug, and monitors the patient in the absence of double checks and other safety measures taken when medications are ordered and administered on the hospital wards. In the list of high-alert medications for acute care settings compiled by Institute for Safe Medication Practices, 15 out of 20 medications on this list are commonly stocked in anesthesia carts. Appropriate safeguards must be in place to prevent

errors with the use of risky medications, especially ones that are in similar-looking containers, are highly concentrated, or need dilution before administration. The ASA Statement on Labeling of Pharmaceuticals for the Use in Anesthesiology recommends color-coded, legible labels consistent with the guidelines of the American Society for Testing and Materials (ASTM) International and the International Organization for Standardization (ISO). The purpose is to enhance visual features in accordance with human factors to prevent errors of syringe swaps.

The CMS and TJC standards require all noncontrolled medications to be locked when a patient care procedural area is not staffed by a health-care professional (CMS §482.25(b)(2)(i), JC MM.03.01.01-EP6). Medications listed in Schedules II–V of the Comprehensive Drug Abuse Prevention and Control Act of 1970 must be locked accurate records of the disposition of all controlled substances must be maintained (CMS §482.25(b)(2)(ii), §482.25(a)(3), JC MM.03.01.01-EP3 and EP-6) by the hospital pharmacy. The hospitals are required to have policy and procedures for reporting diversion, managing recalls and expired drugs, and reporting errors and adverse reactions through a hospital-wide medication safety program (CMS §482.25(b)(7), §482.25(b)(8), JC MM.01.01.03-EP5). The professional staff must have access to Information relating to drug interactions and information of drug therapy, side effects, toxicology, dosage, indications for use, and routes of administration 24 h a day, 7 days a week (CMS§482.25(b)(8), JC IM.03.01.01-EP1, MM.02.01.01-EP4–5).

In the PACU, verbal orders must be minimized to avoid medication errors and should be authenticated promptly according to state law or hospital policy (CMS §482.24(c)(1)(iii), JC RC.02.03.07-EP4).

Environmental and occupational safety

Physical environment and facilities

Most standards in CMS CoP §482.41 Physical Environment apply to the OR environment and pertain not only to physical construction and planning of the perioperative areas but also to emergency preparedness plans and capabilities to insure patient safety and well-being (JC LS.02.01.10). All hospitals participating in Medicare are required to comply with Life Safety Code requirements of the National Fire Protection Association (NPFA), unless state fire and safety codes are more stringent and protect patients adequately (CMS §482.41(b), JC EC.02.03.01). Operating and recovery rooms are required to have emergency power and lighting (CMS§482.41(a)(1), NPFA 101, 2000 edition). The OR must have a fire response and evacuation plan as a part of the larger hospital plan (CMS §482.41(b)(7), JC EC.02.05.03-EP1, EP2, EP3, EP5, EP6). All new staff must be oriented to fire safety and must know how to contain fire, use the fire extinguisher, and evacuate safely. The staff should be able to describe the key safety steps if asked by the JC surveyor.

Infection control and occupational safety

The CDC has published extensive guidelines for infection control in case of both nosocomial and occupational acquired infections. The Occupational Safety and Health Administration (OSHA) in section IV of its manual addresses several occupational hazards in health-care facilities and recommends preventive measures. Exposure to bloodborne pathogens, laser use and laser smoke, multidrug-resistant organisms, surgical instruments/equipment, and anesthesia equipment in the OR make it a unique and high-risk environment for infection control. The ASA's recommendations for infection control and AORN guidelines are specifically directed to the perioperative environment.

Quality assurance and performance improvement

The JC and CMS identify the OR as a high-risk area and require that anesthesia and surgical services be a part of the organization-wide quality assurance performance improvement program (QA/PI). The QA/PI activities that apply to the perioperative environment are broadly categorized below.

Data collection

Leaders are the motivating force behind quality-driven organizations, and CMS requires hospital leaders (governing body) to set priorities and determine the detail and frequency of data collection for performance-improvement activities. Data collection sources can include a variety of sources, such as patient charts, staff, observations, interviews, etc. to identify vulnerable areas and direct performance-improvement activities. Priority is given to high-volume, high-risk, or problem-prone processes,

including perioperative processes. Participation in Medicare requires data collection in the following procedural areas:

- surgery and other procedures that place patients at risk of disability or death;
- significant discrepancies between preoperative and postoperative diagnoses;
- adverse events related to using moderate or deep sedation or anesthesia;
- use of blood and blood components;
- all reported and confirmed transfusion reactions;
- significant medication errors;
- significant adverse drug reactions;
- patient perception of the safety and quality of care, treatment, and services.

The CMS also recommends data collection on staff opinions and needs, their perceptions of risk to individuals, their suggestions for improving patient safety, and their willingness to report adverse events. In addition, the JC requires data collection for its ORYX initiative, which integrates outcomes and other performance measurement data into the accreditation process. The ORYX core measures also include perioperative venous thromboembolism prophylaxis and SCIP. These measures are evaluated by both the JC and CMS and are endorsed by the National Quality Forum.

Data compilation and analysis

Statistical analysis and display of data help in trending and identification of opportunities for improvement. The JC requires that any undesirable trends or variation should include staffing analysis (the JC recommends use of the National Quality Forum Nursing Sensitive Measures). An organization-wide safety program must establish a method of communicating critical information to hospital leaders, so that prompt actions can be taken to resolve any problems identified.

Emergency and disaster response

In 2002, the Joint Commission stressed the importance of developing scalable, sustainable, and community-integrated plans for emergency response. In addition, JCAHO mandates conducting two emergency response drills every year to minimize the impact of a disaster. In 2001, JCAHO published a white paper to help hospitals develop systems to create community-wide emergency

Table 23.1 Emergency management standards by JCAHO

1. Develop a management plan that addresses emergency management. Four phases of emergency management are:
   mitigation;
   preparedness;
   response;
   recovery.

2. Perform a health vulnerability analysis
   Establish emergency procedures in response to a hazard vulnerability analysis
   Define the organization's roles with other community agencies
   Notify external authorities
   Notify hospital personnel when emergency procedures initiated
   Assign available personnel to cover necessary positions
   The following activities must be managed:
   … patient/resident activities;
   … staff activities.
   Staff/family support
   Logistics of critical supplies
   Security
   Evacuation of facility, if necessary
   Establish internal/external communications
   Establish orientation/education programs
   Monitor ongoing drills and real emergencies
   Determine how an annual evaluation will occur
   Provide alternate means of meeting essential building and utility needs
   Identify radioactive and biological isolation decontamination needs
   Clarify alternate responsibility of personnel

3. Involve community-wide response

4. Reestablish and continue operations after disaster

preparedness (Table 23.1). The white paper focuses on three major areas:

1. enlisting community to develop local response;
2. focusing on key aspects of the system that prepare the community to mobilize to care for patients, protect its staff, and serve the public;
3. establishing accountability, oversight, and sustainability of a community preparedness system.

For disaster management, the OR poses great challenges, as not only there would be an increased demand on the OR, but also the OR environment might change entirely.

Although the recommendations from the JC are guidelines, every hospital aspires to the JC accreditation. This chapter will not be complete without a mention of disaster management standards as per the JC. Staffing and compensation models must take into account allowances for this vital, but (fortunately) seldom-used role of the OR.

Ongoing performance improvement

As quality measures evolve, health-care organizations need to be able to adapt and prioritize performance improvement opportunities. The CMS and JC, in particular, evaluate health-care facilities' care processes that enhance safety and produce the best outcomes for their patients. Ever since the JC adopted its mission to "continuously improve health care for the public, in collaboration with other stakeholders, by evaluating health care organizations and inspiring them to excel in providing safe and effective care of the highest quality and value," the cramming mentality before an inspection has become a phenomenon of the past. Instead, the JC standards set benchmarks that accredited institutions must meet or exceed on a continued basis. Creating a culture of safety through leadership involvement, organization-wide safety programs, education of the staff, effective communication of changes and safety tips to frontline providers, and visible evidence of safe practices through posters and pocket cards can help achieve and maintain accreditation.

Summary

The hundreds of standards that are set by organizations such as the JC and CMS should not be viewed as an impediment by health-care institutions. On the contrary, perioperative directors can use these standards to promote quality care across the perioperative continuum and escalate issues appropriately for quick resolution. Hospitals that foster a culture of quality and patient safety embrace these standards and do not fear unannounced JC visits. Instead, they use JC standards, sentinel events program, National Patient Safety Goals, and other JC resources as tools to proactively implement patient safety solutions and comply to CMS standards.

Suggested reading

AORN Standards and Recommended Practices for Inpatient and Ambulatory Settings. Denver, Colorado: Association of periOperative Registered Nurses, 2011.

ASA Standards, Guidelines and Statements, 2008. Park Ridge IL; American Society of Anesthesiologists, 2008.

Comprehensive Accreditation Manual for Hospitals, E-Edition 4.0. Joint Commission Resources Inc.

Facts about The Joint Commission. www.iom.edu/~/media/Files/Activity%20Files/Workforce/ResidentDutyHours/PaulSchyveTestimonyFactsabouttheJointCommission.pdf (last accessed May 10, 2012).

Health-care facilities. In *OSHA Technical Manual*, Washington, D.C.: Occupational Safety and Health Administration, 1999.

Hospital CROSSWALK; Medicare Hospital Requirements to 2011 Joint Commission Hospital Standards & EPs. Joint Commission Resource Inc. [US].

Key Milestones in CMS Programs. www.cms.gov/History/downloads/CMSProgramKeyMilestones.pdf (last accessed May 10, 2012).

National Patient Safety Goals Effective July 1, 2011, Hospital Accreditation Program.

N. P. O'Grady, M. Alexander, L. A. Burns, *et al. Guidelines for the Prevention of Intravascular Catheter-Related Infections*. Atlanta, GA: Centers for Disease Control and Prevention, 2011.

D. O'Leary. Comments presented at: Homeland defense: Blueprints for emergency management Reponses; October 23–25, 2002; Washington D.C. Joint Commission on Accreditation of Health Care Organization: Health Care crossroads: Strategies for creating and sustaining community wide emergency preparedness system (white paper). Available at: www.jointcommission.org/assets/1/18/emergency_preparedness.pdf (last accessed May 11, 2012).

Recommendations for Infection Control for the Practice of Anesthesiology, 3rd edn. Park Ridge, IL: American Society of Anesthesiologists, 2011.

Revised Hospital Anesthesia Services Interpretive Guidelines – State Operations Manual (SOM) Appendix A. January 14, 2011.

L. Sehulster, R. Y. W. Chinn. *Guidelines for Environmental Infection Control in Health-Care Facilities*. Atlanta, GA: Center for Disease Control and Prevention, June 6, 2003; **52**(RR10): 1–42.

J. D. Siegel, E. Rhinehart, M. Jackson, L. Chiarello, the Healthcare Infection Control Practices Advisory Committee. *2007 Guideline for Isolation Precautions: Preventing Transmission of Infectious Agents in Healthcare Settings*. Center for Disease Control and Prevention, 2007.

State Operations Manual (SOM). Appendix A. Revision 47, June 5, 2009.

Chapter

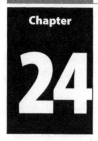

Safety, quality, and pay-for-performance

Richard P. Dutton MD, MBA
Frank Rosinia MD

Introduction   244
Measurement   245
Attribution   247
The OR quality management
plan   247

Mechanics of data acquisition and reporting   248
Outcomes of interest   249
Levels of reporting   250
Pay for performance   251
Summary   251

Introduction

Safety is the most important deliverable in perioperative care, and a critical goal for the manager of any operating room (OR). Broadly defined, safety is the avoidance of any negative outcome from a medical intervention. In the context of surgical procedures, safety implies that everything possible has been done to accomplish the primary goal (completion of the planned surgical procedure) while minimizing the risk of a complication. "Safety" by itself is a Platonic ideal that can be approached, but never 100% achieved. To the credit of anesthesiology, and the profession's decades of effort, routine perioperative care is one of the safest of all medical events. As with the airline industry, the public expects that the safety of anesthesia will always be the highest possible consideration, and that a good outcome is assured.

Quality, on the other hand, begins with patient safety and integrates it with the important clinical concept of risk and benefit. "Risk" includes two potential negatives: the chance that a complication will occur, and the chance that scarce resources will be wasted unnecessarily in trying to prevent one. "Benefit" therefore includes both good patient outcomes and efficient use of resources. A quality anesthetic is therefore one that provides the greatest possible safety with the least possible expense. Whereas safety alone can always be improved by the application of infinitely great resources, quality seeks the point of balance that

represents the most safety for the least cost. This balance can be defined as quality's value equation. At a macro level value is defined as quality outcomes divided by the cost of care [1,2].

By these definitions, it would seem that safety and quality would be opposing concepts, and that pursuit of quality would lead to penny-pinching that endangers safety. In reality this is not so. The value of safety is set very high in the public's opinion, such that safer practices are almost always favored. Further, it has been a consistent finding in the scientific study of medical quality that the safest outcomes are also the most cost-effective. This is true because errors (complications) tend to be much more expensive than uneventful routine care. And both safety and quality are driven by the same management goal: reduction of process variability. The more times a complex procedure is performed, and the more routine it becomes, the less likely it is to become complicated. In perioperative care there is a strong positive correlation between the volume of a given operation performed and the quality of clinical outcomes, especially for rare or infrequent procedures [3].

Forward-thinking OR managers pursue quality outcomes because they know that doing so will guide them to the most efficient business practices. This concept has been noted on the national level, where it has given rise to a tidal wave of regulation intended to force quality improvement in medicine. Although the

OR has been overlooked for many years – surprising given the large proportion of inpatient hospital dollars consumed there – the time is coming when all anesthesiologists and all hospitals will need data showing the quality of their outcomes in perioperative care.

The mild and myopic regulatory incentive programs of today are already transforming into robust "pay-for-performance" mechanisms, in which reimbursement for hospital and providers is directly tied to the outcome achieved. Management of these regulations – in parallel with physical management of the OR – will be an important task for OR leadership going forward, and will impose a strong demand for introspective data.

One variation of pay-for-performance that is going to strongly impact anesthesiologists is increased "bundling" of payment. The concept of the accountable care organization (ACO) is intended to align incentives by paying for health outcomes rather than procedures [4]. In its simplest model, an ACO is paid a lump sum to support the necessary care for a given population of patients for a defined period of time. The ACO, which includes both facilities and health-care providers, must decide internally how best to spend its resources to achieve this goal. The ACO is therefore incentivized to keep its patients healthy by providing preventative care, and to minimize unnecessary spending on tests and procedures that will not contribute to this goal. This is in sharp contrast to the existing fee-for-service model, which generates more money for facilities and providers for each additional test or procedure. Anesthesiologists should be aware of the ACO regulations, and should seek to participate in any institutional effort to create one.

A second, more specific, bundling concept is the surgical or perioperative home. This model proposes a single bundled payment for any patient with a surgical disease, which covers all of their care from the moment of diagnosis until the patient returns to their normal state of health. This bundle would therefore include preoperative testing, the surgery itself, and postoperative recovery and rehabilitation. Because anesthesiologists are the only physicians who care for patients throughout this period and across all surgical disciplines, creation and management of the surgical home is a natural fit. Success in a surgical home model of bundled payment will require a broad perspective on perioperative care, and the ability to find efficiencies throughout the process. The American Society of Anesthesiologists is actively examining the surgical

home model, is proposing demonstration projects to important payers – including the Center for Medicare and Medicaid Innovation – and is developing educational resources to support the membership in this area.

A final note on quality is that the patients are not the only ones who care. Because surgery is so labor intensive, and because the personnel involved require extensive and expensive training, the safety and wellness of the OR staff is also of critical importance to OR management. Replacing an experienced OR circulating nurse with a new graduate requires more than a year of on-the-job training, with associated costs, making metrics of staff satisfaction as important as patient outcomes to the overall quality of the OR.

This chapter will take a close look at the way in which effective OR managers gather data from their work and apply it to improving outcomes. Although the broad principles of OR quality management (QM) are obvious to all, the application of these principles to clinical reality can be challenging. This chapter will seek to connect the dots between lofty principles and day-to-day operations, in a way that can be applied in any kind of surgical facility.

Measurement

Effective QM for an anesthesia practice, an OR suite, or a health-care facility depends on an accurate understanding of the business involved. Human perception is inherently biased by anecdotes, and thus is untrustworthy. Important decisions should be based on objective data whenever possible. *Measurement* is the pursuit of specific data to address aspects of the quality of care, and *measures* are the resulting product. *Quality measures* are specific bits of data that have been statistically processed to provide an accurate picture of some element of patient care. Quality measures may be used for both internal trending over time and for comparison to external standards ("benchmarking") [5].

Quality measures may be further subdivided into *process* and *outcome* measures. Outcome measures (sometime just "outcomes") refer to a tangible change in a patient's condition as a result of the process being studied. For perioperative care, typical outcome measures are shown in Table 24.1. Tangible outcomes include durable changes in patient health (e.g., death, organ system failure, neurologic dysfunction, etc.), changes in financial end points (length of stay, cost of care, etc.), and changes in patient and provider satisfaction.

Table 24.1 Typical outcome measures for perioperative care

Mortality

Unplanned ICU admission

Permanent organ system injury

    Myocardial infarction

    New dysrhythmia

    Stroke

    Peripheral nerve injury

    Visual loss

Allergic reaction

Transfusion reaction

Cardiac arrest

Medication error

Aspiration

Unplanned awareness during procedure

Surgical site infection

Reintubation/respiratory failure

Patient satisfaction (overall)

Postoperative nausea and/or vomiting

Adequacy of pain management

Staff satisfaction

Length of stay in OR/PACU/ICU/facility

Unplanned case cancellation

Process measures examine some element of practice that is strongly associated with a good or bad outcome, and are thus surrogates for the measure that is really desired. Process measures are used when the actual outcome is hard to capture because it is very rare or is difficult to define. For example, occurrence of a postoperative surgical site infection (SSI) is a tangible outcome that results in durable changes to the patient's health and to the expense of their care. However, SSI occurs rarely (<1% of all cases) and is hard to capture within a single department or institution because it occurs days after surgery and may be treated on an outpatient basis at another facility. However, the timely administration of an appropriate prophylactic antibiotic is known to reduce the incidence of SSI; this process measure can be used as a surrogate quality measure for the actual outcome of interest.

Extrapolating from these definitions, it can be seen that an outcome measure is always preferable to a process measure when information about the outcome can be reliably captured. Further, the value of process measures is directly related to the scientific cause-and-effect relationship between the process and the outcome of interest – something that may be a moving target. Process measures must be continually reassessed for relevance, and should be replaced by measurement of the outcome of interest when advancing technology makes this possible. Overinvestment in process measures, and emotional overattachment to them, is one of the most common errors in health-care QM, and contributes substantially to the bureaucratic overhead of modern medicine.

Choosing quality measures for perioperative care should begin with a narrow focus on outcome measures of safety, and then expand over time as interest and resources allow. The typical first question is: How often do patients die or suffer major injury? Sometimes the required data can be found in existing health information technology (HIT) and must merely be abstracted for the QM program. In other cases a specific system of people, paper, and/or software must be established to create the data, link them to the patient's records, and digitize them. The former approach is almost always preferable, as it will be faster and less expensive than creating a new process from scratch [6].

As the QM program matures, new measurement initiatives should be considered. These can be broader views of safety (e.g., examining multiple process measures associated with a single outcome), or broader views of quality (e.g., examining economic indicators such as mean case duration or patient length of stay). In most perioperative QM programs, new measures are added on top of old ones in an iterative fashion, which may lead to substantial measurement clutter. The core outcome measures of mortality and morbidity will remain important and relevant in perpetuity, but many process measures are useful only in the short term and should be retired when no longer of value.

A final consideration in the choice of measures for perioperative QM is the use to which they will be put. This includes both the level of analysis and the level of reporting. If the intention is to measure performance at the individual level, then many outcomes will occur at too low an incidence to be relevant. Even something as common in anesthesia practice as a postdural puncture headache will occur only a few times a year in the practice of most anesthesiologists – too seldom to justify periodic reporting. Timely administration of antibiotics can be observed in almost every OR case, however, and is much more appropriate for individual analysis. Between these examples is a continuum and a principle: the less common an event, the greater the aggregation needed to interpret it and the higher the level for reporting.

Quality management has its greatest value when used internally by a group or facility as a tool to improve care. Internally reported measures are less alarming to the recipients, and require less risk adjustment of the data. They are therefore easier to keep current and relevant. Unfortunately, there is a growing public and regulatory demand for external data reporting. On the one hand, transparency is a desirable goal and a strong motivator of change. On the other hand, perioperative care is a complex multidisciplinary activity in which cause and effect are not always obvious, and public reporting of outcomes has the potential for a number of unintended consequences. Reducing mortality by avoiding high-risk patients or complex cases is one such consequence that may result from public reporting but that does not improve overall health-care quality. Selection of measures for public reporting thus involves different considerations than choosing measures to examine internally. We will consider this point further below.

Attribution

When perioperative QM data are analyzed and reported, one of the critical questions is how the measured outcomes are going to be attributed: Who is responsible for the outcome? At one extreme is an individual practitioner; at the other extreme is an entire facility. In between are teams of individuals, medical or support services, and geographic divisions of the entire hospital. Which level of attribution is appropriate depends on the nature of the measure, the purpose of reporting it, and the intended audience for the report.

Some perioperative measures are rightfully the responsibility of a single practitioner, e.g., the rate of unintended dural puncture when placing an epidural catheter, or the occurrence of vascular injury during surgical dissection. Other events are best examined at a team level, e.g., completion of preoperative documentation by a surgical service, or patient satisfaction with a unit nursing staff. And still other measures reflect multidisciplinary processes or overlapping areas of responsibility and can only be sensibly analyzed in aggregate. One example is the occurrence of perioperative myocardial infarction, which might reflect issues in patient selection and screening, intraoperative anesthetic management, postoperative monitoring, or even pharmacy delivery of medications.

Sometimes the ability to attribute responsibility is limited by the technology of the institution. On many surgical services – especially in teaching hospitals – the providers function as a team, with changing responsibilities on a daily or weekly basis. The admitting physician of record might not be the one who operates on the patient or manages their postoperative care; the anesthesiologist who signs the patient out from the postanesthesia care unit (PACU) may be different from the one who did the case and the one who wrote the postoperative pain-management orders. In these cases it is impossible to reliably attribute events at the individual level, and team reporting is more appropriate.

How outcomes are attributed says a lot about the QM program in question. On the one hand, if all adverse events are attributed to individuals (usually the attending surgeon or admitting physician), then there is insufficient focus on system problems and correctable root causes. On the other hand, attribution of events only at the system or facility level does not meet the public's demand for transparency, and may be seen as an effort to hide poor physicians or services. One approach is to attribute measures differently depending on the audience and the purpose: a central-line-associated bloodstream infection might be reported at the individual level internally (within the anesthesia department, for example) but at the team or facility level in external reporting.

The OR quality management plan

Quality management is the application of finite resources to an infinite problem. The starting point for perioperative QM should therefore be development of an overall strategic plan that indicates which issues will be addressed, in which order. From there the necessary measures can be identified and defined, and technology for data acquisition and analysis put in place. As problems are resolved and resources freed, the next items in priority can be pursued.

The first step in creating a QM plan is assembly of all the necessary stakeholders [7]. Either within the OR committee itself or as a subcommittee, each of the physician, nursing, and support services working in the OR should be represented. Each such group should have input into the allocation of resources (i.e., what is measured and reported) and should participate in the analysis of aggregated data and individual events. The perioperative QM committee should be led by a single individual with the knowledge, time, and enthusiasm to make it a visible and effective instrument for improving patient care.

The committee should begin its work by determining what data will be needed to address the most important issues, as described above, and what resources exist to collect them. Once data collection begins, the committee will be responsible for interpretation and reporting, and for initiating improvement efforts when opportunities arise. These efforts may include changes in OR policy and procedures, acquisition of new equipment and supplies, or focused education.

In addition to "top-down" planning for data collection, analysis, and reporting, the committee should also develop protocols for "bottom-up" QM efforts, of the sort that originate with exceptional cases or events. Familiar to most physicians as the morbidity and mortality process, this is the analysis of individual cases in which something went wrong. The goal is to analyze complicated cases in a detailed and systematic fashion, beginning with a factual description of what happened and proceeding to a creative analysis of ways in which the bad outcome could have been mitigated or prevented. In the complex world of perioperative care, this kind of anecdote-driven QM – done right – will be just as useful for improving outcomes as the more data-driven top-down approach. The key is to create a system and a culture in which adverse events and near misses can be reviewed in an honest, creative, and multidisciplinary fashion, without fear of inappropriate disclosure or individual reprisals. Multidisciplinary review should include members of the team that rendered treatment and if possible the patient involved in the incident or a patient advisor. Patient centeredness adds a new dimension of attention to the traditional morbidity and mortality conferences.

Mechanics of data acquisition and reporting

Techniques for aggregating perioperative data will vary based on institutional resources and the specific measures of greatest interest. The first principle is the most important, however: don't reinvent the wheel. Most institutions already collect a great deal of data, much of them relevant to perioperative care. Before beginning any new effort to create new QM data, the committee should gather everything possible from existing sources. This may include administrative data from hospital and practice billing systems, reports from the facility's admission-discharge-transfer (ADT) system,

supply reports from the instrument room, standing reports from OR management, patient satisfaction surveys from outside consultants, minutes from surgical service morbidity and mortality conferences, and copies of external reports to the Joint Commission, state or federal agencies, or specialty registries such as the National Trauma Data Bank, the National Surgical Quality Improvement Program (NSQIP), the Society for Thoracic Surgeons Registry, or the National Anesthesia Clinical Outcomes Registry. In most facilities, 90% of the data wanted by a perioperative QM program are already in existence somewhere in the system. Finding and validating them, and then synthesizing them, should be an important early task. Internal validation of the data and the reports that are produced with these data are useful exercises before their introduction to a QM committee. The validation process should render an understanding of the data quality and the methodologies used to produce the reports for the committee. This exercise will prepare the committee chair and staff for the inevitable challenges that will occur in committee.

Collecting data specifically for QM should be viewed as a last resort, because it will be expensive for the program, either in the time and money required to hire data collectors or in the good will of the providers who will have to respond to a new form. Because most clinicians are already inundated with documentation requirements, any new request, however well intentioned, will be met with strategies designed to minimize the time required. The unintended consequence is very often "click-through" button punching that may sacrifice accuracy of reporting for speed of completion. This leads to the familiar analytic problem of "garbage-in, garbage-out."

Professionally-trained data abstractors, on the other hand, will generate very accurate data from chart reviews and patient and provider interviews, and will relieve practicing clinicians of this burden. The barrier in this case is the cost of supporting that position. Each abstractor for the NSQIP, for example, can handle about 800 cases per year, at a cost of about $100 000. In some cases, however, the facility will already be supporting data collectors, and it may be possible to add a little bit to their workload without excessive expense.

Wherever possible, data should be collected directly from electronic systems. Most electronic health record (EHR) software comes with a robust reporting tool and a library of preprogrammed reports. Creation of new or customized reports is usually possible as well. The

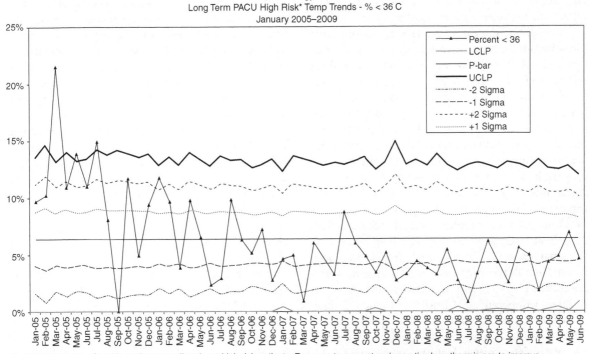

Anaesthesiology Division
Long Term PACU High Risk* Temp Trends - % < 36 C
January 2005–2009

Legend:
- Percent < 36
- LCLP
- P-bar
- UCLP
- -2 Sigma
- -1 Sigma
- +2 Sigma
- +1 Sigma

Goal: Maintenance of perioperative normolhemia on high risk patients. Reasons to prevent perioperative hypothermia are to improve patient comfort, reduce coagulopathy and bleeding. reduce risk of ischemia, prevent wound infection and shorten hospitalization. High risk parients' temperature is measured in the post anesthesia care unit (PACU)

*High Risk includes Thoracolomy, Open Coleclomy, Hepaleclomy, Pancrealeclomy, THR, TKR, Open/AS Shoulder

Figure 24.1. A typical control chart, showing the rate of failure to achieve normothermia in high-risk patients at the time of PACU admission.

goal of the perioperative QM program should be to pull in data from many disparate sources, and synthesize them into a cohesive picture of the business. This occurs through periodic publication of an "OR report" that presents all of the data in a clear and statistically supported fashion. This report should be distributed to all stakeholders in the perioperative process, including the leaders of the surgical, anesthesia, and nursing services. The overall report can then be trimmed or excerpted as needed to provide subreports for particular service lines, to meet regulatory requirements, and for upward reporting within the organization.

Most of the perioperative QM data gathered should be reported as rates (occurrences over cases), and then as trends over time. Especially for internal use, the change in rates over time for a given indicator is the best way to understand it. Is this process stable or deteriorating? Have efforts to improve it had an impact? An initial OR QM report often seems superficial, because it is no more than a snapshot of activities. As repeated measurement occurs, value accumulates, and more

complex analytic techniques become feasible. After 10–12 reports (1 year of aggregation of monthly data) many rates can be expressed on control charts (Figure 24.1), which facilitate differentiation of random up and down variability from truly significant trends.

Outcomes of interest

As above, local circumstances will determine which measures are most relevant to a given practice. In general, however, patient-centered outcomes will always have the greatest impact. This is especially true of safety measures – mortality and serious adverse events – and the perioperative QM program should seek these measures first. Any indication that complications are increasing or are in excess of a national benchmark should be promptly addressed. Early internal detection of adverse safety trends will facilitate prompt correction, and is one of the greatest values of a perioperative QM program.

Fortunately for all, perioperative mortality and serious events are rare, and adverse trends are uncommon.

Day-to-day perioperative QM can therefore focus on other patient-centered measures that are less serious, more common, and easier to measure and improve. These include outcomes such as length of stay, the incidence of postoperative nausea and vomiting, and the adequacy of postoperative pain management. Patient satisfaction might also be included in this category. The federal Consumer Assessment of Healthcare Providers and Systems (CAHPS) project (www.cahps.ahrq.gov) includes a perioperative care satisfaction survey. This is sent to random samples of surgical patients on an ongoing basis and includes questions about the facility, the medical and nursing providers, and the overall experience. These data are publicly reported.

Other outcomes of interest might include various metrics of business performance: billing and collections, payer mix, OR utilization, on-time starts, cancellations, and OR turnover time. Data for these measures are usually easy to obtain in electronic form from the facility's perioperative EHR. As part of the OR quality report this information will be of great value for internal decision making and as a guide to appropriate allocation of resources and return on investment in different service lines.

Staff satisfaction has a strong correlation with efficiency, and can be a leading indicator of future problems with retention and recruitment. Collecting and reporting these data in the QM process is unusual in most systems, but can be of great value when it is done well.

Levels of reporting

As noted above, the OR QM report should serve as the central nexus for perioperative management. Data flow into the report from disparate sources but are then analyzed and presented in a standard format over time. Upward distribution of the report, or selected segments, is important for regulatory and marketing purposes, whereas downward distribution (to providers) is a useful tool for creating change. One decision that must be made is how much of the report to make public within the practice group, at what level of analysis.

On the one hand, transparency and the goal of an open and knowledgeable provider group would suggest that most of the report should be published to all of the anesthesiologists in the group. The more these individuals know about the practice, the better they can make it work. This is certainly true for data reported at the level of the practice as a whole, or for individual facilities covered by the practice. Reporting the patient satisfaction rate, for example, will help emphasize the importance of this metric to the group and will encourage efforts to improve it. Reporting that makes it clear what the problem areas are (with data) will keep all providers aware of the group's active agenda items, and will make them better advocates when talking with surgeons, nurses, patients, and administrators.

More consideration must be given to reports at the individual level that are seen by the entire group. As with any sort of public reporting of QM data, this creates the potential for hurt feelings and unintended consequences. Provider resentment is one concern, especially if the "low outliers" are really the victims of incomplete risk adjustment or random statistical variation. Indiscriminate public embarrassment will reduce individual and group morale and, ultimately, impair recruitment and retention. Gamesmanship is another risk: providers who become competitive with their peers might decline certain cases or patients, or might be motivated to underreport adverse events or bad outcomes. Open reporting at the individual level should therefore be reserved for those metrics that need less risk adjustment, are less professionally embarrassing, and for which some public embarrassment is judged a good tactic to improve group outcomes. One common example that meets these three criteria is "completion of the QM form at the conclusion of a case." This is obviously a necessary process for the perioperative QM program, but might require a change in culture and behavior when first initiated. Monthly publication of an open ranking of compliance – with physician names on it – might be a good motivational tool in the early stages. Once group compliance becomes uniformly good, the public reporting can be abandoned.

A better way to provide individual feedback without public embarrassment is to show results in encrypted form, where providers can see their personal ranking within the group as a whole, but cannot discriminate other individuals. Figure 24.2 shows an example of this reporting principle. A hybrid approach might report results for identifiable service lines, to harness the power of competition, but remain blinded at the individual level. An example would be posting the percentage of on-time starts by a surgical service. This would be appropriate if each service was aiming for the same goal (e.g., patient in the room by 07:30 h) but was free to create its own mechanisms for achieving it (e.g., deciding what time to come to work). If this freedom does not exist, then this kind of reporting is

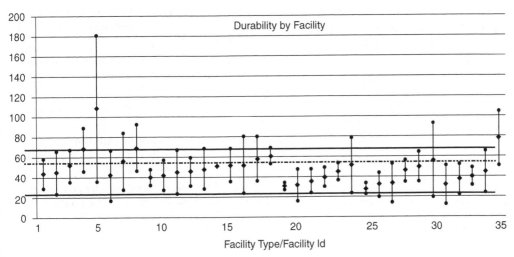

Figure 24.2. An example of anonymous public reporting, showing the mean and standard deviation time required to perform a given surgical procedure, in different surgical facilities. Personnel at each facility know their own ID number, but not the others.

problematic, and the services with more complex setup requirements would feel victimized.

Pay for performance

Pay for performance is a common term in the national health policy debate. In its simplest interpretation this refers to direct incentives for fulfilling certain QM goals. Physicians are offered bonuses and add-ons to the basic physician payment amount that is linked to a measure of performance. Under pay for performance, physicians are paid extra for accomplishing a process measure. Many of the pay-for-performance programs have a local impact and a limited shelf life. In the future performance contracting will shift away from process measures toward outcome measures, overuse and patient-reported outcomes. The Physician Quality Reporting System incentive payment for timely administration of perioperative antibiotics is one such; denial of payment when a "never event" (e.g., wrong-site surgery) occurs is another. The Physician Quality Reporting System will offer financial incentives for participation until 2015, when providers are then penalized for not reporting quality outcomes to the Centers for Medicare & Medicaid Services (CMS). Denial of payment to hospitals for preventable complications is part of the value-based purchasing (VBP) plan enacted by CMS in 2008 [8]. An early goal of the plan is to no longer reimburse hospitals for preventable complications. The VBP seeks to improve quality and efficiency in health care by experimenting with pay-for-performance models that reward higher performing providers and organizations. In the broader sense, however, this term refers to a desired future state of health-care reimbursement: payment for an outcome rather than a process. As taxpayers, it seems sensible to us that physicians should be paid for improving patients' quality of life, rather than for the number of tests ordered or procedures done.

As physicians, however, the change to a pure performance-based system will require nothing less than a revolutionary overhaul of 50 years of health-care finance. Individual providers, and the specialty societies that represent them, are highly attentive to these impending changes, and justifiably agitated about the possibility for reduced income, increased workload, and collateral impacts on patient safety. Optimists believe that the costs of payment reform will be offset by improved operational efficiency; pessimists believe that there will be dramatic winners and losers under any new system. Regardless of individual outlook, however, it is clear that the more data are available to a facility or practice, the more cogent their arguments and advocacy can become. This is one more reason – perhaps the best one – that a robust perioperative QM system is a necessity in today's world.

Summary

A perioperative QM system is a requirement for any effective and efficient OR. Although different institutions will require different structures, the basic concepts of collecting, analyzing, and reporting are universal.

Access to consistent, accurate data will facilitate the work of any OR manager or anesthesiology director. Creating a system that provides these data should be a high priority in any system.

References

1. M. E. Porter. A strategy for health care reform – toward a value-based system. *N Engl J Med* 2009; **361**: 109–12.

2. R. K. Smoldt, D. A. Cortese. Pay-for-performance or pay for value? *Mayo Clin Proc.* 2007; **82**: 210–13.

3. J. F. Finks, N. H. Osborne, J. D. Birkmeyer. Trends in hospital volume and operative mortality for high-risk surgery. *N Engl J Med* 2011; **364**: 2128–37.

4. T. H. Lee, L. P. Casalino, E. S. Fisher, G. R. Wilensky. Creating accountable care organizations. *N Engl J Med* 2010; **363**: e23.

5. L. G. Glance, M. Neuman, E. A. Martinez, K. Y. Pauker, R. P. Dutton. Performance measurement at a "tipping point". *Anesth Analg* 2011; **112**; 958–66.

6. R. P. Dutton. Pro: the AQI model for data collection. *ASA Newsletter* May, 2010.

7. Anesthesia Quality Institute. Quality management in your practice. http://aqihq.org/qm-in-your-practice.pdf (last accessed may 10, 2012).

8. T. J. Hoff, C. Soerensen. No payment for preventable complications: reviewing the early literature for content, guidance, and impressions. *Q Manage Health Care* 2010; **20**: 62–75.

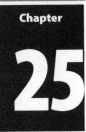

Chapter

25

Sedation
Clinical and safety considerations

Ann Bui MD
Richard D. Urman MD, MBA

Introduction   253
Definitions of sedation   255
Preprocedure evaluation   255
Monitors and equipment   256
Medications   256
Recovery and discharge   257
Regulation   257
Credentialing and competency   260

Education   261
Quality improvement and risk
assessment   261
Outcomes   261
Controversies   261
Future of sedation   262
Summary   262
Appendix: Guidelines and standards   262

Introduction

As health care and technology progress, the need for anesthesia services escalates both in and out of the operating room (OR). Ideally, individuals with the most training and experience with sedation would administer it. Owing to the high volume of cases that require sedation, however, many nonanesthesiologists are providing this service. Today, sedation is administered by both anesthesia professionals (anesthesiologists, certified registered nurse anesthetists, and anesthesiologist assistants) and nonanesthesia professionals (physicians, dentists, registered nurses, physician assistants, etc.). Generally, sedation is optimal for procedures that are quick and/or noninvasive (Table 25.1). Although general anesthesia can be performed for every procedure that could otherwise be done with sedation, sedation is preferred by many patients and health-care providers. Depending on the knowledge and experience of the person providing sedation, sedation may offer a quicker recovery time and may be less invasive compared with general anesthesia.

Medicine advancement has allowed procedures, which typically took place in the OR, to be performed outside of the OR (OOOR). Nowadays procedures done with sedation, both in the OR and OOOR, are increasing in complexity, and the patients receiving these

procedures are having more comorbidities. Despite this, many patients receiving sedation do not necessarily require the presence of an anesthesiologist. The American Society of Anesthesiologists (ASA) Statement on Granting Privileges for Administration of Moderate Sedation to Practitioners Who Are Not Anesthesia Professionals states that "only physicians, dentists, or podiatrists who are qualified by education, training, and licensure to administer moderate sedation should supervise the administration of moderate sedation." The ASA Statement on Granting Privileges to Nonanesthesiologist Supervising Deep Sedation by Individuals Who Are Not Anesthesia Professionals states that "due to a significant risk that patients who receive deep sedation may enter a state of general anesthesia, privileges to administer deep sedation should be granted only to practitioners who are qualified to administer general anesthesia or to appropriately supervise anesthesia professionals." The aforementioned ASA statements address education, training, licensure, supervision, performance evaluation, and improvement requirements for a sedation program involving nonanesthesia providers [1,2,3]. Although the ASA guidelines are generally supported by most regulatory agencies, there are many other professional societies that have their own standards and guidelines on procedural sedation (see Addendum: Society Guidelines

Operating Room Leadership and Management, ed. Kaye A.D., Fox C.J. and Urman R.D. Published by Cambridge University Press. © Cambridge University Press 2012.

Table 25.1 Procedures performed under moderate sedation administered by non-anesthesia trained registered nurses (taken from: E. E. Whitaker, A. Mukherjee, T. Liu, B. Hong, E. S. Heitmiller. Introduction to moderate and deep sedation. In: R. Urman, A. D. Kaye. *Moderate and Deep Sedation in Clinical Practice*, 1st edn. Cambridge University Press, 2012. Chapter 1, pp. 1–7, Table 1.1)

Head and neck	Superficial thoracic	Extremity procedures	Gastrointestinal/abdominal	Vascular	Gynecologic/urologic	Emergency department/radiology
Dental extractions	Breast augmention	Carpal tunnel release	Endoscopic retrograde cholangiopancreatography	Hemodialysis access placement	Dilatation and curettage	Reduction of dislocation or fracture
Blepharoplasty	Breast biopsy	Trigger finger release	Colonoscopy	Pacemaker insertion	Fulguration of vaginal lesions	Complex suturing
Rhytidoplasty	Bronchoscopy	Removal of pins/wires/screws	Endoscopic ultrasound	Angiography	Fulguration of anal lesions	Insertion of elective chest tube
Rhinoplasty	Chest tube insertion	Closed reduction	Gastroscopy	Cardiac catheterization	Cystoscopy	MRI
Laceration				Radiofrequency ablation	Incision and drainage of Bartholin's cyst	Arteriograms
Cataract				Electrophysiologic testing	Vasectomy	Liver biopsy

Table 25.2 Continuum of depth of sedation: definition of general anesthesia and levels of sedation/analgesia

	Minimal sedation	Moderate sedation/analgesia (conscious sedation)	Deep sedation/analgesia	General anesthesia
Responsiveness	Normal	Purposeful[a] response to verbal or tactile stimulation	Purposeful[a] response after repeated or painful stimulation	Unarousable even with painful stimulus
Airway	Unaffected	No intervention required	Intervention may be required	Intervention often required
Spontaneous ventilation	Unaffected	Adequate	May be inadequate	Frequently inadequate
Cardiovascular funtion	Unaffected	Usually maintained	Usually maintained	May be Impaired

Source: American Society of Anesthesiologists Task Force on Sedation and Analgesia by Non-Anesthesiologists. Available online at: www.asahq.org/For-Healthcare-Professionals/Standards-Guidelines-and-Statements.aspx (last accessed May 11, 2012).*a* Reflex withdrawal from a painful stimulus is not considered a purposeful response.

and Standards). For example, the American Nurses Association's (ANA) Procedural Sedation Consensus Statement states that procedural sedation medications can be administered by a registered nurse (RN) only in the presence of a physician, advanced practiced registered nurse or other health-care professional qualified and trained for procedural sedation.

Definitions of sedation

It is important to realize that sedation and general anesthesia are on a continuum. There are different levels of sedation, but they can easily blend with one another and evolve into general anesthesia. Each patient responds differently to sedation medications, and thus, even if the health-care practitioner intended on delivering moderate sedation, a deep sedation or even a general anesthetic can occur. The ASA defines sedation levels according to responsiveness, airway, spontaneous ventilation, and cardiovascular function (Table 25.2). According to the ASA, there are three levels of sedation, which culminate in general anesthesia [4].

Minimal sedation – this is primarily done for anxiolysis. Patients respond normally to verbal commands, are able to maintain a patent airway, are spontaneously breathing and have an unchanged cardiovascular system.

Moderate sedation – this was previously known as "conscious sedation." It is a drug-induced state in which there is a depression of consciousness. However, patients still have a purposeful response to verbal commands, plus or minus light tactile stimulation. Patients continue to maintain a patent airway without any intervention and have adequate spontaneous ventilation. The cardiovascular system is usually unchanged.

Deep sedation – consciousness is depressed significantly and patients require repeated or painful stimuli to evoke a purposeful response. An intervention may be required for patients to maintain a patent airway and spontaneous ventilation may be inadequate. Cardiovascular function is usually unchanged.

General anesthesia – consciousness is lost and patients are unarousable even to painful stimulation. Patients often need assistance in maintaining a patent airway and with ventilation, as this is frequently inadequate. Positive pressure ventilation may be required because of depressed spontaneous ventilation or drug-induced depression of neuromuscular function. Cardiovascular function may be impaired.

Clinically there is not a clear distinction between the levels of sedation and because the levels of sedation can quickly progress into general anesthesia, the ASA standard is that health-care providers should be able to rescue patients from any level of sedation and return them to the original intended level of sedation.

Preprocedure evaluation

Before the procedure, it is imperative to review the patient's medical history, preprocedure labs, diagnostic tests and physically examine the patient. This includes reviewing nil per os (NPO) status, medications and drug allergies, previous anesthesia and/or sedation experiences, and health problems. It is critical

Table 25.3 ASA physical status classification system

ASA physical status 1	A normal healthy patient
ASA physical status 2	A patient with mild systemic disease
ASA physical status 3	A patient with severe systemic disease
ASA physical status 4	A patient with severe systemic disease that is a constant threat to life
ASA physical status 5	A moribund patient who is not expected to survive without the operation
ASA physical status 6	A declared brain-dead patient whose organs are being removed for donor purposes

to recognize the comorbidities that place a patient at higher risk for sedation; these comorbidities include, but are not limited to, morbid obesity, extremes of age, sleep apnea, and an anticipated difficult airway. Patients with multiple systemic comorbidities (ASA physical status 3–5) also are at an increased risk for complications (Table 25.3). The presence of these factors should prompt an anesthesiology consult. The physical examination portion should include obtaining the patient's height, weight, and baseline vital signs along with assessing the airway. The ability to identify a potentially difficult airway is essential. Lastly, before giving any sedation medications, one must ensure that appropriate consents have been completed.

Monitors and equipment

Once sedation has started, proper monitoring of the patient's oxygenation, ventilation, circulation, and level of consciousness must be continually assessed; therefore, it is necessary for the person administrating sedation to be present throughout the entire procedure and to have no other responsibilities. Oxygenation is monitored via continuous pulse oximetry, and every patient should receive supplemental oxygen. Supplemental oxygen along with pulse oximetry can prevent and detect hypoxemia, but neither is ideal for the identification of hypoventilation, airway obstruction, or apnea. In fact, supplemental oxygen can mask problems with ventilation. Ventilation is monitored by continuously observing patient chest movement, evaluating airway patency, and auscultating breath sounds. The ASA Standards for Basic Anesthetic Monitoring state that "During moderate and deep sedation the adequacy of ventilation shall be evaluated by continual observation of qualitative clinical signs and monitoring for the presence of exhaled carbon dioxide unless precluded or invalidated by the nature of the patient, procedure,

or equipment" [5]. Capnography can significantly aid in monitoring ventilation and alerts sedation providers to hypoventilation/apnea much more quickly than clinical observation alone. Evaluation of circulation is done via continuous electrocardiogram and measuring blood pressure at least every 5 min; circulation can also be assessed by palpating pulses and auscultating heart sounds. A patient's level of consciousness is easily monitored by talking to and/or stimulating the patient. The ASA Standards for Basic Anesthetic Monitoring also say that "Every patient receiving anesthesia shall have temperature monitored when clinically significant changes in body temperature are intended, anticipated or suspected" [5]. Although not every procedure done with sedation will require the monitoring of temperature, sedation providers should be cognizant of when it is needed. Before every procedure, it is necessary to ensure the availability of monitors and equipment and that they are functioning correctly (Table 25.4). Despite this, monitors can malfunction at any time during the procedure; thus, no monitor is more valuable than the vigilant health-care provider.

Medications

An important aspect of safely providing sedation is knowing the pharmacologic profiles of the common medications used. Although a plethora of medications exist that will provide sedation and/or analgesia, the agents most commonly used are benzodiazepines and opioids (Table 25.5). Both are easily titratable and their actions can be mitigated by reversal agents. Because benzodiazepines and opioids are commonly given together, one must acknowledge that their actions and side effects are synergistic and must be careful to avoid oversedation and/or respiratory depression. Although benzodiazepines lack analgesic properties, they are anxiolytics, anticonvulsants, sedatives, and amnestics.

Table 25.4 Equipment needed for moderate and deep sedation (taken from: L. Caperelli-White. Nursing considerations for sedation. In: R. Urman, A. D. Kaye. *Moderate and Deep Sedation in Clinical Practice*, 1st edn. Cambridge University Press, 2012. Chapter 8, pp. 103–4.)

Oxygen source
Airway equipment – including a self-inflating oxygen delivery system capable of delivering 100% oxygen
Suction source with suction catheters
Pulse oximeter with audible alarms
Cardiac monitor with audible alarms
Blood pressure device and stethoscope
Capnography
Emergency cart and defibrillator
Medications to be used for the procedure and their reversal agents
Fluid bags of either 0.9% Normal Saline or Lactated Ringer's

Of the benzodiazepines, midazolam is very popular because of its quick onset, short duration of action, and favorable hemodynamic profile. In situations of oversedation, flumazenil is the reversal agent for benzodiazepines. It is usually given in increments of 0.2 mg and is titrated to effect (i.e., desired level of consciousness). It has a quick onset and a half-life shorter than most benzodiazepines; thus, to avoid re-sedation, flumazenil may have to be administered more than once.

Unlike benzodiazepines, opioids are primarily analgesics. Opioids are administered to prevent and alleviate pain and as an adjunct to sedatives/hypnotics, such as benzodiazepines. Of the opioids, fentanyl is very popular because of its quick onset, short duration of action, and favorable hemodynamic profile. In situations of undesired respiratory depression or excessive sedation, naloxone is the reversal agent for opioids. It is usually given in increments of 0.04 mg and is titrated to effect (i.e., respiratory rate over eight breaths per minute). In cases in which long-acting opioids have been given, it may be necessary to readminister naloxone to avoid repeated respiratory depression.

Recovery and disc harge

After receiving sedation, patients should continue to be monitored in a post-sedation recovery area until time of discharge. This is because many complications can occur during the postoperative period, with respiratory depression and aspiration being the most common. How long a patient must spend in the recovery area and how frequent their vital signs should be monitored and recorded are dependent on the institution, but commonly, vital signs are recorded every 10 min for a minimum of 30 min. Before being discharged,

patients must meet certain criteria. These criteria are also dependent on the institution, but generally include adequate oxygenation and ventilation, hemodynamic stability, and return to baseline level of consciousness. The Aldrete scoring system [6] was one of the first sets of objective discharge criteria used (Table 25.6); a minimum score of 9 out of 10 allowed for discharge. Along with the appropriate monitors, the recovery area must also have the same equipment that was available during the time of sedation, in case a patient was to require resuscitation. Many complications occur during the recovery period because of inadequate monitoring, equipment, and personnel training. If a patient is being discharged home, the patient must receive both verbal and written discharge instructions. It is optimal that the person taking the patient home also be present for these instructions, as the patient may not remember everything. Instructions usually include any activity or diet restrictions specific to the procedure performed and any problems the patient should anticipate.

Regulation

Unlike the Center for Medicare and Medicaid Services (CMS), which is a federal agency, the Joint Commission is "an independent not-for-profit organization" (About The Joint Commission, 2012). Although they each have their own regulations and standards, they also operate together to ensure patient safety at an institutional level. The Joint Commission audits and accredits institutions to ensure that they hold up to the regulations and standards put forth by the Joint Commission and CMS. According to the CMS Condition of Participation, "If the hospital furnishes anesthesia services, [the services] must be provided in a well-organized manner under

Table 25.5 Medication chart (taken from: J. Metzner, K. B. Domino. Anesthesia and sedation outside of the operating room: outcomes, regulation, and quality improvement. In: R. Urman, W. Gross, B. K. Philip. *Anesthesia Outside of the Operating Room*, 1st edn. Oxford University Press, 2011. Chapter 8, pp. 62–73.)

Drug	Sedational amnesia	Anxiolysis	Analgesia	Route/dose	Onset (min)	Peak (min)	Duration (min)	Comments
Sedative/ hypnotics*								
Midazolam (Versed)	Yes	Yes	No	IV: 0.5–1 mg (titrate to effect up to 5–10 mg/h)	0.5–1	3–5	10–30	Minimal cardio-respiratory depression
				IM: 0.08 mg/kg	10–15	20–45	60–120	Reduce dose when used in combination with opioids
								Midazolam is benzodiazepine of choice for short procedures
								Antagonist: flumazenil
Diazepam (Valium)	Yes	Yes	No	IV: 2–3 mg (titrate to effect up to 15 mg)	1–2	8–15	15–45	
				PO: 5–10 mg	30–60	45–60	60–100	
Lorazepam (Acivan)	Yes	Yes	No	IV: 0.25 mg (titrate to effect up to 2 mg)	1–2	15–20	60–120	
				PO: 2–4 mg	60–120	120	>480	
Opioids*								
Fentanyl	No	No	Yes	IV: 28–50 μg intermittent boluses	1–2	5	30–40	Respiratory depression decreased
Meperidine (Demerol)	No	No	Yes	IV: 2.5–75 mg	3–5	5–7	63–180	Response to hypercarbia and hypoxia
								Synergistic sedative and respiratory depressant effects (reduce dose with sedatives)
								Nausea, vomiting
								Meperidine: histamine release

Reversal agents (antagonists)							
Flumazenil (Anexate)	No	No	IV: 0.1–0.2 mg (titrate to effect to max of 5)	1–2	5–10	45–90	Short-acting, repeat doses may be required Avoid in patients receiving benzodiazenines for seizure control Caution with chronic benzodiazepine therapy (withdrawal effect) or with tricyclic antidepressants
Naloxome (Narcan)	No	No	IV: 0.02–1.04 mg (titrate to effect)	1–2	2–3	30–60	Antagonist: naloxone Short-acting, repeat doses may be required May cause hypertension and tachycardia Pulmonary edema reported

*Alterations in dosing may be indicated based upon the clinical situation and the practitioner's experience with these agents. Individual dosages may vary depending on age and coexistent diseases. Doses should be reduced for sicker patients and in the elderly. When using drug combinations, the potential for significant respiratory impairment and airway obstruction is increased. Drugs should be titrated to achieve optimal effect, and sufficient time for dose effect should be allowed before administering an additional dose or another medication.

Table 25.6 Aldrete scoring system (adapted from: J. A. Aldrete. The post-anesthesia recovery score revisited. *J Clin Anesth* 1995; 7: 89–91.)

Respiration
  Able to take deep breath and cough = 2
  Dyspnea/shallow breathing = 1
  Apnea = 0

Oxygen saturation
  $SaO_2 > 95\%$ on room air = 2
  $SaO_2 > 90\%–95\%$ on room air = 1
  $SaO_2 < 90\%$ even with supplemental O_2 = 0

Consciousness
  Fully awake = 2
  Arousable on calling = 1
  Not responding = 0

Circulation
  BP ± 20 mm Hg baseline = 2
  BP ± 20–50 mm Hg baseline = 1
  BP ± 50 mm Hg baseline = 0

Activity
  Able to move 4 extremities = 2
  Able to move 2 extremities = 1
  Able to move 0 extremities = 0

Note: Monitoring may be discontinued and patient discharged to home or appropriate unit when Aldrete score is 9 or greater. Taken from: D. E. Morrison, K. Dorn Hare. Patient evaluation and procedure selection, In: R. Urman, A. D. Kaye. *Moderate and Deep sedation in Clinical Practice*, 1st edn. Cambridge University Press, 2012. Chapter 4, pp. 44–56.

the direction of a qualified doctor of medicine or osteopathy. The [hospital's anesthesiology department] is responsible for all anesthesia administered in the hospital," [7] whether it was administered by anesthesia providers or nonanesthesia providers. The CMS and Joint Commission dictate anesthesia/sedation care preoperatively, intraoperatively, and postoperatively (Table 25.7) The CMS orders that patients must be assessed within 48 h of receiving sedation, monitored intraoperatively with proper documentation as proof, and appropriately cared for postoperatively.

Credentialing and competency

Although on a national level, the Joint Commission requires all institutions to verify a practitioner's state license, Drug Enforcement Administration (DEA) number, and education and training prior to granting the privilege of administrating sedation, the specific credentialing and training one must possess is

determined by individual institutions. The ASA has set forth different requirements for practitioners administrating moderate versus deep sedation, which may be viewed in entirety on their website. Owing to the high potential for deep sedation to evolve into general anesthesia, the ASA states that practitioners administrating deep sedation should also be able to provide general anesthesia safely. The CMS additionally adds that only anesthesia providers (anesthesiologists, nurse anesthetists, and anesthesiology assistants), physicians, dentists, oral surgeons, and podiatrists should be granted the privilege of providing deep sedation. A practitioner providing deep sedation must be trained in advanced cardiac life support (ACLS) and/or pediatric advanced life support (PALS), depending on the patient population receiving deep sedation. A physician, dentist, oral surgeon, and podiatrist must be present to supervise moderate sedation, which can be administered by the aforementioned, in addition to anesthesia providers, registered nurses, and physician assistants. A practitioner administrating any level of sedation should possess the skills to rescue a patient in case the patient enters a deeper level of sedation than intended and return the patient to the intended level of sedation. Hence, it is absolutely crucial that the practitioner performing the procedure and the practitioner administering sedation are separate individuals, with the latter solely focused on monitoring the patient and immediately available in case cardiopulmonary compromise were to occur. Generally, "the Joint Commission requires that sedation providers have adequate training to administer the sedative drugs effectively and safely, the skills to monitor the patient's response to the medications given, and the expertise needed to manage all potential complications" [8]. Additionally, practitioners should be able to identify the varying levels of sedation, which will allow them to intervene appropriately when the patient is being under- or oversedated. Not only should the practitioner have comprehensive knowledge about the sedative drugs, but also about the available reversal agents. Anticipating and recognizing patients' varying response to medications is needed and allows the practitioner to maintain patient hemodynamic stability. Understanding the physiology of oxygenation and ventilation and the ability to differentiate between normal and abnormal vital signs and cardiac rhythms and then relate them to the patient's current state is a necessary skill. Also, practitioners providing all levels of sedation should be competent in assessing and managing the

Table 25.7 Summary of the Joint Commission standards for moderate sedation (taken from: M. T. Antonelli, D. E. Seaver. Quality, legal, and risk management considerations: ensuring program excellence. In: R. Urman, A. D. Kaye. *Moderate and Deep sedation in Clinical Practice*, 1st edn. Cambridge University Press, 2012. Chapter 7, pp. 85–101.)

1. Moderate sedation must be administered by a qualified provider.

2. Patients who will receive moderate sedation must be assessed prior to sedation/procedure.

3. The provider must discuss risks and options with the patient or his/her family prior to sedation/procedure.

4. The provider must re-assess the patient immediately before the sedation is initiated.

5. Monitoring of the patient's oxygenation, ventilation, and circulation during sedation is mandatory.

6. Post-sedation assessment in the recovery area is necessary before the patient is discharged.

7. A qualified provider must discharge the patient from the post-sedation recovery area or discharge must be based on established criteria.

airway and be able to determine when an anesthesiology consultation is needed.

Education

To ensure practitioners have the essential knowledge and skills that are crucial to being a competent sedation provider, institutions must develop educational programs that identify and assess these knowledge and skills. Traditionally, knowledge is obtained via lectures and assessed via written tests. Although this method facilitates basic science knowledge, it is not proficient at teaching and validating clinical skills, reasoning, and decision-making behavior. The latter can be done with simulation-based education, which creates real-life clinical scenarios. No matter the method taken, the institution is obligated to routinely validate and assess the knowledge and skills required, as the responsibilities of sedation practitioners change due to the emergence of new technology and procedures.

Quality improvement and risk assessment

Internally, institutions need a process to address quality improvement and risk assessment to ensure the institution's policies and practices are at the best clinical standard to minimize potential risks of injury. This process provides the ultimate goal of delivering patient safety. Through review and evaluation of institutional policies, quality of care, and patient outcomes, the quality improvement processes improve the practice of sedation. This confirms adherence to standards of care and can systematically be done by regularly reviewing charts chosen at random, and by direct observation of care. The risk-assessment processes are responsible for analyzing situations in which an adverse patient

outcome has occurred or almost occurred. By investigating all the factors that contributed to or caused an adverse patient outcome, changes can be made to prevent such events in the future. The Joint Commission mandates that all sentinel events (i.e., wrong-site or wrong-patient surgery) be reviewed with a root cause analysis (RCA).

"The University of HealthSystem Consortium (UHC), an alliance of academic medical centers and affiliated hospitals that focus on excellence in quality, safety, and cost-effectiveness, recommends the following (…) patient outcomes" be monitored and documented: deaths, aspirations, reversal agent used, unplanned transfer to higher level of care, cardiac/respiratory arrest, medications administered other than those approved, inability to complete procedure as planned, and emergency procedures without a licensed independent practitioner present [7].

Outcomes

Examining the ASA Closed Claims Project data on procedures performed with sedation or monitored anesthesia care (MAC), the most common etiology of death or permanent brain damage is respiratory depression due to oversedation [9,10]. The use of propofol in combination with benzodiazepines and/or opioids increased the incidence of respiratory depression. Most of these events were deemed preventable either by better monitoring techniques, in particular capnography, or enhanced vigilance by the sedation provider. As a result, the ASA considers capnography a standard monitor.

Controversies

Because the use of propofol increases the risk of moderate sedation slipping into deep sedation or even general anesthesia, the ASA Statement on Safe Use of Propofol [11] says that when propofol is administered, patients "should receive care consistent with that required for deep sedation" and that the nonanesthesia provider "should be qualified to rescue patients whose level of sedation becomes deeper than initially intended and who enter, if briefly, a state of general anesthesia." Whether or not propofol can safely be administered by nonanesthesia providers remains a topic of controversy. The studies that have been done on propofol administration by nonanesthesia providers have not shown an increased incidence of severe adverse patient outcome, such as airway compromise requiring bag mask ventilation and/or endotracheal intubation, but these studies do not take into account the incidence and magnitude of respiratory obstruction, hypoventilation, or hemodynamic compromise [12–17]. Future studies that completely investigate the safety of propofol administration by nonanesthesia providers are needed.

Future of sedation

Increasing patient safety during procedural sedation may lie in the use of new medications and new medication delivery techniques. Fospropofol, the prodrug of propofol, has been approved by the Food and Drug Administration (FDA) for the sedation of adults. The slower onset and longer duration of action of fospropofol make it possibly advantageous in minimizing the risk of oversedation. The pharmacokinetic profile of fospropofol is still in progress, but its use as a sedative drug is promising. Because fospropofol gets converted to propofol, its package insert also says that it "should be administered only by persons trained in the administration of general anesthesia and not involved in the conduct of the diagnostic or therapeutic procedure." (Lusedra Warnings and Precautions)

Similar to patient-controlled analgesia (PCA), patient-controlled sedation/analgesia (PCSA) enables the patient to control how much sedation/analgesia he or she receives and when. With the push of a button, patients can have medications (i.e., midazolam, fentanyl) delivered; and with the lockout interval, bolus doses, and maximum infusion rate set by the health-care provider, the risk of oversedation is minimized. Such PCSA offers high patient satisfaction, and patients tend to use less medication compared with health-care provider administration of sedation/analgesia.

Computer-assisted personalized sedation (CAPS) is a program that monitors a patient's vital signs and level of responsiveness and then determines if and when a patient receives sedation medications. If a patient is being oversedated, as determined by vital signs and lack of responsiveness, then the delivery of sedation medications will be paused or stopped and the delivery of oxygen will increase. The CAPS is not meant to replace the sedation provider, but instead aid in providing sedation; it has not been approved by the FDA at this time.

Summary

In conclusion, it is important for sedation providers to realize that there are distinctly different levels of sedation, but that clinically it may be difficult to differentiate between them. Each institution offering sedation services must follow the federal and state regulations on moderate and deep sedation, and sedation providers must have the appropriate qualifications. The specific education and training required of sedation providers differs between institutions. Although most institutions adopt the ASA guidelines and standards, each professional society also has its own set of guidelines. In the end, whether sedation is administered by an anesthesia or nonanesthesia provider, patient safety is of utmost concern.

Appendix: Guidelines and standards

American Academy of Pediatrics (AAP) and American Academy of Pediatric Dentistry (AAPD)

Guidelines for monitoring and management of pediatric patients during and after sedation for diagnostic and therapeutic procedures: an update (2006). *Pediatrics* 2006; **118**: 2587–602. Available online at: www.aapd.org/media/Policies_Guidelines/G_Sedation.pdf.

American Association of Critical-Care Nurses (AACN)

Position statement on the role of the RN in the management of patients receiving IV moderate sedation for short-term therapeutic, diagnostic, or surgical procedures (2002). Available online at: www.aacn.org/WD/Practice/Docs/Sedation.doc.

American Association of Nurse Anesthetists (AANA)

Position statement on the qualified providers of sedation and analgesia: considerations for policy guidelines for registered nurses engaged in the administration of sedation and analgesia (2003). Available from AANA: www.aana.com.

Latex allergy protocol (1993). *AANA J* 1993; **61**: 223–4.

American Association of Oral and Maxillofacial Surgeons (AAOMS)

Statement by the American Association of Oral and Maxillofacial Surgeons concerning the management of selected clinical conditions and associated clinical procedures: the control of pain and anxiety (2010). Available online at: www.aaoms.org/docs/practice_mgmt/condition_statements/control_of_pain_and_anxiety.pdf.

Anesthesia in outpatient facilities (2007). In AAOMS Parameters of Care: Clinical Practice Guidelines, 4th edn (AAOMS ParCare 07). 55.PC07-CD. Available from AAOMS: www.aaomsstore.com.

American College of Cardiology (ACC) and American Heart Association (AHA)

ACC/AHA guidelines on perioperative cardiovascular evaluation and care for noncardiac surgery (2007). *J Am Coll Cardiol* 2007; **50**: 159–242.

American College of Emergency Physicians (ACEP)

ACEP policy statement: sedation in the emergency department (2011 revision). Available online at: www.acep.org/policystatements.

Clinical policy: procedural sedation and analgesia in the emergency department (2005). *Ann Emerg Med* 2005; **45**: 177–96. Available online at www.acep.org/clinicalpolicies. Xiv.

Policy statement: delivery of agents for procedural sedation and analgesia by emergency nurses (2005). *Ann Emerg Med* 2005; **46**: 368. Available online at: www.acep.org/policystatements.

American College of Radiology (ACR) and Society of Interventional Radiology (SIR)

ACR–SIR practice guideline for sedation and analgesia (Res. 45, 2010). Available online at: www.acr.org/guidelines.

American Dental Association (ADA)

Guidelines for teaching pain control and sedation to dentists and dental students (2007).

Available online at: www.ada.org/sections/about/pdfs/anxiety_guidelines.pdf.

Guidelines for the use of sedation and general anesthesia by dentists (2007). Available online at: www.ada.org/sections/about/pdfs/anesthesia_guidelines.pdf.

American Nurses Association (ANA)

Procedural sedation consensus statement (2008). Available online at: www.nursingworld.org/NursingPractice.

American Society for Gastrointestinal Endoscopy (ASGE)

Position statement: nonanesthesiologist administration of propofol for GI endoscopy (2009). *Gastrointest Endosc* 2009; **70**: 1053–9.

Sedation and anesthesia in GI endoscopy (2008). *Gastrointest Endosc* 2008; **68**: 815–26.

Guidelines for conscious sedation and monitoring during gastrointestinal endoscopy (2003). *Gastrointest Endosc* 2003; **58**: 317–22.

American Society of Anesthesiologists (ASA)

Standards for basic anesthetic monitoring (2011). Available online at: www.asahq.org/For-Healthcare-Professionals/Standards-Guidelines-and-Statements.aspx.

Statement on anesthetic care during interventional pain procedures for adults (2010).

Available online at: www.asahq.org/For-Healthcare-Professionals/Standards-Guidelinesand-Statements.aspx.

Statement on granting privileges for deep sedation to non-anesthesiologist sedation practitioners (2010). Further information from ASA: www.asahq.org.

Continuum of depth of sedation: definition of general anesthesia and levels of sedation/analgesia (2009). Available online at: www.asahq.org/For-Healthcare-Professionals/Standards-Guidelines-and-Statements.aspx.

Distinguishing monitored anesthesia care ("MAC") from moderate sedation/analgesia (conscious sedation) (2009). Available online at: www.asahq.org/For-Healthcare-Professionals/Standards-Guidelines-and-Statements.aspx.

Guidelines for office-based anesthesia (2009). Available online at: www.asahq.org/For-Healthcare-Professionals/Standards-Guidelines-and-Statements.aspx.

Standards for postanesthesia care (2009). Available online at: www.asahq.org/For-Healthcare-Professionals/Standards-Guidelines-and-Statements.aspx.

Statement on qualifications of anesthesia providers in the office-based setting (2009).

Available online at: www.asahq.org/For-Healthcare-Professionals/Standards-Guidelinesand-Statements.aspx.

Statement on safe use of propofol (2009). Available online at: www.asahq.org/For-Healthcare-Professionals/Standards-Guidelines-and-Statements.aspx.

Statement on nonoperating room anesthetizing locations (2008). Available online at: www.asahq.org/For-Healthcare-Professionals/Standards-Guidelines-and-Statements.aspx.

Guidelines for ambulatory anesthesia and surgery (2008). Available online at: www.asahq.org/For-Healthcare-Professionals/Standards-Guidelines-and-Statements.aspx.

Statement on granting privileges for administration of moderate sedation to practitioners who are not anesthesia professionals (2011). Available online at: www.asahq.org/For-Healthcare-Professionals/Standards-Guidelines-and-Statements.aspx.

Statement on granting privileges to nonanesthesiologist practitioners for personally administering deep sedation or supervising deep sedation by individuals who are not anesthesia professionals (2006). Available online at: www.asahq.org/For-Healthcare-Professionals/Standards-Guidelines-and-Statements.aspx.

Practice guidelines for sedation and analgesia by non-anesthesiologists (2002). *Anesthesiology* 2002; **96**: 1004–17. Available online at: www.asahq.org/For-Healthcare-Professionals/Education-and-Events/Guidelines-for-Sedation-and-Analgesia-by-non-anesthesiologists.aspx.

Practice advisory for preanesthesia evaluation (2002). *Anesthesiology* 2002; **96**: 485–96.

Association of perioperative Registered Nurses (AORN)

The following AORN Position Statements are available online at: www.aorn.org/PracticeResources/AORNPositionStatements/ (last accessed May 16, 2012).

Allied Health Care Providers and Support Personnel in the Perioperative Practice Setting

Care of the Older Adult in Perioperative Settings

Creating a Practice Environment of Safety

Criminalization of Human Errors in the Perioperative Setting

Entry into Practice

Environmental Responsibility

Ergonomically Healthy Workplace Practices

Healthy Perioperative Work Environment

Immediate Use Steam Sterilization

Noise in the Perioperative Practice Setting

One Perioperative Registered Nurse Circulator Dedicated to Every Patient Undergoing a Surgical or Other Invasive Procedure

Operating Room Staffing Skill Mix for Direct Caregivers

Orientation of the Registered Nurse and Certified Surgical Technologist to the Perioperative Setting

Patient Safety

Patients and Health Care Workers with Boodborne Diseases

Perioperative Advanced Practice Nurse

Perioperative Care of Patients With Do-Not-Resuscitate (DNR) Orders

Preventing Wrong-Patient, Wrong-Site, Wrong-Procedure Events

Responsibility for Mentoring

RN First Assistants

Role of the Health Care Industry Representative in the Perioperative/Invasive Procedure Setting

Safe Work On-Call Practices

Surgical Smoke and Bio-Aerosols

Value of Clinical Learning Activities in the Perioperative Setting in Undergraduate Nursing Curricula

Workplace Safety

Policy for Sunset of AOR Position Statements

Recommended practices for managing the patient receiving moderate sedation/analgesia (2002). *AORN J* 2002; **75**: 642–6, 649–52.

Centers for Medicare & Medicaid Services (CMS)

CMS interpretive guidelines for anesthesia and sedation (summary). Available online at: www.cms.gov/ Regulations-and-Guidance/Guidance/Transmittals/ downloads/R74SOMA.pdf.

Activities/Interpretive-Guidelines.aspx.

Emergency medicine and CMS interpretive guidelines. Available online at: www.acep.org/Content. aspx?id=75563.

xvi Guidelines and standards Comp. by: Kkavitha Stage: Revises1 Chapter No.: FM Title Name: Urman&Kaye Page Number: 0 Date:18/10/11 Time:13:24:49.

Society of Critical Care Medicine (SCCM)

Clinical practice guidelines for the sustained use of sedatives and analgesics in the critically ill adult (2002). *Crit Care Med* 2002; **30**: 119–41.

The Joint Commission

Accreditation handbook for office-based surgery: what you need to know about obtaining accreditation (2011). Available online at: www.jointcommission.org/ accreditation/ahc_seeking_obs.aspx.

Comprehensive accreditation manual for hospitals (CAMH): the official handbook (2011 update). Available online at: www.jcrinc.com/Joint-Commission-Requirements/Hospitals.

University HealthSystem Consortium (UHC)

Moderate sedation best practice recommendations (2005). Available from University Health-System Consortium, 2001 Spring Road, Suite 700, Oak Brook, Illinois 60523, USA (www.uhc.edu).

Position statement on the role of the RN in moderate sedation best practice recommendations (2001). Available from UHC (www.uhc.edu).

Deep sedation best practice recommendations (2001). Available from UHC (www.uhc.edu).

References

1. Statement on Granting Privileges for Administration of Moderate Sedation to Practitioners Who Are Not Anesthesia Professionals (2011). American Society of Anesthesiologists. Available online at: http://asahq.org/ For-Healthcare-Professionals/Standards-Guidelines-and-Statements.aspx (last accessed May 10, 2012).

2. Advisory on Granting Privileges for Deep Sedation to Non-anesthesiologist Sedation Practitioners (2010). American Society of Anesthesiologists. Available online at: http://asahq.org/For-Healthcare-Professionals/ Standards-Guidelines-and-Statements.aspx (last accessed May 10, 2012).

3. Statement on Granting Privileges to Non-Anesthesiologist Practioners for Personally Administering Deep Sedation or Supervising Deep Sedation by Individuals Who Are Not Anesthesia Professionals (2006). American Society of Anesthesiologists. Available online at: http://asahq.org/ For-Healthcare-Professionals/Standards-Guidelines-and-Statements.aspx (last accessed May 10, 2012).

4. Continuum of depth of sedation: definition of general anesthesia and levels of sedation/analgesia (2009). American Society of Anesthesiologists. Available online at: www.asahq.org/For-Healthcare-Professionals/ Standards-Guidelines-and-Statements.aspx (last accessed May 10, 2012).

5. Standards for Basic Anesthetic Monitoring. American Society of Anesthesiologists. Available online at: http:// asahq.org/For-Healthcare-Professionals/Standards-Guidelines-and-Statements.aspx (last accessed May 10, 2012).

6. J. A. Aldrete. The post-anesthesia recovery score revisited. *J Clin Anesth* 1995; **7**: 89–91.

7. M. T. Antonelli, D. E. Seaver. Quality, legal, and risk management considerations: ensuring program excellence, Chapter 7, pp. 85–101. In: R. Urman, A. D. Kaye. *Moderate and Deep Sedation in Clinical Practice*, 1st edn, Cambridge University Press, 2012.

8. The Joint Commission. Provision of care, treatment, and services standards, record of care, and improving organizational performance. In: *Comprehensive Accreditation Manual for Hospitals*. Oakbrook Terrace, IL: The Joint Commission, 2011.

9. J. Metzner, K. L. Posner, K. B. Domino. The risk and safety of anesthesia at remote locations: the US closed claims analysis. *Curr Opin Anaesthesiol* 2009; **22**: 502–8.

10. S. M. Bhananker, K. L. Posner, F. W. Cheney, *et al.* Injury and liability associated with monitored anesthesia care: a closed claims analysis. *Anesthesiology* 2006; **104**: 228–34.

11. American Society of Anesthesiologists. Statement on Safe Use of Propofol (2009). Available at: http://asahq.org/

For-Healthcare-Professionals/Standards-Guidelines-and-Statements.aspx (last accessed May 10, 2012).

12. D. Schilling, A. Rosenbaum, S. Schweizer, *et al.* Sedation with propofol for interventional endoscopy by trained nurses in high-risk octogenarians: a prospective, randomized, controlled study. *Endoscopy* 2009; **41**: 295–8.

13. K. R. McQuaid, L. Laine. A systematic review and meta-analysis of randomized, controlled trials of moderate sedation for routine endoscopic procedures. *Gastrointest Endosc* 2008; **67**: 910–23.

14. G. A. Cote, R. M. Hovis, M. A. Ansstas, *et al.* Incidence of sedation-related complications with propofol use during advanced endoscopic procedures. *Clin Gastroenterol Hepatol* 2010; **8**: 137–42.

15. H. Fatima, J. DeWitt, J. LeBlanc, *et al.* Nurse-administered propofol sedation for upper endoscopic ultrasonography. *Am J Gastroenterol* 2008; **103**: 1649–56.

16. D. K. Rex, V. P. Deenadayalu, E. Eid, *et al.* Endoscopist-directed administration of propofol: a worldwide safety experience. *Gastroenteroogy* 2009; **137**: 1229–37.

17. H. Singh, W. Poluha, M. Cheung, *et al.* Propofol for sedation during colonoscopy. *Cochrane Database Syst Rev* 2008; (4): CD006268.

Chapter

26

Medical informatics in the perioperative period

Keith J. Ruskin MD

Introduction   267
Medical information
systems   267

Security and patient confidentiality   270
Communication in the OR   271
Summary   272

Introduction

Although many health-care providers are familiar with an electronic health record (EHR) and use it routinely, anesthesiologists have a unique understanding of how information is used throughout the perioperative period. Anesthesiologists are responsible for knowing all aspects of the patient's medical history, and therefore review all areas of the patient's chart. Most other medical specialties work with only one portion of the record: specialty consultants, for example, may review notes and laboratory data and then write a series of recommendations. Radiologists may view the patient's admitting data, read an X-ray, and then dictate a note into the chart. Anesthesiology, however, is one of the most information-intense medical specialties. Anesthesiologists also produce a highly detailed record of the intraoperative course, which may include imaging (from a cardiac echocardiogram or fluoroscopic images of a nerve block), laboratory data (e.g., arterial blood gas analysis), and consultations.

Health information technology is a broad topic, and anesthesia informatics is the subject of a large textbook. It is, however, possible to summarize key points of health information technology as they pertain to management of the perioperative suite. This chapter discusses anesthesia information management systems and operating room (OR) information systems, with special attention to benefits, implementation, and obstacles to deployment. It also discusses the Health Insurance Portability and Accountability Act (HIPAA) and Health Information Technology for Economic and Clinical Health (HITECH) regulations and how they impact medical care. Lastly, a brief discussion of communication in the perioperative environment explains how technology can facilitate transmission of important information.

Medical information systems

For many years, the medical profession was slow to adopt information technology. While most other industries used computers to track inventory, schedule workers, and bill for products and services, physicians relied on handwritten notes and slips of paper glued into charts. Computers were used mainly for billing and transmitting laboratory results. The first anesthesia information management systems were developed by physicians who were also computer enthusiasts. These early systems were designed for the needs of a specific practice, usually only interfaced with one type of physiologic monitor, and were little more than a record generator. The primary advantages of these early systems were that they relieved the anesthesia provider of the task of writing vital signs down every few minutes and they created a legible replacement of a paper record.

Health-care professionals and institutions are now rapidly incorporating computers into every aspect of medical practice. Information technology is now being rapidly embraced as an aid to OR management. Anesthesia information management systems create a comprehensive, legible record of the patient's course during the intraoperative period. Scheduling systems

Operating Room Leadership and Management, ed. Kaye A.D., Fox C.J. and Urman R.D. Published by Cambridge University Press. © Cambridge University Press 2012.

are used to manage the flow of patients through the OR, postanesthesia care unit, and critical care units. Radiofrequency identification (RFID) technology is used to track patients, equipment, pharmaceuticals, and blood products.

Medical information systems can provide critical information at the point of care, facilitate communication between health-care providers, and track outcomes – all of which have the potential to increase efficiency while making patients safer. Operating room information systems can also integrate information such as guidelines and protocols with patient information, changing clinician behavior by making specific recommendations. Decision support extends the physician's knowledge base by placing information into context with regard to a specific patient.

Anesthesia information management systems

Anesthesia information management systems (AIMS) are a specialized form of an EHR that automatically collects, stores, and presents patient data that are gathered during the perioperative period. Modern AIMS are composed of an integrated suite of hardware and software that can interface with a variety of physiologic monitors and anesthesia machines. These systems can usually be interfaced with other hospital information systems, such as a laboratory reporting system and the patient's EHR, bringing the comprehensive medical record to the point of care within the perioperative suite. Although most of the functionality of an AIMS involves collecting and storing data from the perioperative period, many systems include a preoperative evaluation module, automated paging capabilities, and many other features.

Benefits of AIMS

The promise of AIMS is to improve patient safety and the quality of care, and these benefits are beginning to be realized. The Anesthesia Patient Safety Foundation stated over a decade ago that the Foundation "endorses and advocates the use of automated record keeping in the perioperative period and the subsequent retrieval and analysis of the data to improve patient safety" [1]. Although AIMS are costly and complex to implement and maintain, their advantages are rapidly becoming apparent and these systems are likely, in a few years, to become a de facto standard of care.

The adoption of AIMS has been accelerating over the past several years. Although fewer than 10% of ORs were estimated to have an AIMS installed in 2007 [2], a more recent survey reveals that 24% of ORs had installed a system by 2010, with 13% in the process of installation and another 13% actively evaluating a system [3]. There are several reasons for this rapid growth in the number of planned and installed AIMS, including patient safety, quality management, economic factors, and compliance with government regulations. Given the density of information generated by modern physiologic monitors, AIMS are the only practical way to collect and interpret all of the data generated during the perioperative period. National organizations whose purpose is to analyze perioperative data to detect ways to improve quality, such as the National Surgical Quality Improvement Program and the Anesthesia Quality Institute (AQI), depend upon receiving data in electronic form.

Benefits to individual patients include a legible record that is available as part of the EHR and availability of the entire medical record at the point of care, but there are other benefits as well. Dexter et al. were able to significantly reduce waiting and nil per os (NPO) times of children undergoing endoscopic procedures by analyzing information from an OR information system and applying a statistical model for case scheduling [4].

The AIMS can provide decision support and enhance compliance with guidelines such as those of the Surgical Care Improvement Project (SCIP) and pay-for-performance measures [5]. In an outpatient surgery center, a new antibiotic prophylaxis form combined with prebuilt order sets improved compliance with timely antibiotic administration to over 90% while saving an estimated $8500 per year in pharmacy costs [6]. An AIMS developed by the Massachusetts General Hospital and Vanderbilt University, and General Electric's Centricity, incorporates modules that prompt users to administer an antibiotic prior to surgical incision and then document compliance [7] – compliance with guidelines on antibiotic administration has been shown to decrease surgical infection rate [8]. In addition, AIMS can generate alerts for drug interactions or patient allergies, decreasing the possibility of an adverse event. Lastly, a recent study suggests that automated reminders can reduce the frequency of prolonged gaps in blood pressure management during surgical procedures [9]. Economics is an important factor in the decision to implement perioperative information management systems, and in many cases drives the choice of a specific product. The OR is one of the largest revenue streams within most health-care institutions, and managers can use information generated from AIMS and OR information systems to track outcomes, schedule procedures more efficiently, and formulate strategic plans. Many payers now require electronic documentation of patient encounters as a condition of reimbursement for health-care services, and this is also a significant motivator in the decision to purchase an AIMS.

The primary financial benefits of an AIMS include a reduction in drug costs, improved charge capture, reduced staffing costs, and improved OR and scheduling efficiency. The AIMS probably do not decrease anesthesia time [10], but they can improve OR turnover and scheduling efficiency. Epstein *et al.* were able to infer a patient's correct room location using vital signs transmitted from a monitor to the AIMS, something that could not be done using an AIMS system or OR information management system alone. This enabled them to efficiently track a patient as he or she moved, for example, from a block room to the OR for an orthopedic procedure [9]. By analyzing aggregate data, it is possible to determine actual mean procedure durations for specific surgeons, which can make scheduling ORs more efficient. In one novel application of real-time data analysis, a group of electrical engineers was able to interpret multichannel audio and video recordings to detect the specific phase of surgery. The authors postulate that their technique may be used to automatically detect adverse events [11]. Although this technique remains to be validated and implemented, the use of real-time data analysis is an intriguing possibility.

An AIMS has the potential to offer a significant return on investment through increased payments (and avoidance of withheld payments) from Physician Quality Reporting System (PQRS) initiatives, improved charge capture, and better documentation. The AIMS can automatically search for missing documentation and alert the appropriate provider. At the Massachusetts General Hospital, customized software written for the AIMS automatically identifies missing procedure attestations and alerts the appropriate provider. This system has significantly increased collection of appropriate physician fees for services that had previously not been reimbursed [12].

An AIMS can facilitate clinical research through a large patient database that can be queried in order to find ways to improve clinical practice. Many health-care payers are beginning to offer incentives to institutions that "benchmark" their care to determine the incidence of complications and the quality of their patient outcomes, and this process will probably become a de facto requirement within the next few years. The AQI is a nonprofit foundation that was created by the American Society of Anesthesiologists (ASA) to maintain a comprehensive, national clinical outcomes registry. The AQI relies on AIMS to provide the clinical information needed to objectively evaluate anesthesia practice patterns and ultimately improve patient care. At the present time, the AQI is using this information to provide benchmarking information to participating practices.

Implementation of an AIMS

Despite their benefits, there are significant obstacles to the adoption of an AIMS. Specific challenges include adapting preexisting workflows to the new system, training providers, and tracking errors in charting and billing that may occur during the transition. Many health-care professionals view the implementation of information technology as a goal in and of itself, but successful adaption of an EHR or other information system requires a fundamentally different approach. Information systems should be viewed as a solution to a specific problem or as a way to meet a defined goal. Before choosing a system, it is critically important to identify the problems that must be solved or the needs that must be met. This will make it possible to identify a solution that meets these exact needs.

The cost of installing and maintaining a system is substantial, and includes the "up-front" charges for hardware and software, the costs of customizing the product, and ongoing support and maintenance. This cost has been estimated to be as high as $4000–$6000 per OR and between $14 000 and $45 000 for installation of a server [13]. The return on investment depends upon the financial and management practices at each institution, but usually includes improvements in scheduling, decreased drug costs, improved charge capture, and improved coding.

Because of the high cost of installation, a health-care institution may choose an AIMS as part of the purchase of a larger information system. The benefits to the institution of choosing such a system include compatibility with other parts of the EHR, and possibly a discounted price. The system chosen by the hospital may, however, not be the ideal one for the practice model. The anesthesiologists who will be using the system must therefore be involved with all aspects of the purchase and implementation. An AIMS does not simply replace a paper chart with an electronic one; successful adoption of this complex system requires substantial changes in workflow.

During the purchase process, the initial focus is almost exclusively on clinical implementation, but it is essential to plan for how the product will be used, which types of reports are required, and how the existing workflow integrates with the system. Consideration should be given to the functionality that will be required (e.g., preoperative evaluation or postanesthesia care unit documentation), the anesthetizing locations at which workstations must be installed, support services that will be provided after the initial depolyment, and initial and ongoing training for users. Maintenance and system upgrades should also be considered, as should backups of the data and the purchase of redundant hardware to minimize downtime in the event of a system failure.

It is important for the anesthesia department to identify a clinical champion who will work with the vendor during the initial customization. The champion should have a background in both clinical anesthesia and information technology and work with the vendor and health-care institution information services personnel to facilitate all stages of implementation [14]. A comprehensive plan should be outlined and distributed to all members of the department well in advance of the scheduled implementation. This plan should include the strategy that will be used for the "go-live" ("Big Bang" or a phased implementation), as well as a training schedule and a contingency plan that will be implemented in the event of a system failure [13].

If the goal of purchasing an AIMS is to produce a paper printout of an anesthesia record at the end of an anesthetic, this functionality is likely to be available "out of the box." Reports that have been built into the software are usually generic in nature, however, and generally do not include custom elements have been added to the database. If the goal of implementing an AIMS is to archive electronic medical records, push information to an institutional EHR, track drug usage, or create customized reports, then additional resources and planning will be required, and this will incur additional costs. It is not uncommon to discover that the system does not produce reports that the physicians or institution consider to be essential. Technical or licensing restrictions may not even permit the data to be directly accessible. It is therefore imperative that all of the anticipated requirements be carefully thought out

and clearly specified in the request for proposal (RFP). Additional items that should be considered include "paging modules" that will allow staff to be notified at specific milestones, integration with hospital or laboratory information systems, and the ability to interface with a billing system.

The new system and changes in workflow are a distraction that may temporarily impede patient care. Moreover, the presence of a computer on the anesthesia gas machine may tempt personnel to use it for online shopping, catching up on email, or other extraneous purposes during periods of low workload. Although there are no studies of how computer use affects anesthesia care in the OR, a recent study may provide clues. Observers found that anesthesia providers read books or magazines during periods of low workload in 35% of cases. Although vigilance did not appear to be impaired, performance of manual tasks, record keeping, and interacting with others was decreased [15]. It seems logical that implementing a new, unfamiliar system would have a similar effect. Inappropriate use can be minimized through the implementation of "appropriate use" policies and content filters.

Security and patient confidentiality

HIPAA and HITECH

The HIPAA of 1996 was enacted to protect workers and their families from losing health-care insurance coverage when they change or lose a job. Title II of HIPAA required the establishment of national standards for exchanging health-care information and for the creation of a national identifier for health-care providers, institutions, and insurers. The HIPAA also established sweeping requirements for the security and privacy of health information. These requirements are meant to improve the efficiency of health care by facilitating electronic data interchange between health-care providers, payers, and governmental agencies. Although HIPAA has fundamentally changed the health-care infrastructure in the United States, most physicians are aware of HIPAA because of the Privacy Rule.

The HIPAA Privacy and Security Rules defines protected health information (PHI) as any information that is held by a health-care provider, a payer, or their business associates that concerns health status, medical treatment, or insurance payments and that can be linked to a specific individual. This has been broadly interpreted to cover a patient's entire medical record. The Security Rule describes three types of safeguards that must be put into place by "covered entities." *Administrative safeguards* describe how a covered entity will comply with the rules and include policies and procedures that govern the protection and use of PHI. These policies are developed and enforced by a privacy officer. *Physical safeguards* cover all aspects of the hardware and software used to store PHI. These rules mandate that access to computers be limited only to authorized personnel and that access be closely monitored and controlled. Computers or devices (such as a laptop or tablet computer) that store PHI must be protected against unauthorized use. In general, storing PHI on a personal device should be discouraged because of the possibility that it could be lost or stolen. *Technical safeguards* cover the security of PHI as it is transmitted from one entity to another. Health information must be encrypted if it is transmitted over an open network (e.g., the Internet). Before information is transmitted, both parties must authenticate each other, either by a password system (if computers are used) or by a telephone callback (for a conversation).

The HITECH Act was enacted as part of the 2009 American Recovery and Reinvestment Act (ARRA) and gives the US Department of Health and Human Services (HHS) the authority to establish a set of programs, incentives, and penalties for adoption and use of certified EHR systems (see www.cms. gov/EHRIncentivePrograms/). The requirements of HITECH build upon the HIPAA regulations, which deal primarily with electronic data interchange, security, and privacy. The HITECH regulations cover content of the record, quality management, and transmission of health information. The Centers for Medicare & Medicaid Services (CMS) has proposed a set of requirements for "meaningful use" of electronic records in five areas under HITECH:

- improve quality, safety, and efficiency, and reduce health disparities;
- engage patients and families in their health care;
- improve care coordination;
- improve population and public health;
- insure adequate privacy and security of health information.

The CMS defines a "meaningful EHR user" as a health-care provider who uses a "certified" EHR for purposes such as order entry or e-prescribing; uses electronic transmission of data for the purposes of health-care coordination; and submits clinical quality measures to an approved government agency. Health-care providers who comply with these requirements through 2015 receive a small incentive payment, whereas providers who fail to meet the 2015 deadline for implementation may receive a reduction in Medicare payment as a penalty.

Although no AIMS systems have been certified as meeting "meaningful use" criteria, many of these systems fulfill the functions required in HITECH. For example, many AIMS systems offer decision support for items such as perioperative antibiotic administration. In addition, AIMS have the potential to automatically report disease conditions for which registries exist (e.g., malignant hyperthermia). They also meet many of the goals for quality, safety, and efficiency. Those AIMS that use accepted standards, such as SNOMED or HL-7, may allow devices to communicate with each other and with other AIMS. An AIMS can record vascular access or regional anesthesia techniques performed using ultrasound guidance, or transesophageal echocardiography performed during cardiac surgery. At the present time, however, CMS has not certified AIMS as meeting meaningful use criteria.

Communication in the OR

Anesthesiologists work in a dynamic environment in which information critical to patient care must be quickly and accurately exchanged. Cellular telephones, wireless computers, and other electronic tools can improve patient care by providing rapid access to vital information from any location. Effective communication has been shown to be a critical component of safety in high-risk environments. Failure to convey information quickly and accurately has been shown to be a root cause of medical errors; one study found that communication failures were the second most prevalent cause of medical errors [16]. Reliable information technology tools are critical to patient safety in the perioperative environment. Ideally, a core communication infrastructure should be created that is compatible with new devices. In many cases, such a system can be installed using readily available equipment.

Voice communication

A variety of options are available to facilitate voice communication within a hospital or other health-care institution. It is now possible, for example, to install cellular telephone repeaters that permit the use of ordinary mobile telephones throughout a building.

Telecommunication companies can also install "micro-cells" within the building that are functionally equivalent to any other cellular base station.

Wi-Fi networks can be used to carry voice conversations. A variety of commercial providers now offer telephone service to the public using Voice over Internet Protocol (VoIP) as an alternative to traditional telephone service. Either generic or specialized specialized systems can be installed in the health-care environment. These advantages, combined with the low cost and wide availability of Wi-Fi equipment, make this technology well suited for many health-care applications.

Paging and text messaging

Many communications experts recommend that health-care institutions retain paging systems to transmit extremely urgent information. Despite their "one-way," asynchronous nature, paging systems do offer several advantages: they allow a simple message (e.g., a "Code Blue" page) to be conveyed simultaneously to a group of people. If the paging transmitter is in the hospital, messages can be sent very quickly. If, however, a commercial paging service is used, the latency period is specified in the terms of service and may allow up to an hour for a message to be sent out.

Some OR management systems include modules that can automatically alert specific members of the care team when certain milestones are reached, sending a message to the transport service to bring the next patient to the OR when the previous patient is transferred to the postanesthesia care unit, for example. This has the potential to improve OR efficiency. In one study, an AIMS automatically paged the attending anesthesiologist if allergy information had not been entered into the medical record. This significantly decreased the incidence of incomplete charts [17]. Clinical alerting systems that automatically send laboratory results to alphanumeric pagers have been shown to improve patient care and are installed in a growing number of hospitals [18]. Epstein *et al.* have developed an automated staff recall system that uses short text messages and is accessible from an AIMS. In the event of a mass casualty incident, such a system can potentially reduce the amount of time required for a hospital to mount a response [19].

Advanced communication tools

The advent of low-cost tablet computers combined with high-speed Wi-Fi networks has resulted in the development of systems that provide unprecedented access to information. The Department of Anesthesiology at Vanderbilt University has designed a comprehensive information management and documentation suite called the Vanderbilt Perioperative Information Management System (VPIMS). This system integrates data from physiologic monitors, the hospital information system, and in-room video cameras. This information is presented to anesthesiologists throughout the institution and can be accessed from laptop computers, desktop computers, display boards in the perioperative suite, and tablet computers[20].

Summary

Implementation of a comprehensive information technology program in the OR can improve patient care while maximizing efficiency and helping to capture reimbursement for services. Anesthesiologists have a unique understanding of how information flows through the hospital, and have historically been at the forefront of initiatives to improve patient safety. Using an AIMS in the perioperative period can facilitate efficient scheduling, improve patient care by providing access to critical information, and create a legible record that is available throughout the health-care institution. A well-thought-out communication infrastructure can also improve patient safety by allowing patient information, reference materials, or clinical guidelines to be sent to the point of care. Modern communication tools also allow anesthesiologists to convey information to each other without leaving the patient's bedside. The discipline of anesthesia informatics is relatively new, but it has the potential to make dramatic improvements to the practice of perioperative medicine.

References

1. American Patient Safety Foundation Newsletter. 2001; **16**: 49.

2. R. H. Epstein, M. M. Vigoda, D. M. Feinstein. Anesthesia information management systems: a survey of current implementation policies and practices. *Anesth Analg* 2007; **105**: 405–11.

3. T. L. Trentman, J. T. Mueller, K. J. Ruskin, B. N. Noble, C. A. Doyle. Adoption of anesthesia information management systems by US anesthesiologists. *J Clin Monit Comput* 2011; **25**: 129–35.

4. B. Smallman, F. Dexter. Optimizing the arrival, waiting, and NPO times of children on the day of pediatric

endoscopy procedures. *Anesth Analg* 2010; **110**: 879–87.

5. D. B. Wax, Y. Beilin, M. Levin, N. Chadha, M. Krol, D. L. Reich. The effect of an interactive visual reminder in an anesthesia information management system on timeliness of prophylactic antibiotic administration. *Anesth Analg* 2007; **104**: 1462–6, table of contents.

6. C. C. Braxton, P. A. Gerstenberger, G. G. Cox. Improving antibiotic stewardship: order set implementation to improve prophylactic antimicrobial prescribing in the outpatient surgical setting. *J Ambul Care Manage* 2010; **33**: 131–40.

7. B. Rothman, W. S. Sandberg, P. St Jacques. Using information technology to improve quality in the OR. *Anesthesiol Clin* 2011; **29**: 29–55.

8. J. J. Stulberg, C. P. Delaney, D. V. Neuhauser, D. C. Aron, P. Fu, S. M. Koroukian. Adherence to surgical care improvement project measures and the association with postoperative infections. *JAMA* 2010; **303**: 2479–85.

9. J. M. Ehrenfeld, R. H. Epstein, S. Bader, S. Kheterpal, W. S. Sandberg. Automatic notifications mediated by anesthesia information management systems reduce the frequency of prolonged gaps in blood pressure documentation. *Anesth Analg* 2011; **113**: 356–63.

10. J. Balust, A. Macario. Can anesthesia information management systems improve quality in the surgical suite? *Curr Opin Anaesthesiol* 2009; **22**: 215–22.

11. T. Suzuki, Y. Sakurai, K. Yoshimitsu, K. Nambu, Y. Muragaki, H. Iseki. Intraoperative multichannel audio-visual information recording and automatic surgical phase and incident detection. *Conf Proc IEEE Eng Med Biol Soc* 2010; **2010**:1190–3.

12. S. F. Spring, W. S. Sandberg, S. Anupama, J. L. Walsh, W. D. Driscoll, D. E. Raines. Automated documentation error detection and notification improves anesthesia billing performance. *Anesthesiology* 2007; **106**: 157–63.

13. J. M. Ehrenfeld, M. A. Rehman. Anesthesia information management systems: a review of functionality and installation considerations. *J Clin Monit Comput* 2011; **25**: 71–9.

14. W. S. Sandberg. Anesthesia information management systems: almost there. *Anesth Analg* 2008; **107**: 1100–2.

15. J. M. Slagle, M. B. Weinger. Effects of intraoperative reading on vigilance and workload during anesthesia care in an academic medical center. *Anesthesiology* 2009; **110**: 275–83.

16. M. T. Kluger, M. F. Bullock. Recovery room incidents: a review of 419 reports from the Anaesthetic Incident Monitoring Study (AIMS). *Anaesthesia* 2002; **57**: 1060–6.

17. W. S. Sandberg, E. H. Sandberg, A. R. Seim, *et al*. Real-time checking of electronic anesthesia records for documentation errors and automatically text messaging clinicians improves quality of documentation. *Anesth Analg* 2008; **106**: 192–201, table of contents.

18. E. G. Poon, G. J. Kuperman, J. Fiskio, D. W. Bates. Real-time notification of laboratory data requested by users through alphanumeric pagers. *J Am Med Inform Assoc* 2002; **9**: 217–22.

19. R. H. Epstein, A. Ekbatani, J. Kaplan, R. Shechter, Z. Grunwald. Development of a staff recall system for mass casualty incidents using cell phone text messaging. *Anesth Analg* 2010; **110**: 871–8.

20. P. St Jacques, B. Rothman. Enhancing point of care vigilance using computers. *Anesthesiol Clin* 2011; **29**: 505–19.

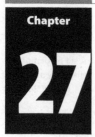

Simulation training to improve patient safety

Valeriy Kozmenko MD
Judy G. Johnson MD
Melville Wyche III MD
Alan D. Kaye MD, PhD

Teaching team-training skills   274   Summary   278

Teaching team-training skills

Patient safety is one of the most pressing challenges of the modern health-care system. According to an Agency for Healthcare Research and Quality (AHRQ) report, "as many as 44 000 to 98 000 people die in US hospitals each year as the result of lapses in patient safety." Patient safety is a multifactorial problem that requires attention on multiple levels, including individual, team, unit/section, and the organization as a whole. Effective team communication is an important contributing factor that affects quality of patient care and safety in the clinical environment. As with many other complex behaviors, team communication skills are best learned in the immersive clinical environment. Using high-fidelity simulation to teach better communication between health-care professionals is an ideal method, because it creates such an environment without putting a real patient in danger. Team training to improve patient safety can be done either in the real clinical environment or at the simulation center. Both methods have their advantages and disadvantages.

In situ simulation creates what is called a mixed-reality immersive environment in which real medical equipment can be used in conjunction with a high-fidelity simulator. As the trainees operate in the accustomed environment, they are quickly immersed in the scenario and are engaged in a dynamic interaction with each other and the simulator. Conducting *in situ* simulation-based team training could reveal organizational breaches in patient safety. For example, when Louisiana State University (LSU) Health Sciences Center in New Orleans conducted a series of team-training simulation sessions at a rural hospital, running a malignant hyperthermia scenario revealed the fact that there was not a designated freezer with cold intravenous fluids that must be used in that life-threatening medical condition. Having training done at the site of daily work makes trainee scheduling easier; however, it creates a challenge of making clinical space available for the activity that does not involve real patient care. Transportation of simulation equipment to the site of training is another challenge.

Teaching team-training skills in the setting of a simulation center has its own advantages, such as no need to move simulation equipment, and the possibility of using higher-fidelity stationary simulators such as the Medical Education Technologies human patient simulator (HPS) rather than its portable versions, which have somewhat lower realism. As the training is done outside of the busy clinical environment, it is easier to schedule as many simulation sessions as needed. Usually, simulation centers have special classrooms for debriefing and are equipped with advanced audio/video systems. However, some trainees might find the simulation center setting very different from the real clinical environment, with different brands of mechanical lung ventilators, anesthesia machines, and surgical equipment, which can make translation of newly learned skills from simulated classroom to real-life patient care more difficult.

Regardless of whether the training is performed at the point of the patient care or in the academic

Operating Room Leadership and Management, ed. Kaye A.D., Fox C.J. and Urman R.D. Published by Cambridge University Press. © Cambridge University Press 2012.

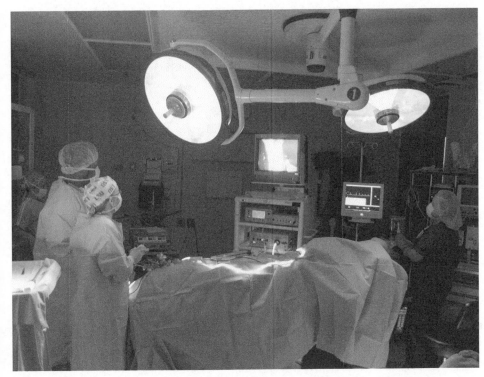

Figure 27.1 Simulated laparoscopic cholecystectomy at Earl K. Long hospital in Baton Rouge, Louisiana.

environment, each simulation session should have clearly defined learning objectives and critical performance indicators. These will help in the evaluation of the trainee and in gauging whether the communicational skills have been learned and successfully used. For example, LSU Health Sciences Center has created and successfully conducted multiple team-training courses and has received several grants funded by the AHRQ and the National League of Nursing (NLN) to train practicing operating room (OR) staff, medical and nursing students, and residents from different fields of health care on how to effectively communicate in a stressful dynamic clinical environment (Figure 27.1).

All simulation courses were administered in the same fashion. Each training session started with a brief introduction, setting ground rules for the course and orientation on how to interact with the simulator. The trainees were instructed to treat the simulator as a real patient and act as they would act in a real-life situation. Using an LSU proprietary technology, called "Clinical Model" greatly enhances the realism of the simulation. It allows verbal communication between the trainees and the virtual patient (Figure 27.2).

After the 10–15 min orientation, we conduct the first scenario, which lasts approximately 40–45 min.

After finishing the first scenario we conduct a focused facilitated debriefing. Participants are encouraged to reflect on the events of the simulation and their relation to relevant individual and team behaviors and actions. These reflections are then linked to specific teamwork competencies. Video replay is used during the debriefing to illustrate key concepts or promote team discussion. During the debriefing, the instructor facilitates the discussion, in such a way that the following principles of an effective team communication are learned:

1. flattened hierarchy to encourage sharing information between the team members;
2. role clarity;
3. cross-monitoring;
4. anticipatory response;
5. closed-loop communication;
6. situational awareness;
7. shared mental model;
8. mental rehearsal;
9. open communication.

The authors' data collected during the AHRQ-funded 2-year-long simulation training course demonstrated that the trainees perceived high-fidelity simulation training as highly realistic and useful (Table 27.1).

Table 27.1 System for Teamwork Effectiveness and Patient Safety (STEPS) training module questionnaire

Item	*Response	Post-training questions Frequency/percentage (#, %)	Mean	SD
Training features				
The training session was conducted in a setting that was convenient for me.	1	0/0	5.553	0.829
	2	1/2.1		
	3	1/2.1		
	4	1/2.1		
	5	12/25.5		
	6	32/68.1		
The training module fit well within my regular workday schedule.	1	0/0	5.319	1.044
	2	2/4.3		
	3	1/2.1		
	4	5/10.6		
	5	11/23.4		
	6	28/59.6		
Authenticity of the training environment and simulation scenarios				
The physical setting of the training was realistic.	1	0/0	5.425	0.773
	2	0/0		
	3	1/2.1		
	4	5/10.6		
	5	14/29.8		
	6	27/57.4		
Patient scenarios reflected realistic situations that teams might face in the OR.	1	0/0	5.59	0.717
	2	0/0		
	3	1/2.1		
	4	3/6.4		
	5	10/21.3		
	6	32/70.2		
Scenarios were effective for examining teamwork and patient safety practices.	1	0/0	5.744	0.440
	2	0/0		
	3	0/0		
	4	0/0		
	5	12/25.5		
	6	35/74.5		
During scenarios, I momentarily forgot about simulation and acted as if the situation were real.	1	2/4.3	4.936	1.186
	2	0/0		
	3	2/4.3		
	4	8/17.0		
	5	18/38.3		
	6	17/36.2		

Table 27.1 (*cont.*)

Item	*Response	Post-training questions Frequency/percentage (#, %)	Mean	SD
The composition of the OR team reflected what I experience in the real-life setting.	1	0/0	5.55	0.717
	2	0/0		
	3	0/0		
	4	6/12.8		
	5	9/19.1		
	6	32/66.7		
Training effectiveness				
I would benefit from participating in future training like today's session.	1	0/0	5.48	0.804
	2	0/0		
	3	0/0		
	4	9/19.1		
	5	6/12.8		
	6	32/68.1		

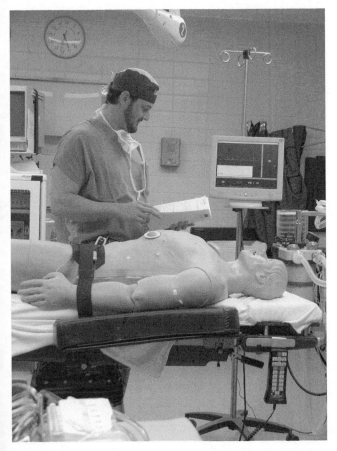

Figure 27.2 Patient interview before the surgical procedure in the OR at Earl K. Long hospital in Baton Rouge, Louisiana.

All other team training courses to improve patient safety were conducted in a similar fashion, and collected data confirmed that this method of training is highly effective regardless of the trainee's level of clinical expertise.

Summary

It appears that high-fidelity simulation may be a useful tool for teaching effective team communication skills to health-care professionals. Simulation is an important tool in the OR on many levels. Major goals of a simulation program include team building, effective communication skills, and education for potentially life-threatening situations. An effective simulation program will be perceived by the participant to be similar to real-life stresses and encountered situations in a real OR.

Suggested reading

S. W. Chauvin, Principal Investigator. *Evaluation of the System for Teamwork Effectiveness and Patient Safety (STEPS)*. 2006. Agency for Healthcare Research and Quality, Grant # U18 HS016680–01, Funding Period: 9/1/2006–8/31/2008.

Medline Plus, Patient Safety. Available online at: www.nlm.nih.gov/medlineplus/patientsafety.html (last accessed May 10, 2012).

Index

Note: page numbers in *italics* refer to figures and tables

academic medicine, 40, 42, 44
accountability, 22, 33
accounts payable, 119
accounts receivable (A/R), 117, 163
accreditation, office-based surgery
    practice, 201–2
Accreditation Council for Graduate
    Medical Education (ACGME),
    residency programs, 139
acid test ratio, 71–2
action plans, strategic planning, 30
activity measures, 78
activity ratios, 71
activity time, 74
acute pain management, 178
adjusted utilization, 48–9
administrators, 6, 8
admission unit design, 87
adult ego, 21
Affordable Care Act (US), 39–40, 220
Agency for Healthcare Research and
    Quality (AHRQ), 22
aggregate conversion factor, *165*
aging patients, risk assessment, 123
airflow models, 86–7
Aldrete score, 187, *192*, *209*
allocated operating room time, 47–8
ambulatory surgery, 108–9
ambulatory surgical centers (ASC),
    108–19
  accounts payable, 119
  accounts receivable, 117
  anesthesia, 109
  anti-kickback provisions, 110–11
  business plan, 111
  capacity, 113
  case volumes, 113
  cash distribution, 119
  Certificate of Need requirement,
    111
  convenience factors, 109
  costs, 109, 114–17
  daily sales outstanding, 117
  design of operating room, 106
  efficiency factors, 110
  entrance/exit, 106
  equipment costs, 115

financial metrics, 117–19
financial proforma, 113–19
financing, 114–15
fixed costs, 114
freestanding, 110
governing board, 111
hospital joint venture, 110
inventory, 117–19
legal structure, 110–11
limited liability companies, 110
managed care contracting strategy,
    112–13
Medicare provider application, 111
Medicare reimbursement, 112
net revenue, 112
numbers, *109*
operating metrics, 115–16
OR utilization, 115–16
out-of-network strategies, 112–13
ownership, 110–11
payer mix, 112
performance monitoring, 115
pioneers, 109
practicalities, 109
practice-based, 110
preferred provider network plans, 112
proforma income statement, 112
regulatory approval, 111
reimbursement level estimation, 112
revenue per case, 113
safe harbor guidelines, 110–11
satisfaction surveys, 119–20
scheduling efficiency, 115–16
staffing management, 116
Stark law, 110–11
supply costs, 116–17
support services, 106
types, 110
variable costs, 114
working capital, 115
American Society of Anesthesiologists
    (ASA)
  Crosswalk, 169, *177*
  physical status classification,
    212–13, *212*, *256*
American Society of PeriAnesthesia
    Nurses (ASPAN), 190, 191

amygdala, emotional pathway, 17
analgesia, postoperative, 109
analytical tools for decision-making,
    35–6
  breakeven analysis, 35–6
  decision tree, 36
  internal rate of return, 35
  net present value, 35
  prioritization matrix, 36
  return on investment, 35
  sensitivity analysis, 36
anchoring bias, 37
anesthesia, 108
  academic departments, 43
  academic program, 42
  ambulatory surgical centers, 109
  costs, 151
  dentist training, 208–9, 214
  intermediate recovery, 187–8
  mobile, 204
  modifiers, 174
  office-based surgery practice, 204,
    208
  out-of-OR, 122–3
  preoperative risk assessment, 122–3
  provider supply/demand, 152
  records, 174–5
  recovery from, 186–7
  retractable utility columns, 102
  risk assessment, 121
  support staff, 43
  transaction code sets, 143
  see also general anesthesia; regional
    anesthesia; sedation
Anesthesia Administration Assembly
    (AAA), 161–3
anesthesia care team model, 140–1,
    151, 154
  anesthesiologist/CRNA mix, 153–4
  anesthesiologists, 140–1, 151
  billing for anesthesia, 144
  non-physician providers, 140–1,
    151
  see also Anesthesiologist Assistants
    (AA); Certified Registered
    Nurse Anesthetist (CRNA)
anesthesia induction rooms, 88–9

anesthesia information management
    systems (AIMS), 267–70
  adoption, 268
  benefits, 268–9
  clinical champion, 270
  clinical research facilitation, 269
  costs, 269–70
  decision support, 268
  economics, 268–9
  goals, 270
  guideline compliance, 268
  implementation, 269–70
  investment return, 269
  workflow changes, 270
anesthesia practice, 139–40
  care delivery models, 139
  group, 140
  independent, 140
  provider employment, 140
anesthesia practice management,
    139–49
  ability/accountability/affability/
    affordability/answerability/
    availability, 145
  anesthesia care team model, 140–1
  anesthesia department evaluation,
    145–7
  benchmarking, 144–5
  billing, 143–4
  codes for billing, 143–4
  communication, 147
  compliance, 144–5
  contracting, 141–2
  evaluation of practice, 145
  financial instability, 148–9
  group ability to respond/adapt,
    147
  group financial strength/stability,
    146–7
  ineffective leadership, 148
  interpersonal conflict, 147
  leadership evaluation, 146
  leveraging of partnership, 149
  marketing, 143
  pain management services, 143
  performance indicators, 145–6
  Physician Quality Reporting
    System, 145
  poor performance, 147
  provider credentials, 146
  quality deficiencies, 147
  quality metrics, 147
  quality outcomes, 146
  reengineering practice, 147–9
  recruiting, 142
  reimbursement, 143–4
  Relative Value Guide, 143–4, 169
  request for proposal (RFP) process,
    141–2
  scheduling, 142–3

Surgical Care Improvement Project
    measures, 144
  underperforming practice, 147–9
  underperforming providers, 148
  underqualified providers, 148
  value-based purchasing, 149
Anesthesia Quality Institute (AQI),
    269
anesthesia services, 41
  accounts receivable, 163
  acute pain management, 178
  ancillary, 176–8
  Centers for Medicare and Medicaid
    Services standards, 238
  compensation for services (CFS)
    agreements, 160–5
  documentation, 238
  information from data, 163
  invasive monitoring lines, 176–8
  Joint Commission standards, 238
  key performance indicators, 163, 166
  monitored anesthesia care, 172–3
  patient assessment, 238
  payer mix, 163
  postoperative evaluation, 238
  pre-anesthesia evaluation, 238
  productivity per FTE, 163–4
  qualifications, 238
  scope, 238
  scope of practice, 238
  sedation, 172
  staffing, 161
  staffing grid, 161, 162
  stakeholders, 160
  standard, 238
  subsidizing by hospitals, 44
  transesophageal echocardiography,
    177
  see also billing, anesthesia services;
    compensation for anesthesia
    services
anesthesia staffing models, 151–8
  ancillary personnel, 157
  anesthesia technicians, 157
  care team model, 151
  challenges, 152–3
  choices, 153–4
  compensation, 154–5, 157
  CRNA only, 154
  evaluation pre-/postanesthesia, 152
  housekeeping staff, 157
  incentive plans, 156–7
  labor law, 158
  management change, 152–3
  nurses, 157
  physician only model, 153
  productivity, 154–6, 156, 157
    ASA units, 155–6
    measurement complications, 155
    measures, 155–6, 156, 157

provider supply/demand, 152
  regulatory issues, 152
  staffing need assessment, 153
  supervision, 152
  unions, 158
anesthesia technicians, 157
anesthesia time, 173–5, 177–8
  discontinuous, 173, 178
Anesthesiologist Assistants (AA),
    140–1, 151, 153–4
anesthesiologists, 6, 7–8, 140–1, 151,
    153–4
  academic setup, 154
  characteristics, 15
  full-time equivalents, 161, 163–4
  leadership to involve surgeons, 43
  patient safety training, 42
  perioperative system, 218
  physician, 151–4
    CRNA supervision, 152
    physician-only staffing model,
      153
    service supervision, 152, 154
    supervision requirement opt-out,
      154
anti-kickback provisions, 110–11, 207
anticoagulant therapy, 239
anxiolysis, office-based surgery
    practice, 207
asepsis/aseptic practices, 232–3
Association of periOperative Registered
    Nurses (AORN), 222–3
  Perioperative Standards and
    Recommended Practices, 222,
    222
Availability Bias, 36–7
average charge per case, 180
average collection per case, 180
average collection per unit, 180
aviation management standards,
    132–3

balance sheet, 69
Balanced Scorecard monitoring tool,
    30
beliefs of organization, 26
benchmarking, 144–5, 179–80, 206
benzodiazepines, 256–7
bias role in decision-making, 36–7
billing
  anesthesia practice management,
    143–4
  anesthesia services, 57, 144, 172–4
    acute pain management, 178
    ancillary, 176–8
    base units, 173
    benchmark measurement,
      179–80
    concurrency, 174–5
    documentation, 174–6, 178

general anesthesia, 173
modifying units, 173–4
obstetric, 178–9
Physician Quality Reporting System, 179
regional anesthesia, 173
time units, 173
average charge per case, 180
average collection per case, 180
average collection per unit, 180
compliance, 180–1
days in accounts receivable, 180
documentation, 174, *177*
gross collection ratio, 180
net collection ratio, 180
office-based surgery practice, 206
surgical services, 171–2
see also coding systems for billing
biological indicator (BI), sterilization, 231
block utilization, 229
blood loss, office-based surgery practice, 210
blood pressure, office-based surgery practice, 209
body substance isolation, office-based surgery practice, 204–5
Bottleneck, 74
breakeven analysis, 35–6
breakeven point, 68
BREEZE™ preoperative evaluation program, 126–7
Building Information Modelling (BIM), 82
buildings
lifespan, 93
migration to new, 94
refurbishment/renovation, 77, 93
bundling
payment, 245
surgical care, 134–5
business performance, quality measures, 250
business plan, ambulatory surgical centers, 111

cabinets, design of operating room, 103
cable communications, 92
call systems, 92
capital, hospital expenses, 41
capital budget, 225–6, *226*
capital structure, 71, 72
care
coordination, 171
surgical bundling, 134–5
see also anesthesia care team model; healthcare; perioperative care quality
care delivery models, 139

care model, design of OR, 82
care team model, 140–1, 151, 154
CareScience Quality Index, 11
cases
cancellations, 53
elective, 46
forecasting time remaining in ongoing, 62–3
mix for hospitals, 40
overlapping, 57
scheduling, 59–61
operating room time release, 60–1
rules, 59–60
sequencing of surgical, 190
urgent, 47, 53, 56
volumes in ambulatory surgical centers, 113
cash distribution, ambulatory surgical centers, 119
cash flow statement, 69–70
ceiling-mounted booms, 86, 102
cell phones, 271–2
Centers for Medicare and Medicaid Services (CMS), 43, 144, 235–8
Conditions of Participation, 144
disaster/emergency response, 241–3
environmental safety, 240–1
infection control, 241
inspections, 236
medication safety, 240
occupational safety, 241
patient rights, 236
performance improvement, 241
quality assurance, 241
safety enhancement, 242–3
sedation regulation, 257–60, 265
standards, 236–43
central line-associated infection, 239
Certificate of Need (CON), ambulatory surgical centers, 111
Certified Registered Nurse Anesthetist (CRNA), 139–41, 152
care team model, 151, 153–4
change, 10
change programs, outcomes/variables, 10
Child Ego, 21
cleanup time, 48
clinical governance, 11
clinical pathways, design of OR, 82
clinical research, facilitation by anesthesia information management systems, 269
clinicians, design of OR, 80–1, 93–4
cloud computing, 92
coding systems for billing, 168–9
abbreviation use, 176
anesthesia practice management, 143–4

ASA Crosswalk, 169
assignment of alternative, 176
Current Procedural Terminology, 168, 171–2, 175
documentation, 175–6
epidural catheters, 178
evaluation and management, 170–1
Healthcare Common Procedure Coding System, 169
ICD-9 (ICD-10) codes, 168–9
National Correct Coding Initiative, 169
Relative Value Guide, 169
Resource-Based Relative Value System, 169
surgical services, 171, 183–5
abbreviations use, 184–5
multiple procedures, 184
process, 184
cognitive decision biases, 36–7
commitment, 26, 33
communication, 10, 16
advanced tools, 272
anesthesia practice management, 147
cable/fiberoptic, 92
design/construction of operating rooms, 97
development of effective skills, 21
failure, 11
improvement, 239
informed consent, 136
IT systems, 100, 271–2
medication information, 239
paging/text messaging, 272
perioperative plan, 128
platforms, 92–3
preoperative risk assessment, 123
voice, 271–2
compensation for anesthesia services, 160–7
aggregate conversion factor, *165*
anesthesia staffing models, 154–5, 157
budget display, *166*
data evaluation, 161–3, 166
implementation, 166–7
information conversion to knowledge, 166–7
information from data, 163
key performance indicators, 163, 166
professional overheads, 164–5
relative productivity display, *164*
revenue projection, 164
strategic planning, 166
utilization benchmarks, 165–6
compensation for services (CFS) agreements, 160–5

competitive analysis, 28–30
  industry analysis, 29–30
  power of buyers, 29
  power of suppliers, 29
  rivalry among existing
    competitors, 29
  threat of entry, 29
  threat of substitutes, 29
complementary transactions, 21
complete enumeration, 54–8
compliance
  billing, 180–1
  federal sentencing guidelines, 180–1
computational flow dynamic (CFD)
  models, 86–7
computer-aided design (CAD), 82,
  84, 85
computer-assisted personalized
  sedation (CAPS), 262
computers, 126, 267–8, 271
concurrency, billing for anesthesia
  services, 174–5
confirmation bias, 37
conflict, fear of, 33
construction of operating rooms, 95
  budget, 97
  commissioning, 98
  communication, 97
  construction documents, 98
  construction phase, 98
  decision, 96
  hybrid ORs, 105–6
  infection prevention, 104
  integrated systems, 105
  interim life safety measures, 104
  new technology, 105
  nurse leader, 97
  operational processes, 98
  planning and design team, 96–7
  planning phase, 98
  project phases, 97–8
  responsibilities, 97
  schematic phase, 98
  strategic planning, 95–6
contribution margin, 50, 53, 68
controllable costs, 68
controlled substances, 205
cooperation, game theory, 7, 8
costs, 50, 67–8
  ambulatory surgical centers, 109,
    114–17
  anesthesia, 151
  anesthesia information
    management systems, 269–70
  cuts, 22
  fixed, 50, 67, 114
  indirect, 67–8
  managerial accounting, 49–50
  operating room efficiency, 42–3
  PACU, 190–1

perioperative care quality, 133–4
  variable, 50, 67, 114
counselling, evaluation and
    management services, 171
crew resource management (CRM),
  132–3
critical incidents, call systems, 92
crossed transactions, 21
Crosswalk (ASA), 169, *177*
cultural competence of workplace, 22
culture, 11–12
  change, 10
  organizational, 9–10
current liquidity ratio, 71
Current Procedural Terminology
  (CPT), 168, 184
  anesthesia reimbursement, 143–4
  coding systems for billing, 171–2,
    175, 179

daily sales outstanding (DSO), 117
data, quality management, 241, 248–9
  acquisition/reporting, 248–9
days in accounts receivable, 180
days of cash on hand, 72
decision making, 12–13, 32–7
  alternatives
    characteristics, 34
    development/evaluation, 34
    evaluation, 34–6
    rules for development, 34
    variables, 34–5
  analytical tools, 35–6
  anesthesia information
    management systems, 268
  bias role, 36–7
  on day of surgery, 62–3
  focus, 37
  framing of decision, 33–4
  goals, 37
  implementation, 37
  leaders, 9
  medical, 171
  operating room efficiency, 50
  operational, 54
  outside opinions, 34
  prioritization matrix, *36*
  team building, 32–3
  team dysfunctions, 32–3
  timeline, 37
decision process, informed consent, 137
decision tree, 36, *36*
deep vein thrombosis risk, 210
defect reduction, 90–1
demographic statistics, design of OR,
  81
dental procedures, office-based
  surgery practice, 214
dentists, anesthesia training, 208–9,
  214

design of operating rooms, 95
  admission unit, 87
  airflow models, 86–7
  ambulatory surgical centers, 106
  ancillary department coordination,
    102
  anesthesia induction rooms, 88–9
  budget, 97
  cabinets, 103
  care model, 82
  ceiling-mounted booms, 86, 102
  clinical pathways, 82
  clinician involvement, 80–1, 93–4
  communication, 97
  communication systems, 100
  computational flow dynamic
    models, 86–7
  computer models, 82, *84, 85*
  configuration, 102–3
  cycle, *80*
  data outlets, 102–3
  delay reduction, 88
  demographic statistics, 81
  design development, 98
  dimensions, 85–6, 102
  documentation systems, 100
  door placement, 102
  efficiency measures, 79
  electrical outlets, 102–3
  evidence-based design, 99
  facility handover, 94
  flexibility, 82
  flows, 85
  functional mapping, 85
  future-proofing, 93
  general principles, 99–102
  holding area, 100
  individual operating rooms, 102
  instrument preparation area, 89
  instrument processing, 87
  interior finish, 103
  issues for decision, 82–5
  lounge area for staff, 101
  materials flow, 100–1
  migration to new building, 94
  mock-up, 85
  nurse leader, 97
  operational processes, 98
  OR of the future, *88*
  outsourced equipment planners,
    103
  parallel working, 88
  patient cubicles, 99–100
  patient flow, 99–100
  personnel involved, 80–1
  planning and design team, 96–7
  planning phase, 98, 100
  plans, 82–5
  postanesthesia care, 87, 100
  preoperative area, 100

process, 80–7
process mapping, 81–2, *83*, *90*
project phases, 97–8
redevelopment, 81
regional block area, 89
responsibilities, 97
restricted area, 99
schedule of accommodation, 82
schematic drawing, 102–3
schematic phase, 98
semi-restricted area, 99
site visits, 81
space requirements, 102
staff movement, 90, *91*
staff support areas, 101
stakeholders, *105*
sterile supplies, 87
strategic planning, 95–6
substerile space, 103
tenders for fixtures, 94
translation from drawing to
        framing, 94
transport flows, 89–90, *91*
unrestricted area, 99
utilities, 86
ventilation systems, 86–7
waiting reduction, 88
wall finishes, 103
waste, 79, *80*
see also equipment
design of post-anesthesia care unit
        (PACU), 87, 189–90
diagnosis, surgical services, 172
Diagnostic Related Groups (DRG)
        reimbursement, 8–9
DICE framework, 10
director, 15, *16*
support, 15
disaster response, 241–3
discharge
    fast track from hospital, 188–9
    office-based surgery practice,
        208–9
    postanesthesia care unit,
        186–90
        criteria, 188, *188*, 189, 192
    sedation, 257
disruptive behavior, 22
documentation
    acute pain management, 178
    anesthesia services, 238
    billing, 174, *177*, 178
    guidelines, 170–1
    integrated care pathways, 124
    medical care, 170
    office-based surgery practice, *202*
    patients, 170
    sedation, 261
    surgical services, 237
    systems, 100, 123–4

education levels, 5
efficiency, operating room, 42–3, 49,
        77–9
    calculations, 54–8
    case scheduling, 59–61
    on day of surgery, 50–2
    forecasts, 58–9
    increasing, 54–61
    inefficiency sources, 75–6
    maximization, 55–6
    operating room time release, 60–1
    scoring system, 78, *78*
    stakeholder group definition, *78*
    urgent cases, 56
efficiency metrics for finance, 226–8
elective case, 46
electrical wiring, office-based surgery
        practice, 204
electronic records, 248–9, 271
emergency referrals, pain
        management services, 197
emergency response, 241–3, *242*
emergent case, 46–7
emotion(s), management, 21
emotional contagion, 17
emotional intelligence, 3, 16–17
    components, *3*, 17–18
    impact on malpractice claims,
        19–20
    importance, 19–20
    improving, 20
    measuring, 18
    performance predictor, 20
    personal competence, 18
    professional interactions, 17
    resonant leadership, 19–20
    self-assessment, 20
    self-awareness, 18
    self-education, 20
    self-management, 18
    social awareness, 18
    social competence, 18
emotional pathways, 17
empathy, 18
employees
    leader impact, 11
    see also staff; staffing
enhanced precautions, 232
environment of OR, successful, 15–23
    dissonant leadership, 19
    emotional pathways, 17
    human resource department, 22
    manager/director, 15
    psychology in, 16, 20
    resonant leadership, 19–20
    structural analysis, 20–2
    team training, 22
    transactional analysis, 20
    see also emotional intelligence
environmental safety, 240–1

epidural catheters, coding systems for
        billing, 178
epinephrine, liposuction, 213
equipment
    capital, 54
    costs for ambulatory surgical
        centers, 115
    data sheet, 104
    hospital expenses, 41
    hybrid operating rooms, 105
    planning, 103–4
    purchasing protocol, 103–4
    sedation, 256, *257*
    storage, 101
    transportation, 89–90
equity
    building, 70–1
    return on equity, 72
evidence-based design, 99
executives, stakeholders, 6

Federal Drug Enforcement
        Administration (DEA), 205
        205
fiberoptic communications, 92
finance, 225–30
    anesthesia information
        management systems, 268–9
    block utilization, 229
    capital budget, 225–6, *226*
    efficiency metrics, 226–8
    operational budget, 225
    PACU, 190–2
    turnaround time, 228–9
financial accounting statements, 69–70
financial instability, anesthesia
        practice management, 148–9
financial performance, 67–76
    contribution margin, 68
    costs, 67–8
    measures, 70–2, 117–19
    operational performance
        relationship, 68–70
financial proforma for ambulatory
        surgical centers, 113–19
    case volumes, 113
    costs, 114
    financial metrics, 117–19
    key components, 113
    location, 112
    site plan, 112–13
financing, ambulatory surgical centers,
        114–15
fire safety, 240–1
Five Competitive Forces That Shape
        Strategy (Porter), 28
fixed costs, 50, 67, 114
flash sterilization, 230
flow rate, 74, 75
    maximum, 74

flow time, 74
fospropofol, 262
framing, decision-making, 33–4

game theory, 6–8
    application to OR suites, 7–8
    concepts, 7
    cooperation, 7, 8
    game types, 7
    mutual defection, 8
    outcomes, 7
    players, 7
    punishments/rewards, 7
    stakeholders, 6
general anesthesia, 173, 255, *255*
Germany, OR management, 8–9
governing board, ambulatory surgical
        centers, 111
graduate medical education, 43–4
    costs, 43
gross collection ratio, 180

hand hygiene, 239
harm to patient, preventability, 11
Health Information Technology for
        Economic and Clinical Health
        (HITECH) Act (2009), 271
Health Insurance Portability and
        Accountability Act (HIPAA,
        1996), 270–1
Health Quiz program, 126
health care
    changes, 39–40
    costs in medical malpractice, 42
    delivery system, 123–4
    economics, 40
    leadership, 4
    literature, 4–5
    patient decisions, 129
    variability in, 79
    waste, 79
Healthcare Common Procedure
        Coding System (HCPCS), 169
HealthQuest score, 126
hospitals
    admissions, 40, 211
    capital expenses, 41
    case mix, 40
    economics, 40
    expenses, 41–2, 44
    inpatient care, 40
    labor expenses, 41
    medical advances in surgery, 108
    medical equipment expense, 41
    medical malpractice costs, 42
    pain management services, 199, *199*
    payer mix, 40, 112
    profitability, 40
    revenue, 40–1, 44
    supply expenses, 41

support staff, 43
    teaching, 44
    utilization, 39
housekeeping staff, 157
human behavior, 16
human resource department, 22
HUMANE steps for cultural
        competence, 22
hybrid operating rooms, construction,
        105–6
hypothermia, office-based surgery
        practice, 209

ICD-9 (ICD-10) codes, 168–9
immediate-use steam sterilization, 101
income generation, preoperative
        evaluation/management,
        128–9
income statement, 69
    proforma, 112
indirect costs, 67–8
industry analysis, 29–30
infection control, 232–4
    aseptic practices, 233
    Centers for Medicare and Medicaid
        Services standards, 241
    central line-associated infections,
        239
    engineering practices, 232–3
    enhanced precautions, 232
    hand hygiene, 239
    Joint Commission standards, 241
    multidrug-resistant organisms,
        204–5, 239
    office-based surgery practice,
        204–5, *205*
    standard precautions, 232
    Surgical Care Improvement Project
        measures, 144, 233–4
    surgical site infection, 133, 239, 246
    universal precautions, 204–5, 232
    work practices, 233
Infection Control Risk Assessment
        (ICRA), 104
infection prevention, 104, 239–40
information systems, 267–72
    communication, 100, 271–2
    computers, 267–8
    HIPPA, 270–1
    meaningful use criteria, 271
    patient confidentiality, 270–1
    security, 270–1
information technology (IT), 92–3,
        267
informed consent, 136–8
    Centers for Medicare and Medicaid
        Services standards, 237–8
    common law standards, 137
    communication, 136
    decision process, 137

elements, 137
    history, 136–7
    Joint Commission standards, 237–8
    medical staff responsibilities, 236
    patient rights, 236
    patient understanding, 137
    surgical services, 237–8
    surrogates, 138
instruments/instrumentation
    design of operating room, 100–1
    hybrid operating rooms, 105
    preparation area, 89
    processing, 87
    transportation, 89–90
insurance coverage, office-based
        surgery practice, 202–3
integrated care pathways, 124
    documentation systems, 123–4
    preoperative risk assessment, 123–4
integrated systems, construction of
        operating rooms, 105
integrity, 12
intensive care units (ICU), 53–4, 187
internal rate of return (IRR), 35
Internet resources, 126–7
interpersonal conflict, 16, 147
invasive monitoring lines, 176–8
inventory, 74, 91–2, 117–19

Joint Commission (TJC), 132, 235
    anesthesia services, 238
    disaster response, 241–3
    emergency response, 241–3, *242*
    environmental safety, 240–1
    infection control, 241
    informed consent, 237–8
    medication safety, 240
    National Patient Safety Goal
        program, 238–40
    occupational safety, 241
    patient rights, 236
    performance improvement, 241
    quality assurance, 241
    safety enhancement, 242–3
    sedation regulation, 257–61, 265
    standards, 236–43
    surgical services, 236–8
just-in-time sterilization, 230

ketorolac, 109
key performance indicators, anesthesia
        services, 163, 166

labor
    hospitals expenses, 41
    productivity, 73
    see also staff; staffing
labor cost, 49–50, 73
    not changing service-specific
        staffing, 62

number of allocated rooms, 62
reduction, 56
reduction of surgical/turnover
times, 61–2
unit, 73–4
labor law, 158
labor services (obstetric), 179
laboratory specimens, transportation,
90
leaders
aloneness, 9
circles of influence, 10
decision making, 9
manager differences, 3–4, 5
predispositions, 6
traits of successful, 6
leadership
challenges, 8–12
characteristics, 12–13
competency areas, 5
dissonant, 19
effectiveness, 6
emergence, 6
evolution, 1–6
failure, 11
health-care literature, 4–5
organizational structures, 8
patient safety impact, 11–12
positions, 9
quality initiatives impact, 11–12
significance for healthcare
organizations, 4
structures, 9
styles, 1–3, 12
Lean and Six Sigma, 77, 79, 90–1
legislation, office-based surgery
practice, 207
leveraging of partnership, 149
life support systems, office-based
surgery practice, 204
limbic system, emotional pathway, 17
Limited Liability Companies (LLCs),
110
liposuction, 213
advisory, 213
complications, 210
epinephrine, 213
infiltrate solutions, 213
office-based surgery practice,
213–14
techniques, 213–14
liquidity, 71–2
liquidity ratios, 71–2
Little's Law, 74

malpractice claims, 19–20
managed care contracting strategy,
112–13
management
leadership differences, 3–5

tactical *versus* operational decisions,
52–4
manager, 15, *16*
support, 15
managerial cost accounting, 49–50
meaningful use criteria, 271
Medicaid, 40, 196, 235–6
medical centers, academic, 40, 44
medical conditions, previously
unrecognized, 122
medical direction, 174–5
modifiers, 174–5
medical errors, 22
medical gases, 204
Medical Group Management
Association (MGMA), 161–3
medical malpractice
claims, 42
financial risk, 42
healthcare costs, 42
preventable errors, 42
sentinel events, 42
medical records, 170, 202
medical services, necessity, 170
Medicare, 40, 112, 235–6
certification for office-based surgery
practice, 211
pain management services, 196, 199
patient age, 134
provider application in ambulatory
surgical centers, 111
Resource-Based Relative Value
System, 169
medications
current, 126
handling, 240
information communication, 239
labeling, 239–40
safe use, 239–40
sedation, 256–7, *258*, 261–2
storage, 240
minimally invasive surgery (MIS)
room design, 85–6
mission statement, 26
goals, 26
parts, 26
structure, 26
mixed-reality immersive environment,
274
mobile communications, 92
mobile phones, 271–2
monitored anesthesia care (MAC),
172–3
monitoring tools, 30
motivation, 13
multidrug-resistant organisms, 204–5,
239

National Correct Coding Initiative
(NCCI), 169

National Fire Protection Association
(NFPA), 104, 203, 240–1
National Health Service (UK), clinical
governance, 11
National Patient Safety Goal (NSPG)
program, 238–40
National Quality Forum (US), culture
dimensions, 11–12
nausea management, 213
needs analysis, design/construction of
OR, 96
needs of organization, 26
negotiation, 13
net collection ratio, 180
net patient costs, 73
net patient revenue, 73
Net Present Value (NPV), 35
net revenue, 112
new technology
construction of operating rooms,
105
perioperative system, 219
nitrous oxide, 108
non-operative time reduction, 89
non-zero-sum games, 7
nurses
anesthesia staffing models, 157
leader for design/construction of
operating rooms, 97
PACU, 190–1
perioperative system, 218–19
sedation administration, 255
stakeholders, 6
nursing, 222–34
inventory, 225
organizational structure/design, 222
resource management, 223–5
staffing levels, 222–3, *224*

obesity risks, 123, 211
obstetric anesthesia, billing, 178–9
obstructive sleep apnea, 211
occupational hazards, 203–4
occupational safety, 241
office-based surgery practice, 201–14
accreditation, 201–2
adverse events, *203*
Aldrete score, *209*
anesthesia, 204–6, 208
anxiolysis, 207
availability, 205–6
backup power, 204
billing, 206
blood loss, 210
blood pressure, 209
body substance isolation, 204–5
classification, 207
clinical care, 207–8
comorbidity identification, *208*, 211
controlled substances, 205

office-based surgery practice
  dental procedures, 214
  dentist anesthesia training, 208–9,
    214
  discharge from care, 208–9
  documentation, *202*
  duration of surgery, 210–11
  electrical wiring, 204
  evacuation plans, 203–4
  facility standards, 211–12
  fast-tracking criteria, *209*
  hospital admission, 211
  hypothermia, 209
  infection control, 204–5, *205*
  insurance coverage, 202–3, *203*
  legislation, 207
  life support systems, 204
  liposuction, 210, 213–14
  medical gases, 203–4
  Medicare certification, 211
  multidrug-resistant organisms, 204–5
  nausea and vomiting management,
    213
  non-participating provider, 206
  obesity risk, 211
  obstructive sleep apnea, 211
  occupational hazards, 203–4
  OSHA standards, *205*
  pain management, 212
  patient records, 202
  patient selection, 207, 211
  payment plans, 206–6
  physical classification of patients,
    212–13, *212*
  physical examination, 211
  physiologic stressors, 209–10
  plastic surgery advisories, 208–9
  postoperative care, 208–9
  postoperative recovery, 211
  practice management, 205–6
  preoperative history, 211
  preoperative tests, 212
  procedures performed, 209
  professional liability
    insurance, *203*
  provider participation, 206
  provider qualifications, 211–12
  quality improvement plan, 202
  risk management, 203–4
  sedation, 207–8
  sentinel events, *203*
  thromboprophylaxis, 210
  universal precautions, 204–5
  utilization benchmarking, 206
  vicarious liability, 202–3
operating margin ratio, 72
operating metrics, ambulatory surgical
  centers, 115–16
operating room (OR)
  activity measures, 78

allocations, 54–7, 61–3
services, 53
utilization, 41, 49, 57–8
workload, 48
see also efficiency, operating room;
  productivity of operating room
operating room (OR) time, 47
  adjusted utilization, 48–9, 52
  allocation, 52, 61
  inefficiency of use, 49
  non-operative time reduction, 89
  open access, 53, 54
  overutilized, 49–50, 52–3
  reduction, 61–3
  releasing, 60–1
  surgical time reduction, 61–2
  turnover, 47–8, 61–2
  underutilized, 48, 50, 52, 59
operational budget, 225
operational indicators, 70
operational performance, 73–6
  financial performance relationship,
    68–70
  process capacity, 74–6
  process performance, 74
operational processes, design/
  construction of operating
  rooms, 98
operations management, 67–76
  contribution margin, 68
  financial performance relationship
    operational performance, 68–70
opioids, 257
organizational chart for OR
  management, *16*
organizational structures, 8
organizations
  informal, 9–10
  large, 8
  small, 8
out-of-network strategies, ambulatory
  surgical centers, 112–13
outcomes
  adverse operative, 128
  measures, 245–6, *246*, 261
  sedation, 261
  unexpected, 42
outpatient services, revenue, 74
overconfidence bias, 36
overheads, 67–8
overprocessing/overproduction, waste
  management, 92
owners, stakeholders, 6

paging, 272
pain, postoperative, 109
pain management services
  acute pain, 178
  administrative staff, 196–7
  anesthesia practice management, 143

anesthesia services, 178
availability, 196–7
charging, 199
emergency referrals, 197
financial considerations, 196
free-standing, 199
hospital-based services, 199, *199*
inpatient consultations, 197
interface with existing services, 194–5
Medicare, 196, 199
offering, 194
office-based surgery practice, 212
operation hours, 196–7
outpatient appointments, 197
patient types, 196
personnel for quality care, 195
phone calls from patients, 197
physician-referred patients, 197–9,
  197
referrals, 197–9
self-referred patients, *196*, 197–9
support services, 195
support staff, 195, 197
time management, 197
time to care provision, 195, 197
types offered, 195–6
pain practice management, 194–200
parallel working, 88–9
parent ego, 20
patient(s)
  age in Medicare, 134
  documentation, 170
  examination, 170–1
  healthcare decisions, 129
  identification, 239
  prevention of harm, 11
  stakeholders, 6
  systems review, 170
  understanding for informed
    consent, 137
patient assessment, 237–8
patient confidentiality, 270–1
patient-controlled sedation/analgesia
  (PCSA), 262
patient cubicle design, 99–100
patient flow, design of operating room,
  99–100
patient information, access to, 92
patient rights, 236
  informed consent, 236
  restraint use, 236
patient safety, 11–12, 22, 268, 274
  simulation training, 274–8
  training, 42
pay-for-performance, 245, 251, 268
payer mix for hospitals, 40, 112
payment, 134, 206
  bundling, 245
  reforms in perioperative system,
    220

people alignment, 10
performance
  improvement, 241
  indicators, 145–6
  management, 10
  measurement, 134
  monitoring, 115
perioperative care quality, 133–6
  care delivery, 134
  change drivers, 135–6
  costs, 133–4
  delivery system redesign, 136
  measurement, 133–4
  payment, 134
  performance measurement, 134
  stakeholders, 135
  surgical care bundles, 134–5
  values, 135
  variation, 134
perioperative medicine, future of,
    216–20
perioperative plan, communication,
    128
perioperative standards, 132–8
  care quality, 133–6
  focus areas, 133
  informed consent, 136–8
  purpose, 132
  surgeon level of experience, 133
  surgical site infection, 133
  tools, 133
  wrong-site surgery, 133
perioperative system, 217
  anesthesiologists, 218
  critical role of leadership, 5
  current system, 217
  nurses, 218, 219
  payment reform, 220
  primary care providers, 218–19
  reimbursement, 216–17, 220
  sedation care provision, 218
  specialties, 218–19
  structure, 216
  subsystems, 217
  systems theory research, 217–18
  technology, 219
  telemedicine, 219–20
personal competence, 18
personality dimensions, 6
personnel costs, 68
Physician Quality Reporting System
    (PQRS), 145, 179, 251, 269
  modifiers, 179
physicians
  barriers to leadership roles, 5
  employed, 40–1
  leadership evaluation in anesthesia
      practice management, 146
  satisfaction, 42–3
  subsidized, 40–1

  see also anesthesiologists, physician
physiologic stressors, office-based
    surgery practice, 209–10
planning
  design of operating room, 100
  purposeful, 25–6
  see also strategic planning
planning and design team, 96–7
plastic surgery advisories, 208–9
political savvy, 12
population diversity, 22
postanesthesia care area design, 100
postanesthesia care unit (PACU),
    186–92
  Aldrete score, 187, 192
  bypass, 188–9
  control chart, 249
  cost-reduction strategies, 190–1
  design, 87, 189–90
  discharge, 186–90
    criteria, 188–9, 188, 192
  early recovery, 186–7
  finances, 190–2
  late recovery, 188
  length of stay, 191–2
  patient flow, 190
  recovery phase, 186–9
  staff wages, 191
  staffing, 190, 192
  time minimizing, 190
  White–Song score, 187–9, 187
Postanesthesia Discharge Scoring
    System (PADSS), 187–8, 187
postoperative care, office-based
    surgery practice, 208–9
power of buyers, 29
power of suppliers, 29
power system backup, 204
practice management, 205–6
  see also anesthesia practice
      management
preference cards, 224–5
preferred provider network plans, 112
prefrontal cortex, emotional pathway,
    17
preoperative care delivery models,
    124–5
preoperative clinics, 124–5
  appointments, 127
  communication of plan, 128
  health history, 127
  Medical Director, 127
  medical record review, 127
  perioperative evaluation/
      management, 129
  physician-directed, 127–8, 128
  plan development, 127–8
  triage, 127
preoperative evaluation/management,
    121–9

care delivery models, 124–5
  computer programs, 126
  current medication, 126
  day-of-surgery, 125
  early remote triage, 125–7
  economics, 128–9
  inadequate, 128
  income generation, 128–9
  internet resources, 126–7
  physician-directed clinic, 127–8
  primary care providers, 125
  risk assessment, 121–4
  systems review, 126
  waiting time, 129
preoperative risk assessment, 121–4
  anesthetic management, 122–3
  communication, 123
  health-care delivery system, 123–4
  integrated care pathways, 123–4
  patient factors, 121–2
  postoperative complications
      prediction, 122
  surgical factors, 122
preventable errors, 42
primary care providers, 125, 218–19
principal agent problem, 10
prioritization matrix, 36, 36
problem solving, team approach, 1
process analysis, 74–5
process capacity, 74–6
process measures, 246
process performance, 74
process utilization, 75
productive potential measure, 78–9
productivity of operating room, 46–63
  case scheduling, 59–61
  efficiency, 54–61
  forecasts, 58–9, 62–3
  low workloads, 58
  number of allocated rooms, 62–3
  service-specific staffing, 62
  time reduction impact, 61–3
professional goals, 10
professional group tensions, 10
professional liability insurance, 203
profit, 50
profit margin, 67
profitability ratios, 71
project phases, design/construction of
    operating rooms, 97–8
propofol, 261–2
prospective payment system (PPS),
    8–9
protected health information (PHI),
    270–1
provider credentials, anesthesia
    practice management, 146
psychology in OR, 16, 20
pulmonary complications risk
    assessment, 122

pulmonary embolism risk, *208*, 210
purpose, 12, 25–7

quality, 244–5
quality assurance, 241
quality initiatives, 11–12
quality management, 246–7
  bottom-up planning, 248
  data, 248
  data acquisition/reporting, 248–9
    rates/trends, 249
  data collection, 248–9
  individual level reporting, 250–1,
    251
  internally reported, 247
  new measures, 246
  open reporting, 250–1
  outcomes of interest, 249–50
  plan, 247–8
  reporting levels, 250–1
  responsibility for outcome, 247
  sedation, 261
  stakeholders, 247–8
  see also pay-for-performance
quality measures, 245–7
  anesthesia practice management, 147
  anonymous public reporting, *251*
  attribution, 247
  business performance, 250
  choosing, 246
  control chart, *249*
  internally reported, 247
  new, 246
  outcome measures, 245–6, *246*
  patient-centered, 249–50
  process measures, 246
  staff satisfaction, 250
  uses, 246–7
quality outcomes, 11, 146, 244–5
Queuing Theory, 79

reengineering of OR function,
  77–94
  see also design of operating rooms
recency effect, 36–7
regional anesthesia, 173, 192
regional block area, 89
regulatory approval, ambulatory
  surgical centers, 111
reimbursement, 143–4, 220
  level estimation, 112
  rules, 168
relationship management, 18
Relative Value Guide (RVG), 143–4,
  169, 178–9
release time, 230
reliability, sustainable transformation
  to higher state, 11
remodeling/renovation of operating
  room, 95–6, 102

request for proposal (RFP) process,
  141–2
resonant leadership, 19–20
Resource-Based Relative Value System
  (RBRVS), 169
resource management
  inventory, 225
  nursing, 223–5
  preference cards, 224–5
restraint use, patient rights, 236
restricted area of operating room, 99
results, inattention to, 33
return on equity, 72
Return on Investment (ROI), 35
revenue, 50
  generated by facility per patient, 73
  hospitals, 40–1, 44
  net patient revenue, 73
  outpatient services, 74
  per case, 113
Revised Cardiac Risk Index (RCRI),
  122
risk management, 203–4, 261
rivalry among existing competitors,
  29

safe harbor guidelines, 110–11
safety, 244
  interim measures during
    construction, 104
  performance improvement, 242–3
  staff, 245
  see also patient safety
satisfaction surveys, 119–20
scheduling
  block, 229–30
  block utilization, 229
  cases, 59–61
  efficiency in ambulatory surgical
    centers, 115–16
  efficiency metrics for finance, 226–8
  open, 229–30
security, information systems, 270–1
sedation, 253–62
  administration, 253–5, *254*, 262
  anesthesia services, 172
  care provision, 218
  comorbidities, 255–6
  competency, 260–1
  complexity of procedures, 253
  computer-assisted personalized
    sedation, 262
  conscious, 207
  controversies, 261–2
  credentialing, 260–1
  deep, 207–8, 253, 255, *255*, 260
  definitions, 255
  discharge, 257
  documentation, 261
  education, 261

  equipment, 256, *257*
  guidelines, 262–5
  knowledge, 261
  levels, 253, 255, *255*
  medications, 256–7, *258*, 261–2
  minimal, 255, *255*
  moderate, 253–5, *254*, *255*
  monitors, 256
  non-anesthesia providers, 253–5, *254*
  office-based surgery practice, 207–8
  outcomes, 261
  patient-controlled sedation/
    analgesia, 262
  patient outcome monitoring, 261
  preprocedure evaluation, 255–6
  propofol, 261–2
  quality improvement, 261
  recovery, 257
  regulation, 257–65, *261*
  risk assessment, 261
  skills, 261
  standards, 262–5
  training, 260–1
self-assessment, 20
self-awareness, 18, 21
self-management, 18
selfish actions, 7–8
semi-restricted area of operating
  room, 99
semi-variable costs, 67
sensitivity analysis, 36
sentinel events, medical malpractice,
  42
setup time, 48
simulation training, 274–8
  course administration, 275–8
  critical performance indicators, 274–5
  laparoscopic cholecystectomy, *275*,
    277
  learning objectives, 274–5
  mixed-reality immersive
    environment, 274
  team training skills, 274, *274*
site plan, 112–13
situational leadership, 3
social awareness, 18
social capital, 10–11
social competence, 18
Social Security Act (1965), 235–6
staff
  individual level quality management
    reporting, 250–1, *251*
  leader impact, 11
  movement, 90, *91*
  safety, 245
  satisfaction, 250
  wellness, 245
staff scheduling, 46–8, 52
  matching workload, 52
  service-specific, 52–3

staff support areas, 101
staffed assignment, 46
staffed hours, 46
staffing
  anesthesia services, 161
  calculated, 56
  efficiency, 54–6
  grid for anesthesia services, 161, *162*
  management in ambulatory surgical centers, 116
  nurses, 222–3, *224*
  post-anesthesia care unit, 190–2
  service-specific, 56
  surgical case sequence, 190
  see also anesthesia staffing models
stakeholders, 6, 15
  anesthesia services, 160
  design of operating rooms, *105*
  perioperative care quality, 135
  quality management, 247–8
  salience, 6–7
standard precautions, 232
Stark law, 110–11, 207
sterile supplies, 87
sterilization, 230
  biological indicator, 231
  critical variables, 231–2
  cycles, *232*
  flash, 230
  immediate-use, 101
  just-in-time, 230
  mechanisms, 230–1
  moisture, 230
  residual air in vacuum cycle, 231
  steam, 230–1
  surgical sterilizing departments, 87, 89–90
  temperature, 230
  time, 230
storage, 91–2
strategic planning, 25–31
  action plans, 30
  compensation for anesthesia services, 166
  competitive analysis, 28–30
  design/construction of operating room, 95–6
  goals, 30
  mission statement, 26
  monitoring, 30
  objectives, 30
  process, 27–30
  purpose development, 26–7
  SWOT analysis, 28
  targets, 30
  timeline, 27–8, *28*
  values statement, 27
  vision statement, 26–7
structural analysis, 20–2

structural change, 10
substerile room, design of operating room, 103
sunk-cost effect, 36
suppliers, 6
supplies
  costs, 68, 116–17
  design of operating room, 100–1
  inventory, 225
support services, ambulatory surgical centers, 106
surgeons, 6
  level of experience, 133
  satisfaction, 43
  selfish actions, 8
surgery
  case sequencing, 190
  mistakes prevention, 240
  pre-procedure verification process, 240
  procedure site marking, 240
  technology advances, 219–20
  time-out performance, 240
  see also wrong-site surgery (WSS)
surgical care bundles, 134–5
Surgical Care Improvement Project (SCIP), 144, 233–4, 268
surgical centers, freestanding, 123
surgical procedures, simulation training, *275, 277*
surgical services, 47
  billing, 171–2
  Centers for Medicare and Medicaid Services standards, 236–8
  coding systems for billing, 171, 183–5
    abbreviations use, 184–5
    multiple procedures, 184
  Current Procedural Terminology, 184
  diagnosis, 172
  documentation, 183–4, 237
  informed consent, 237–8
  Joint Commission standards, 236–8
  patient assessment, 237
  provider qualifications, 237
  scope, 236–7
surgical site infection (SSI), 133, 239, 246
surgical sterilizing departments, 87, 89–90
surrogates, informed consent, 138
SWOT analysis, 28
  compensation for anesthesia services, 166
  opportunities, 28
  strengths, 28
  threats, 28
  weaknesses, 28

System for Teamwork Effectiveness and Patient Safety (STEPS), *274*
system theory research, 217–18
systems review, 126, 170

Tax Relief and Health Care Act (2006), 179
team building, 32–3
  dysfunctions, 32–3
team training, 22
  simulation training, 274–5
TeamSTEPPS program, 22
telemedicine, perioperative system, 219–20
telephone interviews, 125
text messaging, 272
Theory X, 1–3
Theory Y, 1, 3
threat of entry, 29
threat of substitutes, 29
thromboprophylaxis, 210
time allocation
  release time, 230
  see also scheduling
total margin ratio, 72
training
  dentists for anesthesia, 208–9, 214
  patient safety, 42, 274–8
  sedation, 260–1
  simulation, 274–8
  team, 22, 274–5
trait theory, 6
transactional analysis, 20
  complementary transactions, 21
  crossed transactions, 21
  structural analysis, 20–2
transesophageal echocardiography (TEE), 177
transformational leadership, 4
transportation, 89–90, *91*
  equipment, 89–90
  instruments, 89–90
  laboratory specimens, 90
  patients, 89
  surgical sterilizing departments, 89–90
triage
  early remote, 125–7
  before preoperative clinic appointment, 127
  Web-based, 126–7
trust
  absence of, 33
  building, 11
turnaround/turnover time, 47–8, 228–9

underperforming providers, 148
underqualified providers, 148

unions, anesthesia staffing models, 158
universal precautions, 204–5, 232
unrestricted area of operating room, 99
urgency, stakeholders, 6–7
urgent case, 47, 53, 56
utilities for OR, 86
utility columns, retractable for anesthesia, 102
utilization benchmarking, 206

Value-Based Purchasing (VBP), 149, 251
values statement, 27
Vanderbilt Perioperative Information Management System (VPIMS), 272
variable costs, 50, 67, 114
ventilation system design, 86–7
vicarious liability, 202–3

vision, 12
vision statement, 26–7
Voice over Internet Protocol (VoIP), 272
vomiting management, 213–12

waiting time, 74, 88, 129
wall finishes in OR, 103
waste
    design of operating rooms, 79, 80
    in healthcare, 79
waste management
    communication platforms, 92–3
    defect reduction, 90–1
    instrument preparation area, 89
    inventory, 91–2
    non-operative time reduction, 89
    overprocessing/overproduction, 92
    parallel working, 88–9

reengineering of OR function, 87–93
    regional block area, 89
    staff movement, 90
    storage, 91–2
    transportation, 89–90
    waiting, 88
wellness of staff, 245
White–Song score, 187–9, 187
Wi-Fi networks, 272
wireless communications, 92
working capital, 71, 115
workload, 56, 58
    forecasts, 58–9
wrong-site surgery (WSS), 133
    drivers, 133
    prevention, 12, 133

zero-sum games, 7